Johannes Ring · Allergy in Practice

Johannes Ring

Allergy in Practice

With a Foreword by Thomas Platts-Mills

With 149 Figures in 175 Parts and 186 Tables

Springer

Prof. Dr. med. Dr. phil. Johannes Ring
Klinik und Poliklinik für Dermatologie und Allergologie am Biederstein
des Klinikums rechts der Isar der Technischen Universität München
Biedersteiner Straße 29, D-80802 München

ISBN 3-540-00219-7 Springer-Verlag Berlin Heidelberg New York

Library of Congress Control Number: 2004110368

This work is subject to copyright. All rights are reserved, whether the whole or part of the material is concerned, specifically the rights of translation, reprinting, reuse of illustrations, recitation, broadcasting, reproduction on microfilm or in any other way, and storage in data banks. Duplication of this publication or parts thereof is permitted only under the provisions of the German Copyright Law of September 9, 1965, in its current version, and permission for use must always be obtained from Springer-Verlag. Violations are liable to prosecution under the German Copyright Law.

Springer-Verlag Berlin Heidelberg New York
Springer is a part of Springer Science+Business Media
http://www.springeronline.com

© Springer-Verlag Berlin Heidelberg 2005
Printed in Germany

Title of the German edition:
Johannes Ring, Angewandte Allergologie. 3., neu bearbeitete Auflage
Urban & Vogel Medien und Medizinverlagsgesellschaft mbH & Co KG,
München 2004
ISBN 3-89935-128-2

The use of general descriptive names, registered names, trademarks, etc. in this publication does not imply, even in the absence of a specific statement, that such names are exempt from the relevant protective laws and regulations and therefore free for general use.
Product liability: The publishers cannot guarantee the accuracy of any information about the application of operative techniques and medications contained in this book. In every individual case the user must check such information by consulting the relevant literature.

Editor: Marion Philipp
Desk Editor: Irmela Bohn
Production Editor: Joachim W. Schmidt
Cover design: eStudio Calamar, Spain
Typesetting: FotoSatz Pfeifer GmbH, D-82166 Gräfelfing
Printed on acid-free paper – 24/3150 – 5 4 3 2 1 0

Preface

μηδεν αγαν (ancient Greek)
"Avoid overreactions" (principle of applied allergology)

Allergy is "in," and has been for some years now. The term "allergy" is no longer a foreign word. In spite of this, allergies are still not adequately appreciated either by the general population or by the physicians' community. On the one hand, allergy is like a "fashionable disease" and any disturbance of well-being is regarded as allergy; on the other hand, very severe allergic conditions remain neglected, being left undiagnosed and untreated. It is difficult to find the right balance between the extremes.

After the first two editions of this book (1982 and 1988) sold over 20,000 copies, the publisher and author decided to collaborate on a new and totally rewritten third edition. In this endeavor the original aim of a very brief and precise booklet containing relevant information for allergy practice was not forgotten. The book started as a collection of short information leaflets for residents rotating through the Allergy Division at Munich. It was Dr. J. Aumiller, chief editor of the *Munich Medical Weekly*, who then persuaded me to write a series of short chapters on allergy in practice, and I am still thankful for the brutality with which he forced me rigorously to shorten the text! In this third edition, which is published in both German and English, the author again had a fight to find the most logical method of classification, a difficulty for every complex medical field. There are different possible criteria which can be followed for a classification:

- According to organs (e.g., allergy of the nose, eye, skin)
- According to symptoms (e.g., urticaria, eczema, asthma)
- According to pathomechanisms (e.g., types according to Coombs and Gell)
- According to allergens (e.g., food allergy, animal protein allergy, nickel allergy)
- According to the clinical course and prognosis (e.g., acute or chronic allergies, life-threatening emergencies)
- According to genetic parameters (e.g., familial allergies, sporadic allergies)
- According to age (e.g., childhood allergies, adult allergies)
- and many more

If one pushed these classifications to their logical extent, many overlaps and repetitions would result. The living organism is not necessarily logical, and even less so in its pathophysiological variants.

Nevertheless, we need to stress the importance of a precise terminology in the individual chapters; this is not a sophisticated philosophy but rather reflects the inherent problems, which may be overlooked at a superficial glance, but which are the daily bread and butter of serious allergists.

Furthermore, it was important in the selection of references not only – as is so often seen nowadays – to look through "three years of Medline" but also to include important work from the past. Therefore, I politely ask the reader – maybe like on a holiday trip – to trust the more or less experienced guidance of the author; this guided tour will be subjective, but I promise to relate the most important points in a short and precise way.

Here I want to thank many people. Firstly my clinical and experimental teachers and mentors, Prof. Dr. med. Dr. h.c. mult. Otto Braun-Falco, the master of exact clinical description, the unforgettable Prof. Dr. med. Walter Brendel, who gave me the spirit of enthusiasm for immunology, Prof. Dr. med. habil. Erich Fuchs, the grand old man of German allergology for many discussions, fruitful critical remarks and always enlightening exchanges of ideas over the decades. Prof. Dr. med. Alain de Weck has given me much scientific input and has supported me on my way into the international allergy community. Dr. Eng Tan was my teacher as a "post doc" at the Scripps Clinic and Research Foundation in La Jolla. To my predecessors at university chairs, Prof. Dr. Karlheinz Schulz and Prof. Dr. Theodor Nasemann in Hamburg-Eppendorf, Prof. Dr. med. Dr. phil. Siegfried Borelli at the Department of Dermatology, Biederstein in Munich. I am thankful for the excellent tradition of clinical allergology which I was allowed to continue.

I also want to thank my co-workers in allergology, Prof. Dr. med. Bernhard Przybilla, Priv.-Doz. Dr. med. Dieter Vieluf at the Ludig Maximilians University, and in Hamburg, and Prof. Dr. Jürgen Rakoski and Priv.-Doz. Dr. Ulf Darsow in the daily work now at the Technical University of Munich. The following co-workers have helped in the preparation of single chapters:

Prof. Dr. Torsten Schäfer (epidemiology), Prof. Dr. Heidrun Behrendt (allergy and environment, allergens), Priv.-Doz. Dr. Thilo Jakob, Dr. Martin Mempel, Prof. Dr. Markus Ollert (pathophysiology, diagnostics, immune complex reactions), Dr. Gregor Wildi and Mr. Jan Al (rhinitis, asthma), Dr. Anke Gauger (urticaria), Dr. Knut Brockow (anaphylaxis), Dr. Volker Grimm and Mrs. Claudia Kugler (food allergy), Priv.-Doz. Dr. Ulf Darsow (eczema), Priv.-Doz. Dr. Bernadette Eberlein-König (photoallergy, "eco syndrome"), Dr. Stephanie Weissenbacher and Dr. Matthias Möhrenschlager (therapy and prevention), and Dr. Theresia Ring (Department of Ophthalmology, LMU, "Allergy and the Eye"). Many thanks to Johanna Grosch and to the nurses of the Department of Dermatology and Allergy at Biederstein for their continuous and enthusiastic work for our patients!

I want to thank Mrs. Marion Philipp and Mrs. Gabriele M. Schröder (Springer, Heidelberg) for their professional help with the publishing and printing and to Dr. Thomas Platts-Mills from Charlottesville for the kindness of his foreword!

Finally I want to thank my wife, Prof. Dr. med. Heidrun Behrendt, head of the "Centre for Allergy and Environment" ("ZAUM – Zentrum Allergie und Umwelt"), for manifold support, beautiful electron microscope pictures and her everlasting contagious critical enthusiasm for allergy research!

Munich, am Biederstein
January 2005

Prof. Dr. med. Dr. phil. Johannes Ring

Foreword

Allergic disease has become a major aspect of Western Society, both in terms of medical management and quality of life. However understanding diagnosis and management becomes complex because not only are there multiple allergen sources involved but also a large number of diseases. Hay fever, perennial rhinitis, chronic sinus disease, urticara, atopic eczema, anaphylaxis, food allergy, and asthma each affect large numbers of patients. Because of the overall numbers (15%–20% of the population) there are inevitably a large proportion of patients who are allergic or think they are allergic and attribute other symptoms to this mechanism. One of the striking features of allergy is that each disease varies from very serious to trivial with no clear distinction. Thus for each of the major allergic diseases there are many individuals whose symptoms are not sufficient to go to a doctor and also patients whose lives are made miserable and even threatened by the diseases. Understanding the factors which contribute to such a spectrum of allergic disease is a major challenge.

As this book explains accurate diagnosis of sensitization is essential. Without this, it is not possible to make a realistic assessment of the role of allergy in the disease nor to plan treatment. For each disease there are multiple potenzial allergens involved and the management strategies are different. It is not surprising that assessment and management of allergic disease becomes confusing to many of the health care professionals who have to cope with this problem.

Professor Ring is well known internationally as an allergist and dermatologist who has contributed to research on allergy for at least 25 years (He is also famous for a wonderful sense of humor which sadly, but wisely, doesn't come through in the book). He has now published a book which covers a wide range of diseases which are either allergic or immunological and which provides a comprehensive approach to management. In addition the book provides a complete reference to causes for each of the conditions associated with "Allergie". Overall it is a useful and very helpful contribution to the literature of a still evolving problem.

Johannes has a very broad view of allergic disease but brings special expertise to several areas which are often ignored or glossed over. He has made major contributions to our knowledge of the role of allergens in atopic eczema. In addition he has a profound knowledge of other forms of skin disease. This adds depth and excellent judgment to the opinions expressed. He also includes a really useful chapter on pseudo-allergic reactions. This is an important part of drug allergy and one to which he has often contributed. It is perhaps the awareness of other rashes, pseudo-allergic reactions and anaphylactoid reactions that adds the greatest strength to the book.

In the last few years Johannes and his colleagues have established the "Center for allergy and environment" (ZAUM – Zentrum Allergie und Umwelt) in Munich. This institute which is only five years old has already made its mark. Dr. Behrendt's work on the interaction between air pollutants and allergen particles is well known but this group's work on a group of leukotriene like molecules derived from pollen has opened up a new area of allergy research. All this adds further depth to Dr. Ring's understanding which is clearly evident in the book. Certainly those chapters are a pleasure.

Not unexpectedly, Johannes Ring has written an excellent book which covers a wide range of allergic disease. The book provides a comprehensive but very well planned description of the diseases that are either very common or just common. His pragmatism comes through in all he writes resulting in a really useful guide to an increasingly complex field.

Thomas A.E. Platts-Mills, MD, PhD, FRCP
Oscar Swineford Jr Professor of Medicine
Division Head of Asthma and Allergic Disease

Table of Contents

1	**Clinical Manifestation and Classification of Allergic Diseases**	1
1.1	History	1
1.2	Clinical Manifestation and Definition of Allergy	2
1.3	Classification of Allergic Diseases	5
	References	7
2	**Pathophysiology of Allergic Reactions**	8
2.1	The Immune Response	8
2.2	Antibodies	15
2.3	IgE-Mediated Reaction	16
2.3.1	Mast-Cell Activation	16
2.3.2	IgE and Atopy	17
2.4	Cytotoxic Reactions (Type II)	18
2.5	Immune Complex Reactions (Type III)	19
2.6	Cellular Hypersensitivity (Type IV)	19
2.7	Less Frequent Types of Allergic Reactions (Types V and VI)	20
2.8	Pseudo-allergic Reactions	20
2.9	Mediators of Allergic Reactions	20
2.9.1	Histamine	20
2.9.2	Eicosanoids	20
2.9.3	Leukotrienes	23
2.9.4	Platelet-Activating Factor	23
2.9.5	Serotonin	24
2.9.6	Complement System	24
2.9.7	Mediators from Neutrophil Granulocytes	25
2.9.8	Mediators from Eosinophil Granulocytes	25
2.9.9	Kallikrein-Kinin System	25
2.9.10	Tachykinins	26
2.10	Synopsis of Mediator Release and Inactivation	26
	References	27
3	**Genetics and Environment in the Development of Allergy**	30
3.1	Genetics of Allergy	30
3.1.1	Classical Genetics	30
3.1.2	Molecular Genetics	31
	References	32
3.2	Epidemiology of Allergic Diseases	33
3.2.1	Atopic Diseases	33

3.2.2	Epidemiology of Contact Allergies	35
	References	35
3.3	Allergy and Environment	36
3.3.1	Environment and Health	36
3.3.2	Allergotoxicology	36
3.3.3	Conclusions	40
	References	41
3.4	Allergens	42
3.4.1	"Allergenic Potency"	43
3.4.2	Standardization of Allergen Extracts	44
3.4.3	Terminology of Allergens	44
3.4.4	Aeroallergens	44
	References	57
4	**Allergy Diagnosis**	**60**
4.1	History	60
4.2	Skin Tests	61
4.2.1	Patch Test	61
4.2.2	Friction Test	61
4.2.3	Prick Test	61
4.2.4	Scratch Test	61
4.2.5	Intradermal Test	61
4.2.6	Complications	62
4.2.7	Reading of Skin Tests	63
4.2.8	Pharmacologic Influence	63
4.2.9	Special Skin Test Procedures	63
4.3	In Vitro Allergy Tests	64
4.3.1	Serologic Methods	64
4.3.2	Cellular Tests	67
4.3.3	In Vitro Detection of Allergens	68
4.4	Provocation Tests	68
4.4.1	Conjunctival Provocation Test	68
4.4.2	Nasal Provocation Test	69
4.4.3	Bronchial Provocation Test	69
4.4.4	Oral Provocation Test	71
4.4.5	Parenteral Provocation	72
4.5	Transfer Tests	72
4.6	Unconventional Methods in Allergy Diagnosis	72
4.7	Comparison of Different Diagnostic Procedures	72
	References	73
5	**Allergic Diseases (and Differential Diagnoses)**	**76**
5.1	Diseases with Possible IgE Involvement ("Immediate-Type Allergies")	76
5.1.1	Allergic Rhinitis	76
	References	80
5.1.2	Bronchial Asthma	80
	References	88
5.1.3	Urticaria and Angioedema	89
	References	96

5.1.4	Anaphylaxis	97
	References	103
5.1.5	Food Allergy and Other Adverse Food Reactions	104
	References	112
5.1.6	Insect Venom Allergy	114
	References	120
5.1.7	Allergy and the Eye	122
	References	125
5.2	Allergic Diseases by Cytotoxic Antibodies (Type II)	125
5.2.1	Mechanisms of Antibody-Mediated Cytotoxicity	125
5.2.2	Allergic Diseases of the Blood	128
5.2.3	Allergic Cytotoxic Organopathies	130
	References	130
5.3	Allergic Diseases due to Immune Complexes	131
5.3.1	Immune Complex Anaphylaxis	131
5.3.2	Serum Sickness	131
5.3.3	Allergic (Immune complex) Vasculitis	133
	References	135
5.4	Hypersensitivity Pneumonitis (Allergic Alveolitis)	136
5.4.1	Definition	136
5.4.2	Clinical Symptoms and Diagnosis	136
5.4.3	Pathophysiology	138
5.4.4	Allergens and Common Forms of Hypersensitivity Pneumonitis	139
5.4.5	Allergic Bronchopulmonary Mycosis	141
5.4.6	Therapy of Hypersensitivity Pneumonitis	141
	References	141
5.5	Dermatitis/Eczema	143
5.5.1	Definition and Classification	143
5.5.2	Contact Dermatitis	144
5.5.2.1	Pathophysiology	144
5.5.2.2	Clinical Manifestations of Classic Contact Dermatitis	145
5.5.2.3	The Patch Test	147
5.5.2.4	Therapy	149
	References	149
5.5.3	Atopic Eczema	151
5.5.3.1	Clinical Manifestation	151
5.5.3.2	Pathophysiology	157
5.5.3.3	Therapy	159
	References	162
5.5.4	Topical Glucocorticosteroid Therapy	164
5.5.4.1	Mechanisms of Action	164
5.5.4.2	Practical Application of Topical Glucocorticoids	166
5.5.4.3	Side Effects of Topical Glucocorticosteroids	167
	References	169
5.6	Photoallergy/Photosensitization	170
5.6.1	Classification	170
5.6.2	Clinical Manifestations of Photohypersensitivity	171
5.6.3	Photosensitizers	172
5.6.4	Diagnosis	173

5.6.5	Prophylaxis and Therapy	174
	References	174
5.7	Adverse Drug Reactions	175
5.7.1	Drug Allergy: General Procedures	175
5.7.1.1	Classification	175
5.7.1.2	Pathophysiology	176
5.7.1.3	Risk Factors	177
5.7.1.4	General Diagnosis of Drug Allergy	177
5.7.1.5	Hyposensitization in Drug Allergy	180
5.7.1.6	Adverse Reactions to Special Drugs	180
5.7.1.7	Rare Drug Reactions	183
5.7.1.8	HIV Infection and Drug Allergy	183
	References	184
5.7.2	Pseudo-allergic Drug Reactions	185
5.7.2.1	Definition and Elicitors	185
5.7.2.2	Radiographic Contrast Media	188
5.7.2.3	Plasma Protein Solutions	188
5.7.2.4	Gelatine Volume Substitutes	188
5.7.2.5	Intravenous Anesthetics	188
5.7.2.6	Muscle Relaxants	189
5.7.2.7	Local Anesthetics	189
5.7.2.8	Acetylsalicylic Acid and Non-steroidal Anti-inflammatory Drugs (NSAIDs)	190
5.7.2.9	Additives	191
5.7.2.10	Other Pseudo-allergic Reactions	191
5.7.2.11	Therapy and Prophylaxis	191
	References	191
5.7.3	Exanthematous Drug Eruptions	193
5.7.3.1	Prevalence	193
5.7.3.2	Clinical Classification of Exanthematous Drug Eruptions	194
5.7.3.3	Pathophysiology of Cutaneous Drug Eruptions	202
5.7.3.4	Special Forms of Drug-Induced Skin Diseases	204
	References	205
5.8	Granulomatous Reactions	207
5.8.1	Clinical Examples	207
5.8.2	Pathophysiology	208
5.8.3	Therapy	209
	References	209
5.9	Type VI Reactions (Stimulating/Neutralizing Hypersensitivity)	210
5.9.1	Clinical Examples of Autoimmune Diseases	210
5.9.2	Stimulating Hypersensitivity in Bacterial Infection	211
5.9.3	Stimulating Neutralizing Reactions in Classic Allergic Diseases	211
5.9.4	Therapy	212
	References	212
5.10	"Eco-syndrome" ("Multiple Chemical Sensitivity," MCS)	212
5.10.1	Classification	212
5.10.2	Differential Diagnoses	213
5.10.3	Pathophysiological Concepts	214

5.10.4	Management of Patients with "Eco-syndrome" 215
	References 216

6	**Allergy Prevention and Therapy** 218
6.1	General Concept of Allergy Treatment 218
6.2	Antiallergic Pharmacotherapy 220
6.2.1	Inhibition of Histamine Synthesis 220
6.2.2	Mast Cell Stabilizers 220
6.2.3	Antihistamines 220
6.2.4	Leukotriene Inhibitors 221
6.2.5	Glucocorticosteroids 221
6.2.6	Sympathicomimetics 222
6.2.7	Anticholinergics 223
6.2.8	Phosphodiesterase Inhibitors 223
6.2.9	Secretolytics 223
6.2.10	Preparations with Doubtful Efficiency 223
6.2.11	New Developments 223
6.2.12	Antipruritic Treatment 224
6.2.13	Antiallergic Pharmacotherapy and Pregnancy 225
	References 225
6.3	Immunotherapy 227
6.3.1	Allergen-Specific Immunotherapy (Specific Hyposensitization) 227
	References 234
6.3.2	Other Immunotherapeutic Procedures 236
	References 238
6.4	Unconventional Procedures in Allergy 239
	References 240
6.5	Allergy Prevention 241
6.5.1	Definition 241
6.5.2	Primary Prevention 241
6.5.3	Secondary Prevention 243
6.5.4	Tertiary Prevention 243
6.5.5	Strategies for Aeroallergen Avoidance 243
	References 245

7	**Psyche and Allergy** 248
7.1	The Problem of "Allergic Personality Traits" 248
7.2	Stress 249
7.3	Influence of Psyche upon Allergy 249
7.4	Psychoneuroallergology 250
7.5	Clinical Conditions 252
7.6	Therapy 253
	References 254

8	**Outlook** 257
8.1	Pathophysiology 257
8.2	Clinical Studies 258
8.3	Diagnosis 259
8.4	Therapy 260

8.5	Prevention	260
8.6	Controversies	261
8.7	Role of Allergology	261

9	**Appendix**	**263**
9.1	Societies	263
9.2	Allergy Journals	263
9.3	Position Papers of the European Academy of Allergology and Clinical Immunology (EAACI)	264
9.4	Allergy Textbooks	266

Subject Index 269

Abbreviations

AC	acetylcholine
ADCC	antibody-dependent cell-mediated cytotoxicity
AE	atopic eczema
ANCA	antineutrophil cytoplasmic antibodies
APC	antigen-presenting cells
APT	atopy patch test
B	B lymphocytes
BAL	bronchoalveolar lavage
BAU	biological activity unit
BDNF	brain-derived neurotrophic factor
BHR	bronchial hyperreactivity
BK-A	basophil kallikrein of anaphylaxis
BRI	building related illness
BSA	bovine serum albumin
CAST	cellular allergen stimulation test
CAT	contact allergy time
CD	cluster of differentiation
CGRP	calcitonin gene-related peptide
COLAP	colonoscopic allergen provocation
COPD	chronic obstructive pulmonary disease, chronic bronchitis
CRF	corticotropin releasing factor
CRIE	crossed radioimmunoelectrophoresis
CRP	C-reactive protein
DC	dendritic cells
DNCB	dinitrochlorbenzol
DNCG	disodium cromoglycate
DTH	delayed-type hypersensitivity
EAA	exogen allergic alveolitis
EAC	equivalent allergen concentration
ECP	eosinophil-cationic protein
EEMM	erythema exsudativum multiforme majus
EGF	epidermal growth factor
EIA	enzyme immunoassay (= PRIST)
EMS	eosinophil-myalgia syndrome
ENU	ethylnitrosourea
EOS	eosinophil
EPX	eosinophil protein X
ESR	erythrocyte sedimentation rate

ETS	environmental tobacco smoke
FEV	forced expiratory volume
FEV1	forced expiratory volume in 1 s
G-6-PDH	glucose-6-phosphate dehydrogenase
GC	glucocorticosteroid
GMCSF	granulocyte-macrophage colony-stimulating factor
GPC	giant papillary conjunctivitis
GVH	graft-versus-host reaction
HAART	highly active antiretroviral therapy
HEP	histamine-equivalent potency
HETE	hydroxyeicosatetraenoic acid
HIT	heparin-induced thrombocytopenia
HLA	human leukocyte antigen
HSV	herpes simplex virus
IFN	interferon
IEI	idiopathic environmental intolerances
IGF	insulin-like growth factor
IL	interleukin
IPEC	intragastral provocation under endoscopic control
ITP	idiopathic thrombocytopenic purpura
LATS	long-acting thyroid-stimulating factor
LPR	late phase reaction
LTT	lymphocyte transformation test
MBP	major basic protein
MC	mast cell
MCDP	mast cell degranulating peptide
MCS	multiple chemical sensitivity
MED	minimal erythema dose
MHC	major histocompatibility complex
MIRR	multi-subunit immune recognition receptors
MPL	monophosphoryl lipid
MPO	myeloperoxidase
MPS	mononuclear phagocyte system
NAT	*N*-acetyltransferase
NCA	neutrophil chemotactic activity
NK	natural killer cells
NP	neurophysin
NSAID	non-steroidal anti-inflammatory drugs
ODTS	organic dust toxic syndrome
OPTI	oral provocation test for idiosyncrasy
PAF	platelet-activating factor
PBHRT	photobasophil histamine release test
PCA	passive cutaneous anaphylaxis
PEF	peak expiratory flow
PLA	platelet antigen
PMN	polymorphonuclear neutrophil
PRIST	paper disk radioimmunosorbent test
PRU	Phadebas-RAST unit
PUVA	psoralen ultraviolet A
RAST	radioallergosorbent test

RCM	radiographic contrast media
RIA	radioimmunoassay
ROAT	repeated open application test
SBS	sick building syndrome
SJS	Stevens-Johnson syndrome
SOD	superoxide dismutase
SRS-A	slow-reacting substance of anaphylaxis
SSSS	staphylococcal scalded skin syndrome
STAI	state trait anxiety inventory
T	T-lymphocyte
TCR	T-cell receptor
TEN	toxic epidermal necrolysis
TENS	transepidermal nerve stimulation
TGF	transforming growth factor
TRUE	thin layer rapid use epicutaneous (test)
TNF	tumor necrosis factor
UV	ultraviolet
VIP	vasoactive intestinal peptide
VOC	volatile organic compounds

CHAPTER 1

Clinical Manifestation and Classification of Allergic Diseases

1.1 History

Allergic diseases have been known for centuries, and allergic diseases such as asthma, urticaria and eczema were described in the ancient medical literature of China, Egypt, and Greece (Table 1.1) [7, 22, 24]. The first allergic individual in world history might have been the Egyptian pharaoh Menes, who – according to the hieroglyphs – died in the year 2,641 B.C. after a wasp sting [1].

The first family history of atopy syndrome with asthma, rhinoconjunctivitis and atopic eczema can be found in the Julian-Claudian imperial family of Augustus, Claudius, and Britannicus [20] (Fig. 1.1). In the middle ages, "rose fever" with hay-fever-like symptoms was a well-known entity. Richard III of England was allergic against strawberries according to Shakespeare.

The first clinically exact description of hay fever was given by John Bostock in 1819. C.H. Blackley was the first to prove pollen as the cause of hay fever using skin and provocation tests [2].

The term "allergy" was born on 24 July 1906 in issue no. 30, page 1,457 of the *Munich Medical Weekly* [18], coined by the Viennese pediatrician Clemens von Pirquet to differentiate between protective and noxious immunity (Fig. 1.2). Von Pirquet understood "allergy" as the specifically altered reactivity of the organism. Linguistically, the term should read "allourgy" since the Greek words "αλλος" = "different" and "εργον" = "work" combine in this way. Von Pirquet's definition includes not only hypersensitivity reactions, but also decreased immune reactions; this aspect has been lost today. We define allergy as "specific immunological hypersensitivity leading to disease." A new

Table 1.1. Allergic diseases in the ancient medical literature

Year	Author	Disease
2698 B.C.	Huang Ti	"Noisy breathing"
2641 B.C.	Hieroglyphs	Death by wasp sting (Pharaoh Menes)
460 B.C.	Hippocrates	Hypersensitivity against goat's cheese
25 B.C.	A. Celsus	Description of asthma
120–180	Aretaeus of Kapadokia	Term "asthma"
600	Aetius of Amida	Term "eczema"
865	Rhazes	Rose fever in Persia
1135–1204	Moses Maimonides	Treatment of asthma
1565	L. Botallus	Rose fever in Pavia
1783	Philipp Phoebus	Hay fever (monography)
1802	W. Heberden	"Summer catarrh"
1819	J. Bostock	Self-description of hay fever
1837	J.L. Schoenlein	Purpura rheumatica
1853	J.M. Charcot	Crystals in asthma sputum
1886	E. van Leyden	Crystals in asthma sputum
1868	H.H. Salter	Different asthma elicitors
1872	H.I. Quincke	Angioedema
1872	Wyman	Autumnal catarrh (from ragweed)

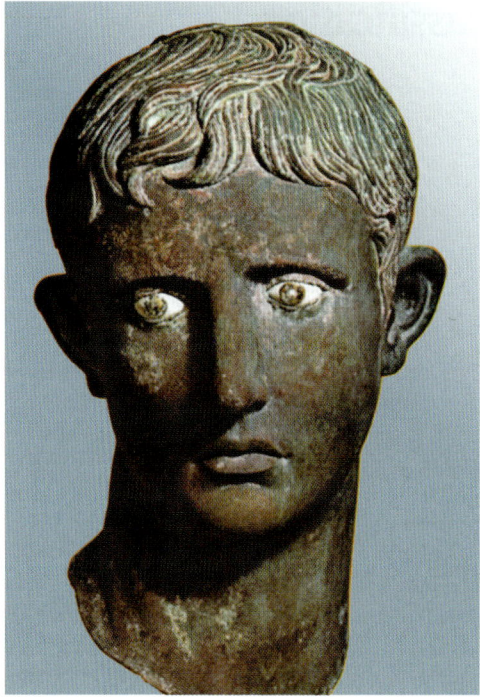

Fig. 1.1. Allergies were already known in ancient times. The Roman Emperor Augustus suffered from atopic syndrome (bronze sculpture, around 14 A.D., British Museum, London)

Mostly, this hypersensitivity is directed against exogenous non-infectious agents. Autoimmune reactions may be included when they are induced through exogenous substances (see Chap 5, Sects. 5.2, 5.7, 5.10).

Table 1.2 lists the historical milestones in the development and understanding of allergy.

The specialty of allergology saw a major advance in the discovery of immunoglobulin E as the carrier of immediate type hypersensitivity. IgE seems to be the most important immunoglobulin in allergology; at some congresses, one gains the impression that allergists would like to change their names to "IgEologists"! We should remember, however, that allergic diseases include many more clinical entities than IgE-mediated reactions.

1.2 Clinical Manifestation and Definition of Allergy

In clinical practice, allergy manifests as various different conditions such as anaphylactic shock, hay fever, allergic conjunctivitis, urticaria, angiooedema, serum sickness, allergic vasculitis, hypersensitivity pneumonitis, contact dermatitis, granulomatous reactions, allergic bronchial asthma, as well as the colorful spectrum of food- or drug-induced adverse reactions [8]. The most important definitions are given in Table 1.3.

consensus of the World Allergy Organization (WAO) on terminology in allergy has been published recently [12].

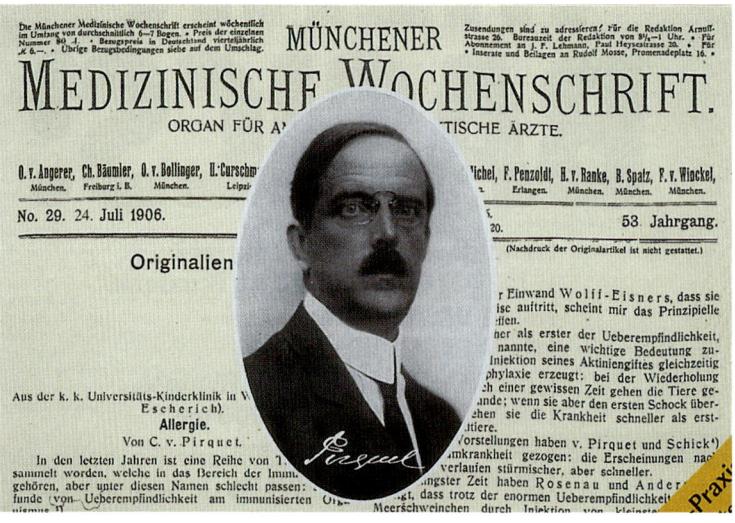

Fig. 1.2. The word "allergy" made its debut in the medical literature on 24 July 1906 in an article written by Clemens von Pirquet, a pediatrician practicing in Vienna, for the *Münchener Medizinische Wochenschrift (Munich Medical Weekly)*

Table 1.2. Milestones in allergy research

Year	Author	Condition
1873	Ch. Blackley	Skin and provocation tests (grass pollen)
1877	P. Ehrlich	Mast cells
1895	J. Jadassohn	Patch test
1900	S. Solis-Cohen	Suprarenal extracts in asthma/hay fever
1902	Ch. Richet, P. Portier	Anaphylaxis
1903	M. Arthus	Local anaphylaxis
1903	Th. Smith	Anaphylaxis against horse serum
1905	von Pirquet, B. Schick	Serum sickness
1906	von Pirquet	Allergy
1906	A. Wolff-Eisner	Hay fever/urticaria correspond to anaphylaxis
1910	W. Dunbar	Pollen extract and antiserum (pollantin)
1910	H. Dale, Laidlaw	Histamine
1911	L. Noon, J. Freeman	Prophylactic inoculation (hyposensitization)
1921	C. Prausnitz, F. Küstner	Humoral hypersensitivity is transferable
1923	A. Coca, R. Cooke	Atopy
1924	K.K. Shen, C.F. Schmidt	Ephedrine (from Ma Huang)
1927	Th. Lewis	Triple reaction of histamine
1928	W. Storm van Leeuwen	House dust allergy/climate chamber
1928	H. Kämmerer	Allergic diathesis
1937	Bovet/Staub	Antihistamines (Phenergan)
1939	H.H. Donally	Food allergens in breast milk
1940	M. Loveless	Blocking antibodies
1941	K. Hansen	Shock fragment
1949	P.L. Hench, E.C. Kendall	Cortisone
1952	Z. Ovary	Passive cutaneous anaphylaxis (PCA)
1953	J.F. Riley, G. West	Histamine in mast cell granules
1954	W. Frankland	First placebo-controlled immunotherapy trial
1956	W. Gronemeyer, E. Fuchs	Bronchial provocation in routine diagnosis
1958	F. Dixon	Immune complex reaction
1960	B.B. Levine, A. de Weck	Penicillin allergy (bivalent hapten)
1961	J. Pepys	Farmer's lung
1963	R.R.A. Coombs, P. Gell	Type I–IV classification
1964	L. Lichtenstein, A. Osler	Histamine release
1966	K. Ishizaka	Immunoglobulin E
1967	S.G.O. Johansson	Immunoglobulin E
1967	R. Vorhoorst, F. Spieksma	House dust mites
1967	R. Altounyan	Cromoglycate
1969	E. Macher, R. Chase	Contact allergy kinetics (mouse)
1977	B. Halpern	Lymphocyte transformation test in allergy
1978	P. Kallós	Pseudo-allergy
1979	B. Samuelsson	Leukotrienes
1984	H. Metzger	IgE receptor
1987	T. Mossmann	Th_1-Th_2 concept
1988	V. Coffmann	Interleukin-4
1989	H. Behrendt	Allergotoxicology
1989	D. Kraft, Baldo	Recombinant allergens
1987	K. Mullis	Polymerase chain reaction (PCR)
1987	P. Piper	Leukotriene antagonists
1996	C. Heusser	Anti-IgE in therapy

Table 1.3. Definitions

Sensitivity	Normal response to a stimulus	Allergy	Immunologically mediated hypersensitivity leading to disease
Hypersensitivity	Abnormally strong response to a stimulus	Idiosyncrasy	Non-immunological hypersensitivity without relation to the pharmacological toxicity
Toxicity	Normal harmfulness of a substance		
Intoxication	Reaction to normal pharmacological toxicity	Intolerance	Hypersensitivity in the sense of pharmacological toxicity
Sensitization	Development of increased sensitivity after repeated contact	Pseudo-allergy	Non-immunological hypersensitivity with clinical symptoms mimicking allergic reactions

Table 1.4. Clinical manifestations of allergic diseases in various organs (examples)

Organ	Symptoms[a]	Differential diagnosis
Cardiovascular	Anaphylaxis, vasculitis	Other cases of shock, vasovagal reaction, vascular diseases
Lung	Bronchial asthma, allergic bronchitis, hypersensitivity, pneumonitis	Bronchitis, chronic obstructive pulmonary disease, irritative toxic asthma, pneumonia
Upper airways	Rhinitis, sinusitis, pharyngitis, laryngeal edema, laryngitis	Vasomotor rhinitis, infection
Eye	Conjunctivitis, atopic keratoconjunctivitis, blepharitis, lid edema	Irritation, infectious conjunctivitis rosacea, psoriasis, seborrheic dermatitis, Melkersson-Rosenthal syndrome
Ear	Otitis externa, serous otitis media? tinnitus? vertigo?	Psoriasis, infection, microcirculatory disturbance
Blood	Hemolytic anemia, thrombocytopenia, agranulocytosis	Hematologic disease, toxic reactions
CNS	Fever	Infectious diseases
	(Cramps)	Neurological diseases
	(Migraine?)	
Skin	Urticaria, angioedema	Hereditary angioneurotic edema
	Vasculitis	Non-inflammatory purpura
	Contact dermatitis and atopic eczema	Other forms of dermatitis
	Drug-induced exanthematous eruptions	Viral exanthematous eruptions
	Granulomatous reactions	Infectious or foreign body granuloma
Oral/genital mucosa	Gingivostomatitis, erythema multiforme, vulvovaginitis (aphthae?)	Infection, morbus Behçet
Gastrointestinal	Food allergy with nausea, gastritis, enteritis	Malabsorption syndromes, infectious gastroenteritis, ulcus pepticum, enzyme deficiency
Musculoskeletal	Arthralgia	Other forms of arthritis and myositis
Kidney	Immune complex nephritis	Other kidney diseases

[a] These symptoms can also be elicited by pseudo-allergic mechanisms

Table 1.5. Classification of pathogenic immune ("allergic") reactions (modified after Coombs and Gell [5])

Type	Pathophysiology	Clinical examples
I	IgE	Anaphylaxis Allergic rhinitis Allergic bronchial asthma Allergic conjunctivitis Allergic urticaria Allergic gastroenteritis (Atopic eczema?)
II	Cytotoxic	Hemolytic anemia Agranulocytosis Thrombocytopenic purpura
III	Immune complexes	Serum sickness Immune complex anaphylaxis Vasculitis Hypersensitivity pneumonitis Nephritis Arthritis
IV	Cellular hypersensitivity	Type IVa (TH1) allergic contact dermatitis Type IVb (TH2) atopic eczema Type IVc (CD8) drug-induced exanthematous eruptions (purpura pigmentosa progressiva) Bullous drug eruptions
V	Granulomatous reactions	Granulomas after injections (e.g., bovine collagen)
VI	"Stimulating" ("neutralizing") hypersensitivity	Autoimmune thyreoiditis Myasthenia gravis Reverse anaphylaxis Insulin resistance Chronic urticaria? (subpopulation with autoantibodies against $Fc_\varepsilon RI$)

Allergies are seen in almost every organ (Table 1.4). Most frequently, however, it is the skin and the mucous membranes that are involved and that represent the interface between the individual organism and its environment [1–27].

1.3 Classification of Allergic Diseases

The multitude of symptoms of allergic diseases (Table 1.4, Fig. 1.3) need a classification. Coombs and Gell [5] were the first to bring some order to the field of clinical immunology and allergology when in 1963 they proposed a classification of pathogenic immune reactions into four types; this classification has tremendous didactic qualities even today. Pathophysiologically oriented, it can be supplemented by the additional type V category for granulomatous and type VI for specific pathogenic antibody effects (stimulating/neutralizing hypersensitivity) (Table 1.5).

Type I. This type comprises IgE-mediated reactions (classical immediate-type allergic reactions), allergic rhinoconjunctivitis, allergic bronchial asthma, urticaria, angioedema, and anaphylaxis. The pathophysiological principle is the release of vasoactive mediators after the bridging of at least two IgE molecules on the surface of mast cells and basophil leukocytes by the allergen. This reaction does not need complement activation. Atopic eczema is characterized by elevated serum IgE levels.

Type II. The not so frequent reactions of type II (mostly hematologic diseases) develop through the action of cytotoxic antibodies directed against surface determinants of cells (after a drug, for instance, has been attached as a hapten to the surface of leukocytes, platelets, or erythrocytes and leads to allergic agranulocytosis or thrombocytopenia).

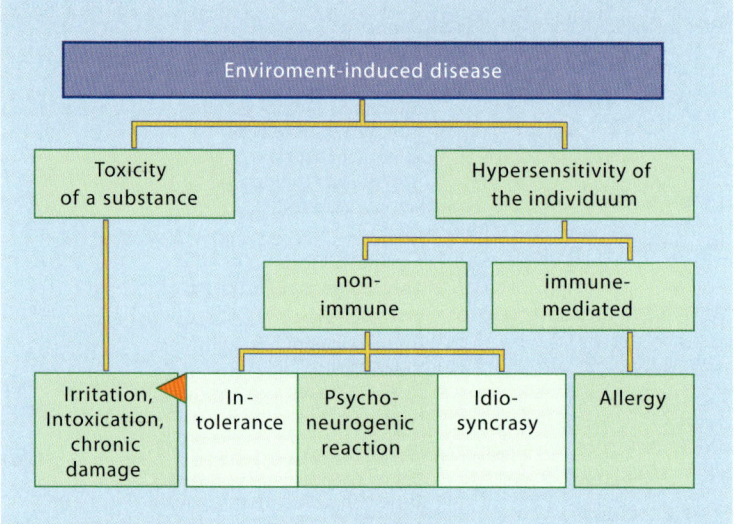

Fig. 1.3. Classification of environmentally related health disorders

Type III. Circulating immune complexes may activate the complement system as well as neutrophil granulocytes and platelets. Clinically, one can distinguish two types according to the kinetics: immune complex anaphylaxis as an immediate reaction has been observed in dextran anaphylaxis and xenogeneic serum therapy. A clinically different entity is the condition of serum sickness, which gave rise to von Pirquet's definition of allergy and accompanies fever, vasculitis, nephritis, arthritis, and urticaria as a consequence of deposits of circulating immune complexes in moderate antigen excess.

It is questionable whether some forms of drug reactions such as erythema nodosum or erythema multiforme which accompany vasculitis and immune-complex deposits may be included here.

Type IV. Reactions mediated through sensitized lymphocytes comprise allergic contact dermatitis, the chronic phase of atopic eczema and many drug-induced exanthematous eruptions. Some forms of purpura pigmentosa progressiva can perhaps be mentioned here. The tuberculin reaction as well as organ transplant rejection follows similar mechanisms. According to modern immunology, predominantly TH1 cells play a role in delayed-type hypersensitivity (DTH), whereas TH2 reactions are important in the early phase of atopic eczema.

Type V. The recently suggested type V category describes granulomatous reactions (such as after injection of foreign material) (e.g., zirconium or soluble bovine collagen) after 2–5 weeks characterized histologically by epithelioid cell granulomas.

Type VI. Pathogenic hypersensitivity reactions occurring through the specific antibody action have been called "stimulating/neutralizing hypersensitivity" (I. Roitt) and occur in autoimmune diseases such as thyreoiditis (LATS, long-acting thyroid-stimulating factor) or myasthenia gravis with antibodies against the acetylcholine receptor in the motoneuron. So-called "reverse anaphylaxis" after injection of antibodies (e.g., anti-IgE or antibodies against the IgE receptor) might also be mentioned here; there is some overlap with type II reactions.

Generally, it should be stressed that every classification is predominantly of a didactic nature. In the living organism – unlike in a textbook – different types of reactions occur and influence each other in parallel. In everyday practice, type I reactions such as allergic rhinoconjunctivitis, allergic asthma, urticaria, and anaphylaxis as well as type IV reactions such as allergic contact dermatitis are the most important manifestations of allergy. Atopic eczema can be regarded as a mixture between type I and type IV reactions.

References

1. Avenberg KM, Harper DS, Larsson BL (1986) Footnotes on allergy. Pharmacia, Uppsala
2. Blackley C (1873) Experimental researches on the cause and nature of hay fever. Ballière, Tindall & Cox, London
3. Bostock J (1819) Case of a periodical affection of the eyes and chest. Med-Chir Trans 10:161
4. Cooke RA (1947) Allergy in theory and practice. Saunders, Philadelphia
5. Coombs RRA, Gell PGH (1963) The classification of allergic reactions underlying disease. In: Gell PGH, Coombs RRA (eds) Clinical aspects of immunology. Davis, Philadelphia, p 317
6. Denburg J (ed) (1998) Allergy and allergic diseases. Humana Press, Totowa
7. De Weck A (1997) A short history of allergological diseases and concepts. In: Kay B (ed) Allergy. Blackwell, Oxford, pp 3–22
8. Fuchs E, Schadewaldt H (1993) Portraits: Karl Hansen. Allergo J 2:80–81
9. Fuchs E, Schulz KH (eds) (1987) Manuale Allergologicum. Dustri, München-Deisenhofen
10. Hansen K, Werner M (eds) (1960) Lehrbuch der klinischen Allergie. Thieme, Stuttgart
11. Holgate S, Church M, Lichtenstein L (eds) (2001) Allergy, 2nd edn. Mosby, London
12. Johansson SGO, Bieber T, Dahl R, Friedmann PS, Lanier BQ, Lockey RF, Motala C, Ortega Martell JA, Platts-Mills TAE, Ring J, Thien F, Van Cauwenberge P, Williams HC (2004) A revised nomenclature for allergy for global use. Report of the Nomenclature Review Committee of the World Allergy Organization, October 2003. J Allergy Clin Immunol 113:832–836
13. Kaplan A (ed) (1986) Allergy. Churchill, Livingstone
14. Kämmerer H (1928) Allergische Diathese. Bergmann, Munich
15. Kay B (ed) (1997) Allergy and allergic diseases, 2 volumes. Blackwell, Oxford
16. Middleton E, Reed CE, Ellis EF (eds) (1998) Allergy. Principles and practice, 5th edn. Mosby, St. Louis
17. Mygind N, Dahl R, Pedersen S, Thestrup-Pedersen K (1996) Essential allergy. Blackwell, Oxford
18. Pirquet C von (1906) Allergie. Münch Med Wochenschr 30:1457
19. Ring J, Behrendt H, Vieluf D (eds) (1997) New trends in allergy IV. Springer, Berlin Heidelberg New York
20. Ring J (1985) Erstbeschreibung einer "atopischen Familien-Anamnese" im Julisch-Claudischen Kaiserhaus: Augustus, Claudius, Britannicus. Hautarzt 36:470–474
21. Roitt I (1998) Essential immunology, 9th edn. Blackwell, Oxford
22. Schadewaldt H (1980–1984) Geschichte der Allergie (4 vols). Dustri, München-Deisenhofen
23. Schultze-Werninghaus G, Ring J (2001) 50 Jahre Deutsche Gesellschaft für Allergologie und klinische Immunologie (DGAI). Allergo J 10:377–382
24. Simons E (ed) (1994) Ancestors in allergy. Global Med Com, New York
25. Urbach E (1935) Klinik und Therapie der allergischen Krankheiten. Maudrich, Vienna
26. Vaughan WT, Black JH (1948) Practice of allergy. Mosby, St. Louis
27. Wahn U, Seger W, Wahn V (eds) (2004) Allergien im Kindesalter, 4th edn. Fischer, Stuttgart

2 Pathophysiology of Allergic Reactions

2.1 The Immune Response

In order to understand allergy as a pathogenic immune reaction, some knowledge of the normal human immune system is crucial. Recently "innate" and "acquired" immunity have been distinguished: "innate" describes primitive defense phenomena after the intrusion of microbes or parasites, involving phagocytes (neutrophils, macrophages), natural killer cells, lysozymes, and the complement system without the involvement of antibodies [24, 46]. These processes often involve the same cytokines and chemokines as those in end phase allergic reactions.

True specific immunity (acquired immunity) enables the organism to distinguish between "self" and "foreign." The recognition of "self" is a prerequisite for the recognition of "foreign" [14, 84] and takes place in approximately 10^{12} lymphocytes.

Figure 2.1 is a scheme of antigen interactions. The antigen – or the hapten after binding to a carrier protein – is recognized by an antigen-presenting cell (i.e., macrophage) from a lymphocyte, which produces a complementary structure (antigen-binding determinant) while proliferating in a "clone" of lymphocytes. This antigen-binding determinant represents the individually specific characteristic of an antibody – or an antigen-specific cell ("idiotype"). Here, the axiom "1 cell = 1 specificity" is valid.

In the process of lymphocyte maturation, several populations have to be distinguished (Fig. 2.2): first, B and T cells, B cells differentiating into antibody-forming plasma cells, and then T cells as carriers of cellular hypersensitivity. The maturation of T cells takes place in the thymus, leading to cytotoxic cells, suppres-

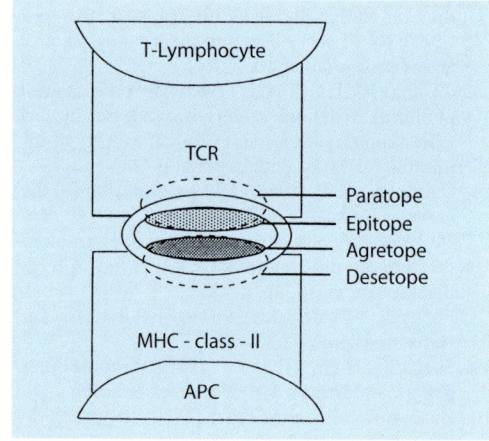

Fig. 2.1. Interaction of T lymphocytes, T-cell receptors (*TCR*) and antigen-presenting cells (*APC*) prior to the production of antibodies. *MHC*, major histocompatibility complex

sor cells (regulatory cells), killer cells, helper cells, effector cells of delayed-type hypersensitivity (DTH) and memory cells. Mature T cells recognize two specificities, one of the foreign antigen and one of a surface marker of its own organism ("self") genetically coded by the major histocompatibility complex (MHC). This phenomenon of MHC restriction originally discovered by Zinkernagel und Doherty [84] means that in the maturation of the immune system self-recognition precedes recognition of foreign. The specificity for self-transplantation antigens differs according to the function of the T cells: cytotoxic T cells (CD8) recognize the classic transplantation antigens of class I (HLA-A, B and C), while helper (CD4) or DTH-

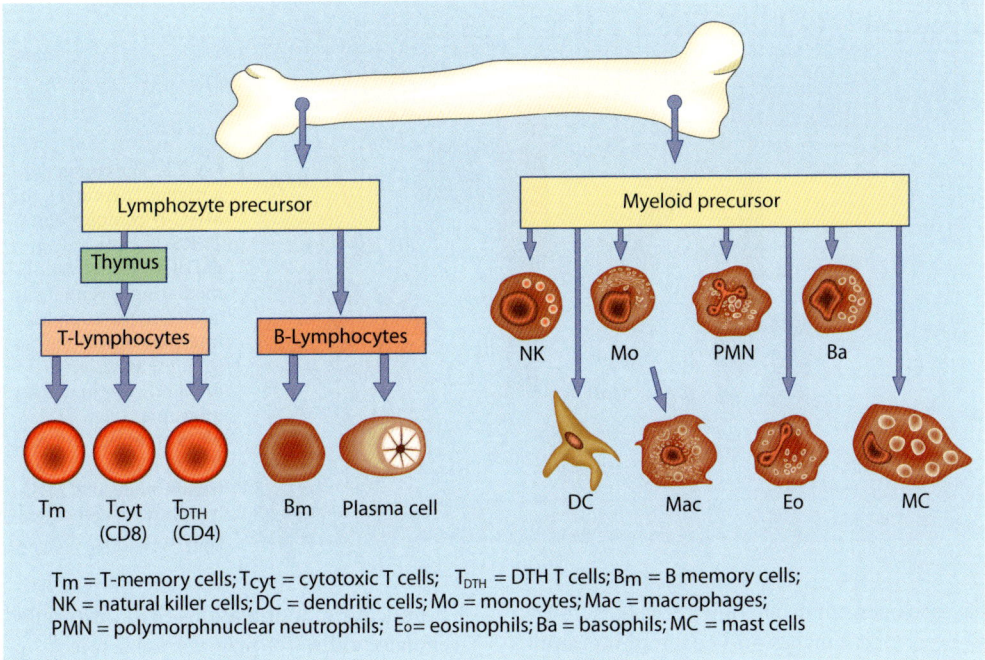

Fig. 2.2. Simplified representation of the formation of blood and immune cells

T cells recognize MHC-class II antigens (HLA-D) [14].

After renewed contact with an antigen, a specifically sensitized T cell proliferates and differentiates into T-effector cells. Cytotoxic T cells kill cells infected by intracellular microbes (e.g., cytopathic virus). DTH cells induce an inflammatory reaction via soluble cytokines.

In the development of an immune response after contact with a foreign substance, the distinction needs to be made between an afferent (induction) and an efferent phase (elicitation).

The early activation of specific T-helper cells occurs as "priming" of naive T cells after antigen presentation through dendritic cells (DCs) expressing MHC class II. DCs are "sentinels" of the immune system in the epidermis (Langerhans cells), but also in every other tissue [29, 62, 65]. During antigen processing, peptides of 8–20 amino acids are formed, which fit in the groove of the MHC complex (like a "sausage on the grill"), allowing optimal presentation to the T-cell receptor (TCR).

Antigen-bearing DCs migrate in the lymph to regional lymph nodes or in parenchymatous organs in the blood to the spleen, where the actual T-cell activation takes place.

While the first contact (primary immune response) takes an interval of some days, after repeated contact (secondary immune response), when there are already activated memory cells, the proliferation of specific lymphocytes in the tissue occurs much faster. The contact of antigen (peptide), MHC II complex, and TCR is the central signal of T-cell activation which mediates specificity. In addition to this first signal, a complex interaction of various cytokines, adhesion factors and co-stimulatory molecules (e.g., CD28) takes place (Fig. 2.3).

Activated T cells function via production of cytokines, direct cell contact using apoptosis-inducing factors [41] or through production of cytotoxic products (e.g., granzymes, perforin). Within effector T-cells, subpopulations are distinguished according to the cytokine secretion pattern, originally described for T-helper cells TH1 and TH2 (Fig. 2.4) [13, 27, 30, 42, 49, 59, 60]. In the meantime, CD8 cells have also been described with different cytokine secretion patterns. Recently, the concept of dichotomy

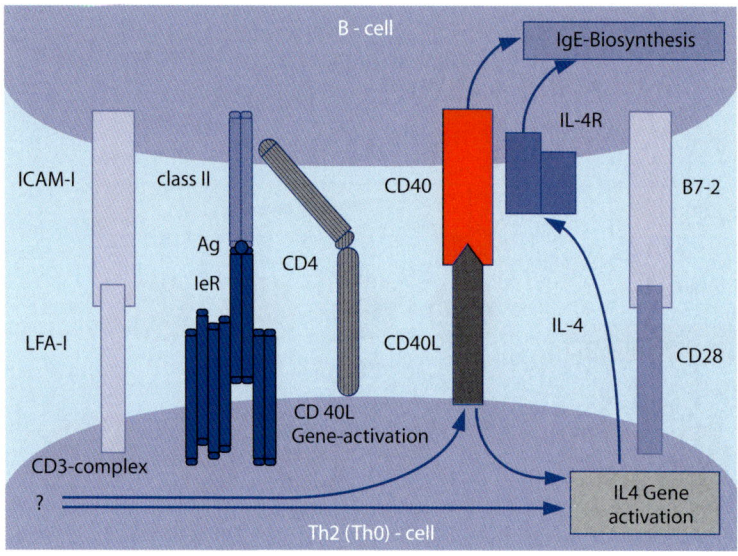

Fig. 2.3. The contact of antigens (peptides), the MHC-II complex and TCR is the central signal of T-cell activation-mediating specificity. In addition, the complex interplay of various cytokines, adhesion factors and co-stimulatory molecules (e.g., CD28) plays an important role. *ICAM*, intercellular adhesion molecule; *LFA*, lymphocyte associated function

has also been applied to other cells (e.g., to DCs or even macrophages and eosinophil granulocytes) [36].

A crucial factor in deciding in which direction a TH0 cell travels is the presence of either interleukin-4 (TH2) or interleukin-12 (TH1) in the microenvironment. While intracellular parasites induce predominantly IL-12 and TH1, extracellular parasites or parasites of a particular nature induce IL-4 or IL-13 production via mechanisms which have not yet been clearly established, either with or without dendritic cells. The origin of the "early" IL-4 (T cell versus mast cell) is still controversial.

In rodent transplantation experiments, IL-10-producing subpopulations (T3) (also called T-regulator cells, Tr) play a crucial role in inducing long-term tolerance [42, 74]. High antigen concentrations enhance T1 patterns, while low antigen doses lead to T2 reactions as well as the presence of IL4 [7].

Table 2.1 shows the most important cytokines for allergy [75], and Table 2.2 lists a selection of relevant surface markers.

There are also B-memory cells which survive through minimal concentrations of antigen stimulation present in lymph follicles and in the bone marrow.

Most T cells carry a receptor with a central α-/β-chain (Table 2.3). In mucous membranes and in the skin, there are T cells with a γ-/δ-receptor [6], recognizing a more limited antigen repertoire (Fig. 2.5). These cells are often directed against microbial cell components (e.g., mycobacteria), but also against nonspecifically damaged cell components (e.g., expression of stress proteins).

Apart from the specific activation of T cells via MHC peptide TCR complex, certain glycoproteins can activate the MHC and the β-chain of the TCR, directly leading to signal transduction (superantigens) (Fig. 2.6).

Activated T cells not only give help to B cells in antibody production but also activate macrophages (e.g., via IFN-γ) to oxygen radical, en-

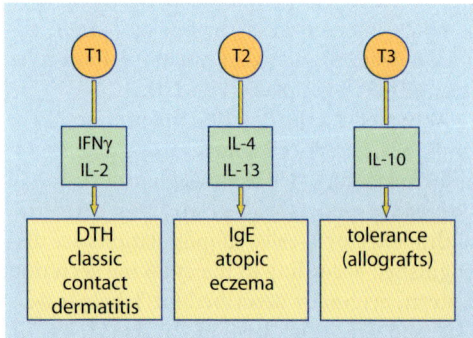

Fig. 2.4. Subpopulations of T-helper cells and their pathophysiological significance (T3 may also be called T-regulator cells)

Table 2.1. Cytokines, cytokine receptors and functions (selection). IL, interleukin; T, T lymphocytes; B, B lymphocytes; CD, cluster of differentiation; DC, dendritic cells; EOS, eosinophils; PMN, polymorphonuclear neutrophil granulocytes; NK, natural killer cells; TNF, tumor necrosis factor; MC, mast cells; IFN, interferon

Name	Formation	Receptor	Function
Interleukin-1	Epithelium, fibroblasts	M, DC receptors CD121	Thymocyte maturation, fever, epithelium activation
Interleukin-2	T	CD25 (α-chain)	Proliferation of T, activation NK
Interleukin-3	T, EOS, MC	CD123	Growth, priming
Interleukin-4	T (CD4+-TH2), MC	CD124	B-cell maturation, IgE formation
Interleukin-5	T (CD4+-TH2), MC	CD125	B and EO activation
Interleukin-6	M, T, endothelium	CD126	B-proliferation, acute inflammation
Interleukin-7	Fibroblasts	CD127	B- and T-growth
Interleukin-8	T, M epithelium	CD128	Chemotaxis of PMN
Interleukin-9	T	CD129	Mast cell growth
Interleukin-10	T, M	?	Inhibition of M, T (IL-12)
Interleukin-11	Stroma cells		Platelet formation, acute phase proteins
Interleukin-12	M, DC	?	TH1 promotion, IFN-γ
Interleukin-13	T	?	IgE formation
Interleukin-14	T		B-proliferation
Interleukin-15	M, epithelium, fibroblasts	CD123	B-, T-, and NK-proliferation
Interleukin-16	T	(CD8+ receptor + CD4)	Chemotaxis of CD4
Interleukin-17	Memory T	(CD4+)	IL-6, IL-8, and GMCSF formation
Interleukin-18	M, K, stroma		IFN-γ formation
Interferon-α	M	CD118	Antiviral, antiproliferative
Interferon-β	Fibroblasts, epithelium	CD118	Antiviral, antiproliferative
Interferon-γ	T (CD4+), TH1, NK	CD119	M, NK, endothelium activation
TNF-α (cachectin)	M, T	CD120	Activation of PMN, M, EOS, endothelium, fever
TNF-β (lymphotoxin)	T	CD120	PMN, NK, endothelium
Stem cell factor (SCF)	Stroma	CD117 (c-kit)	Stem cell, mast cell growth

Table 2.2. Selection of CD (cluster of differentiation) surface markers (for abbreviations see Table 2.1)

CD	Expression on	Function
CD1a	DC, LC, Thy	Antigen presentation
CD2	T, Pan-T-cell marker	Associated with T-cell receptor
CD3	T	TCR
CD4	Helper T, DC, M	Binding to MHC II
CD8	Cytotoxic/suppressor-T	Binding to MHC I
CD11	M, PMN, EOS	Integrin, cell adhesion
CD14	M, PMN	Endotoxin receptor
CD16	PMN, M	Fcγ receptor
CD25	T	Activation marker ("Tac")
CD28	T-subpopulation	Ligand for CD80, co-stimulation
CD30	T, B, NK	M. Hodgkin (Reed-Sternberg cells) (Ki-1)
CD34	Blood, endothelium	Binding of L-selectin
CD40	B, DC	Co-stimulation for B-activation (binding of CD154)
CD45 RO	Memory T, M	
CD45 RA	Naive T, M	
CD63	Basophils	Activation marker
CD64	PMN, M	Fcγ I receptor
CD80	B, DC	Co-stimulation (binds CD28 and CD152)
CD86 (also B7-1 and 2)		
CD95 (= Fas, APO1)	T, B, many cells	Apoptosis
CD152 (= CTLA-4)	T	Binds CD80 and CD86, T-regulation

Receptor	Units	Antigen recognition
B-cell receptor (BCR)	Immunoglobulin	(Secondary) antibody production
T-cell receptor (TCR)	α/β or γ/δ plus ε, ζ η	(Primary) cellular response
Fc-receptors		
Fcγ I, II, III	α, β, γ	Antibody-dependent effects (PMN, M, EOS)
Fcε R I	α, β, γ	Activation of mast cells and basophils
Fcε R I	α, γ	Activation of LC, M, EOS
Fcε R II	Two chains, soluble part	Possible inhibition by sCD23+, T, M, LC, B

Table 2.3. Immune recognition receptors (multi-subunit immune recognition receptors, MIRR)

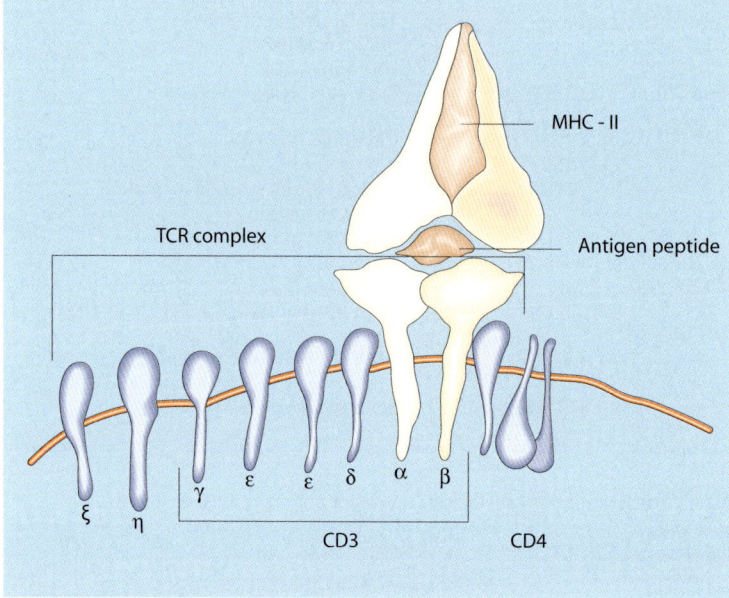

Fig. 2.5. Complex consisting of a T-cell receptor (*TCR*), antigen peptide and MHC class II

zyme, and NO release. In the amplification of inflammation, a complex interaction of cytokines [71], chemokines [3, 35, 85] (Table 2.4), and adhesion molecules [69] (Table 2.5) takes place.

Apart from cytokine secretion, certain T cells – namely CD8+ cytotoxic T cells (T_{cyt}) – can destroy cells [38], e.g., in the defense of intracellular organisms. In allergy, T_{cyt} play a pathogenic role in drug-induced exanthematous eruptions. Depending on the microenvironment, CD8 cells have different cytokine secretion patterns, for instance a TH2 pattern in the presence of IL-4. In this context, clinically well-known phenomena such as the occurrence or exacerbation of allergic symptoms on skin and mucous membranes during infections ("infect allergy") may be explained.

The most important cytokine in the activation and maturation of TH1 cells is IL-12. In the activation of B cells via T cells, co-stimulatory molecules (CD40 and B7 = CD80 and CD86 binding to CD28, CDIS2, or CD154 on the B-cell surface) are crucial (Fig. 2.7); in hyper-IgM syndrome, CD154 is mutated. Without co-stimulatory signals there is no T-cell activation but rather specific inactivation ("clonal anergy"). IL-10 inhibits the expres-

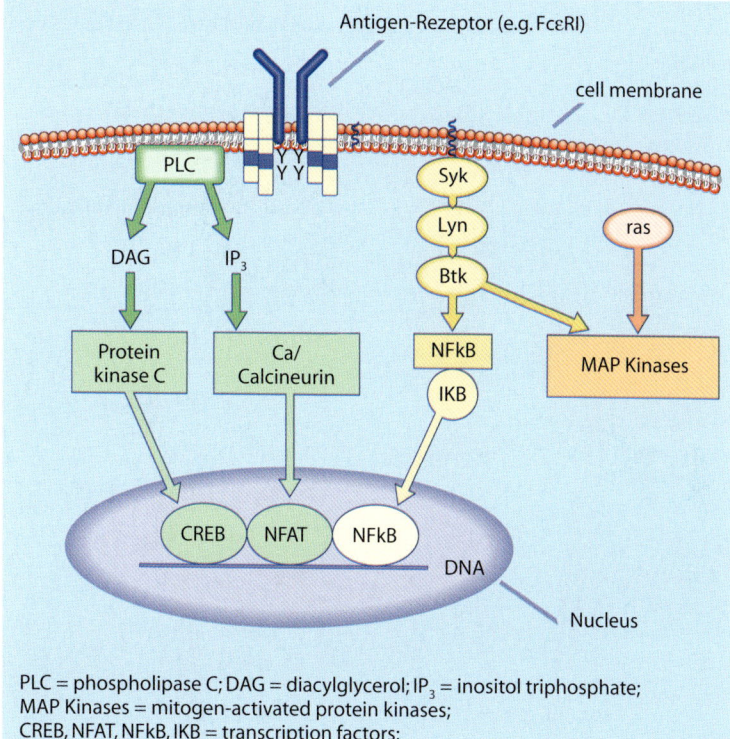

Fig. 2.6. Signal transduction following activation of the receptor of an immune recognition cell

PLC = phospholipase C; DAG = diacylglycerol; IP$_3$ = inositol triphosphate; MAP Kinases = mitogen-activated protein kinases; CREB, NFAT, NFkB, IKB = transcription factors; Syk, Lyn, Btk, ras = protein kinases

Table 2.4. Chemokines and receptors

Chemokine	Synonym	Formation	Receptor
CC chemokines			
CCL1	(TCA-3)	T, MC	CCR 8
CCL2	(MCP-1) (monocyte chemotactic protein)	M, Ly, F, EP	CCR2, CCR4
CCL3	MIP-1α (macrophage inflammatory protein)	M, Ly, PMN, F, MC	CCR1, CCR4, CCR5
CCL4	MIP-1β	M, Ly, PMN, F, MC	CCR5, CCR8
CCL5	RANTES	T, M, F	CCR1, CCR3–5
CCL7	(Monocyte chemotactic protein, MCP)	Platelets, M, MC, F	CCR13
CCL11	Eotaxin	Epithelium, EOS, lung	CCR3
CCL24	Eotaxin 2	T, M	CCR3
CCL26	Eotaxin 3	Epithelium	CCR3
CXC chemokines			
CXCL2	GROβ (growth-related oncogene β)	MC, heart	CXCR2
CXCL4	PF-4	Platelets	?
CXCL7	(Neutrophil-activating peptide) NAP-2	Platelets	CXCR2
CXCL8	Interleukin-8	T, M, epithelium	CXCR1–2
CXCL10	(Interferon-inducible protein) IP-10)	M, PMN, epithelium, fibroblasts	CXCR3
XC chemokines			
XCL1	Lymphotactin	T	XCR1
CX3C chemokines			
CX3CL1	Fraktalkine, neurotactin	Epithelium, T, DC, brain	XC3CR1

Table 2.5. Important adhesion molecules

	Synonyms	Binding
Selectins		
P-Selectin	CD62P	Leukocyte oligosaccharides
E-Selectin	CD62E	Leukocyte oligosaccharides CLA
L-Selectin	CD62L	Specific sugars on naive T cells
Integrins		
β1-Integrins (with seven different α-chains)	CD 29 (CD49a+f)	Collagen, fibronectin, laminin, etc.
β2-Integrin	CD11/CD18	ICAM-1, -2
β3-Integrin	CD61	Fibrinogen, fibronectin, etc.

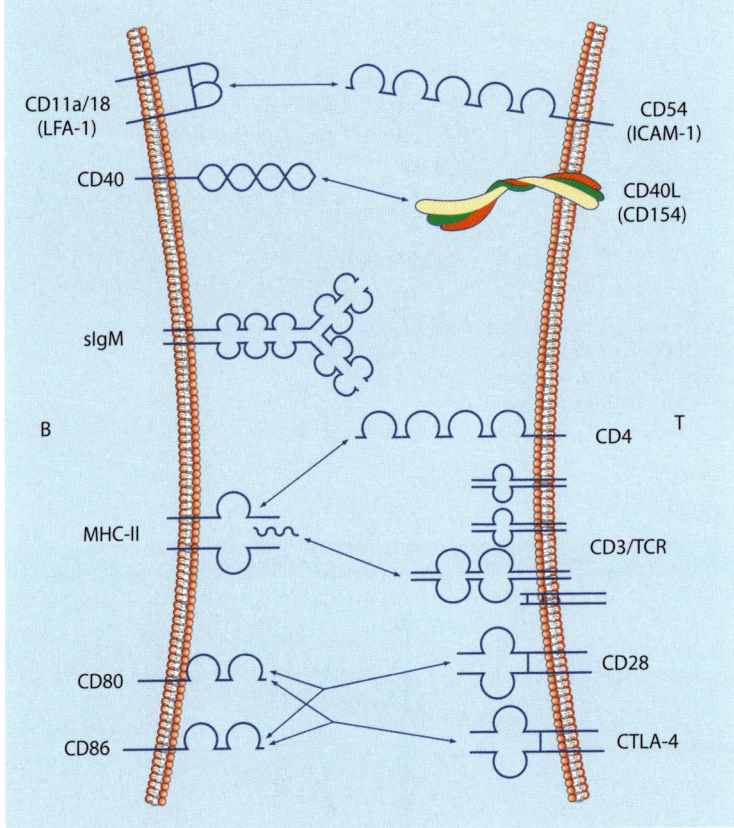

Fig. 2.7. Interaction between the surface markers of B and T cells

sion of co-stimulatory molecules and may induce a specific tolerance by downregulating TH1 responses.

TH1/TH2 reactions influence each other ("yin yang theory"): IFN-γ inhibits IgE production while IL-4 decreases the formation of IL-12 in macrophages. These interactions, also called minimal cellular immunodeficiency or immune deviation, may explain the well-known susceptibility to certain infections in atopics.

B-cell maturation takes place in the bone marrow and in lymphoid organs along the GI tract, corresponding to the bursa of Fabricius in birds. B cells differentiate to antibody-secreting plasma cells (humoral immunity). In the plasma and in lymph fluid, an estimated 10^{20} antibody molecules are present.

A complex interaction between B and T cells regulates B-cell differentiation. T-helper cells (TH = CD4) enhance antibody formation while T-suppressor cells (CD8) inhibit the immune response. Certain antigens (particularly carbohydrates) are able to activate B cells without the help of T cells (so-called T-independent antigens).

2.2 Antibodies

Antibodies are immunoglobulins of five different classes (isotypes) with varying amino acid sequences and heavy chains (see Fig. 2.8), the heavy chains determining the isotype and the name of the immunoglobulin class.

The immunoglobulin molecule may be split into fragments by enzymatic digestion. The Fab fragment contains the hypervariable regions important for antigen binding. The Fc fragment contains the constant part of the antibody molecule, consisting of parts of the heavy chains and mediating important biological functions such as activation of the complement system and binding to cells. The different immunoglobulin classes differ in size, half-life, and biological function (Fig. 2.9).

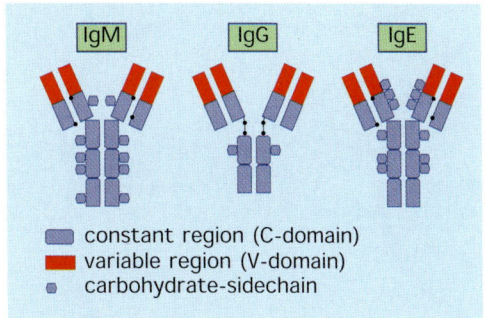

Fig. 2.9. Schematic representation of the different classes of immunoglobulins

Immunoglobulin E as carrier of the immediate-type allergic reactivity differs from IgG by an additional domain in the Fc part, allowing binding to mast cells and basophil leukocytes.

Figure 2.10 shows schemes of the reaction types I, II, and III according to Coombs and Gell [15].

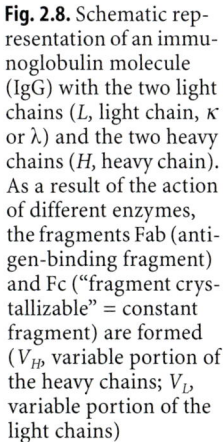

Fig. 2.8. Schematic representation of an immunoglobulin molecule (IgG) with the two light chains (L, light chain, κ or λ) and the two heavy chains (H, heavy chain). As a result of the action of different enzymes, the fragments Fab (antigen-binding fragment) and Fc ("fragment crystallizable" = constant fragment) are formed (V_H, variable portion of the heavy chains; V_L, variable portion of the light chains)

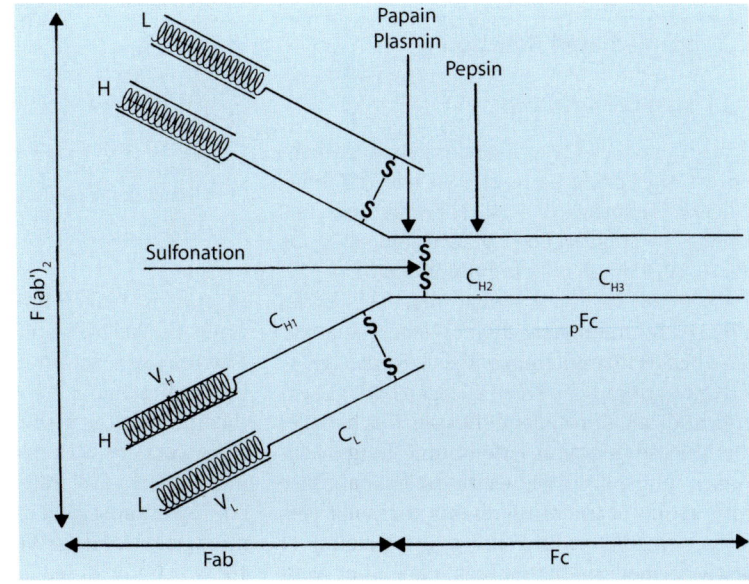

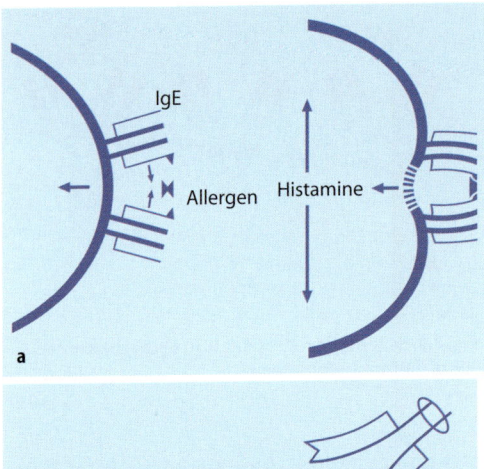
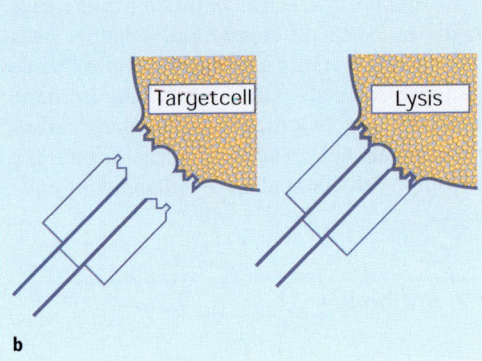
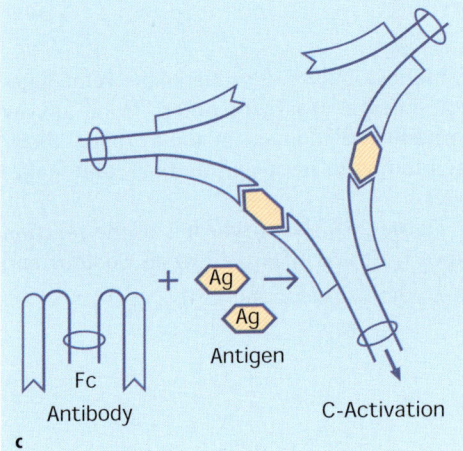
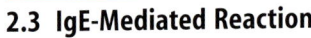

Fig. 2.10a–c. Schematic representation of the pathogenic immune reactions type I, II and III. **a** Type 1: The IgE-mediated reaction involves bridging between the allergen and at least two IgE molecules on the surface of mast cells or basophilic leukocytes. **b** Type II: In the cytotoxic reaction, pathogenic antibodies are aimed at cell surface determinants. **c** Type III: Immune complex reaction: As a result of antigen binding, complement-activating structures are released at the Fc end

Table 2.6. Elicitors of histamine release reactions

- IgE (or cytophilic IgG) (divalent antigen, dimeric IgE, anti-IgE, concanavalin A, anti-IgE receptor, anti-idiotype)
- Complement (C5a, C3a)
- Calcium ionophore
- Basic peptides (48/80, cationic peptides, Synacthen, polymyxin, MCD peptide)
- Opiate alkaloids (e.g., codeine, morphine)
- Tachykinins (e.g., substance P)
- Other direct histamine liberators (relaxants, radiographic contrast media, etc.)
- Enzymes (chymotrypsin, thrombin, phospholipase)
- Cytokines (histamine-releasing factor)
- Detergents
- Physicochemical irritants
- Hypoxia

2.3 IgE-Mediated Reaction

2.3.1 Mast-Cell Activation

The IgE-mediated reaction (classic anaphylaxis) occurs after bridging of at least two IgE molecules on the surface of mast cells or basophil leukocytes by an allergen (Fig. 2.10a) [2, 8, 20, 28, 45, 70, 80, 83]. IgE is an immunoglobulin of MW 190,000 [28, 32, 70]. A human mast cell carries 10^4–10^5 IgE receptors [39, 48]. There is a balance between circulating and cell-bound IgE.

After bridging between allergen and IgE, energy and calcium-dependent signaling induces the release reaction. Membrane-bound enzymes (phospholipase, serine esterase) induce contraction of microtubuli and release of preformed mediators parallel to production of newly formed mediators (e.g., platelet-activating factor, leukotrienes, and prostaglandins) [2, 9, 19, 20, 28, 44, 45, 63, 79] (see Sect. 2.9). The release reaction not only can be triggered by allergen but also by other stimuli activating the IgE receptor within the cell membrane (anti-IgE, anti-FcɛRI). Apart from IgE-dependent mechanisms, a variety of immunological and non-immunological stimuli are able to induce mediator secretion (Table 2.6, Fig. 2.11) [44, 55].

2.3 IgE-Mediated Reaction

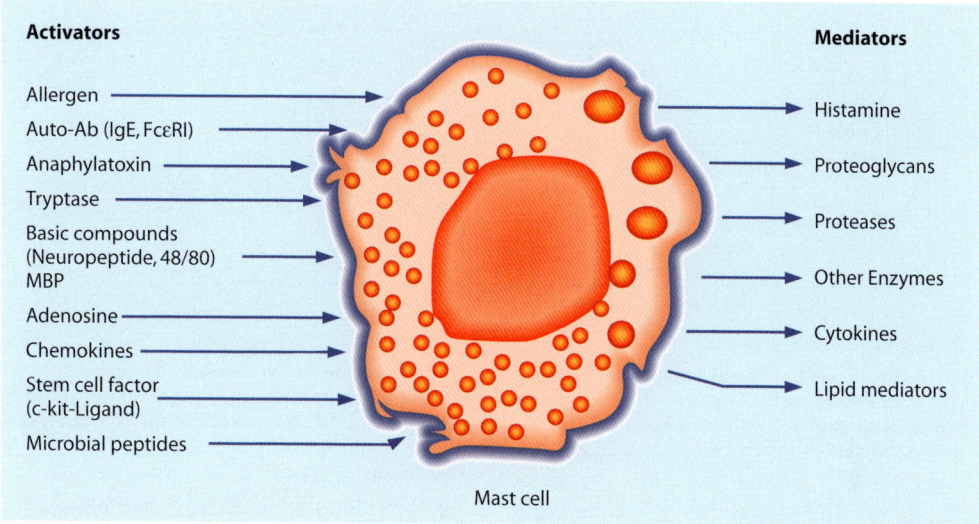

Fig. 2.11. Activators and mediators of the mast cell

The release of mediators is regulated through the second messenger system of cyclic nucleotides cAMP and cGMP (cyclic 3–5-adenosine monophosphate, cyclic 3–5-guanosine monophosphate). cAMP elevation (e.g., by β-adrenergics, prostaglandin E, histamine via H_2 receptor) inhibit mediator release [33] while cGMP elevation enhances mediator secretion (e.g., cholinergic influences) (Fig. 2.12) [2, 19, 20, 34, 58, 64, 72].

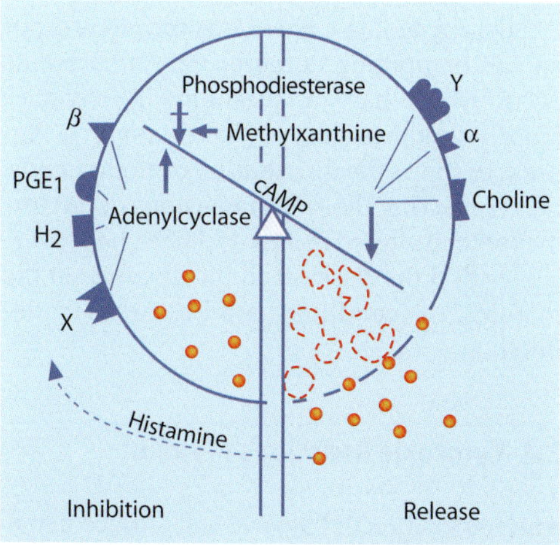

2.3.2 IgE and Atopy

While in normal organisms only minimal amounts of IgE are produced, atopic individuals are characterized by increased IgE production, which is partly genetically determined (see Sect. 3.1). IL-4 and IL-13 induce enzyme activation in the nucleus of B cells (recombinase), leading to the isotype switch between ε-chain and the junction piece (J) and secretion of IgE antibodies [42, 59, 60] (Fig. 2.13).

Although few diseases are characterized by similarly activated IgE levels in the blood, the equation "atopy = IgE" is too simple. Elevated IgE levels are also present in parasitic infestation [12, 22, 30], certain tumors and other T-cell regulatory disturbances (Fig. 2.14).

Apart from increased IgE production, atopic diseases are characterized by unspecific alterations of skin and mucous membrane reactivity (e.g., against autonomic neurosystem transmitters). On the other hand, there are clear-cut IgE-mediated diseases (e.g., anaphylaxis) which do not belong to atopic diseases (Fig. 2.15).

Fig. 2.12. Regulation of histamine release by cAMP. Factors that increase the cAMP concentration (e.g., β-adrenergic stimuli, prostaglandin E, histamine via the H_2-receptor, other =x) inhibit the release of histamine. In contrast, histamine release is promoted by α-adrenergic, cholinergic and other (y) stimuli that lower the cAMP concentration (and usually simultaneously increase the cGMP concentration)

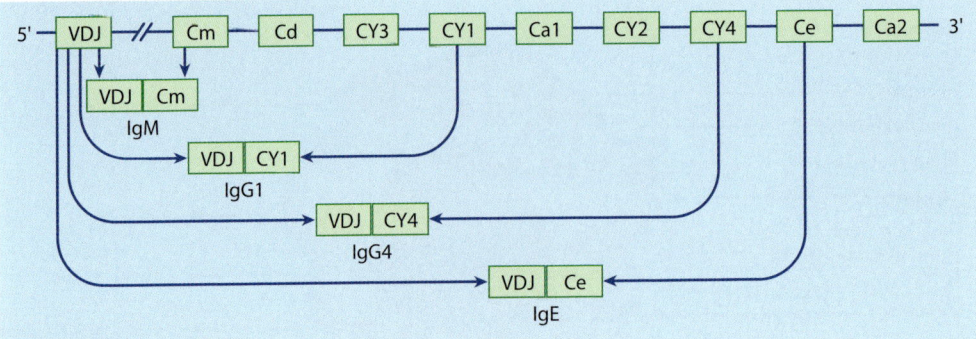

Fig. 2.13. Creation of functional antibody diversity in human beings via the "isotype switch." The gene in the C-region is located below the displaced V-region gene complex (*VDJ*). During antibody production the VDJ segment can be recombined with various genes in the C-region in order to produce antibodies with a certain specificity but different isotypes

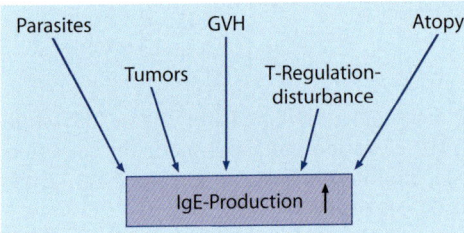

Fig. 2.14. States with heightened IgE formation

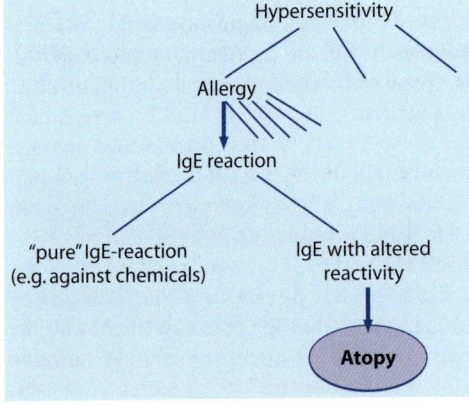

Fig. 2.15. Positioning of atopy within a classification of various forms of hypersensitivity

We define "atopy" as:

- A familiar tendency to develop certain diseases (rhinoconjunctivitis, asthma, eczema) on the basis of hypersensitivity of the skin and mucous membranes to environmental substances
- Being associated with increased IgE production and/or
- An altered nonspecific reactivity (Ring [86])

This definition is derived from the viewpoint of the clinician, who sees the patient and his symptoms first. A new (WAO) definition stresses the laboratory findings of increased IgE formation as a first prerequisite for "atopy" (ref. [12] in Chap. 1). This will have implications with regard to "intrinsic" and "extrinsic" types of atopic diseases (asthma, eczema).

Like any biologic phenomenon, atopy is not an "all or nothing" process. Marginal events occur which have a questionable or rather loose relation to atopy ("latent atopy"). Figure 2.16 shows the distribution of atopic conditions reflecting the two dimensions of IgE formation and altered reactivity. When both overlap we find the classical atopic diseases. At the margins, the conditions are less precisely defined.

2.4 Cytotoxic Reactions (Type II)

Antibodies directed against cell surface determinants (Fig. 2.10b) destroy target cells via complement activation. Clinical examples are allergic agranulocytosis or thrombocytopenia when drugs bind, e.g., at the leukocyte or platelet surface, as well as blood transfusion incompatibility and certain forms of hemolytic anemia (see Sect. 5.2).

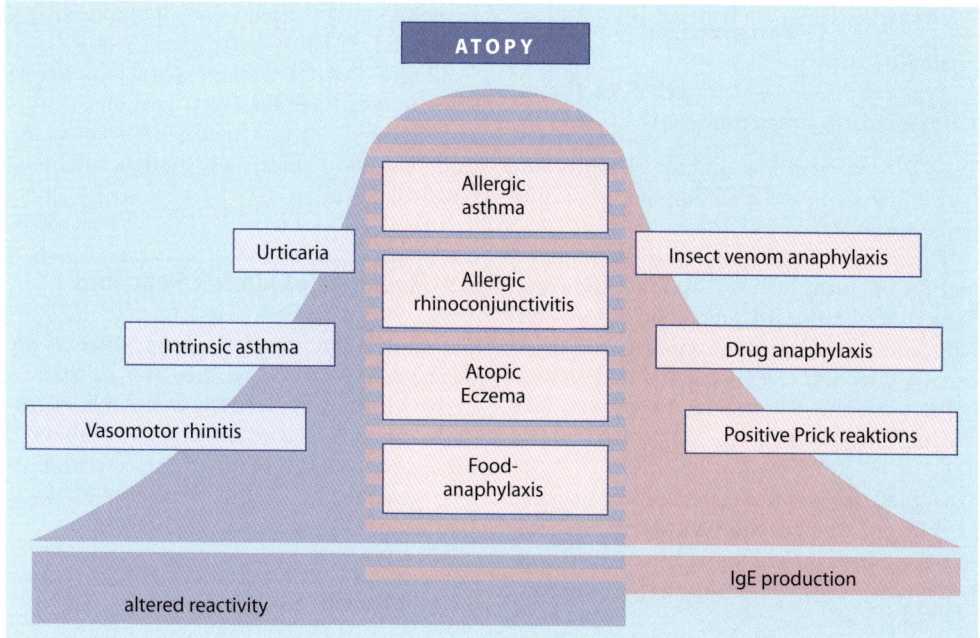

Fig. 2.16. Various manifestations of atopic disorders between altered reactivity and IgE formation

2.5 Immune Complex Reactions (Type III)

Circulating antigen antibody complexes lead to activation of the complement system and neutrophil granulocytes (Fig. 2.10c) [17]. Clinically two types of immune complex reactions have to be distinguished, an acute type with immune complex anaphylaxis (e.g., dextran anaphylaxis) [58] and the slower developing (1–2 weeks) serum sickness after antigen application which occurs with nephritis, vasculitis, arthritis, and urticaria as well as lymph node swelling [17] and fever.

2.6 Cellular Hypersensitivity (Type IV)

Pathogenic immune reactions not transferable by serum but through sensitized effector T lymphocytes have been called cellular hypersensitivity. Cellular immunity as a protective mechanism is essential for life; congenital or acquired defects occur with serious diseases.

However, under certain conditions, cellular immune reactions may also induce disease, when, e.g., effector cells are directed against a target virus which is not necessarily cytopathic (e.g., lymphocytic choriomeningitis of the mouse). In hepatitis B infection, tissue destruction needs a functioning cellular immune reaction, which no longer take places in AIDS.

In certain autoimmune diseases, cellular immune reactions are considered to be pathogenic (e.g., in multiple sclerosis, ulcerative colitis, M. Addison, type I diabetes).

Allergic contact dermatitis represents the classical clinical manifestation of cellular hypersensitivity type IV. Low molecular weight exogenous substances (e.g., metal salts) are bound to protein carriers or lead to alterations of the tertiary structure of the MHC on antigen-presenting cells leading to specific T-cell activation (TH1 reaction) [36, 40, 74] (see Sect. 5.5.2).

Our understanding of T-cell reactivity has been greatly enhanced since the days of Coombs and Gell. Today type IV reactions may be further subdivided (see Table 1.5):

- Type IVa = TH1-triggered reaction (e.g., allergic contact dermatitis)

- Type IVb = TH2 triggered reaction (e.g., atopic eczema)
- Type IVc = T_{cyt}(CD8)-triggered reaction (e.g., bullous drug eruptions)

Type IVb represents a mixture of type I and type IV, since in the eliciting phase IgE antibodies play a role.

The route of application of antigen is important for the manifestation of the reaction: epidermal application of tuberculin (Moro test) induces eczematous skin reactions, while intradermal injection (Mendel Mantoux reaction) induces a dermal papule with the same kinetics starting after 24–48 h, reaching a maximum at 72 h.

Organ transplant rejection can be grouped in the type IVc reactions, while hyperacute rejection in xenografts represents an antibody and complement-mediated reaction [11, 50].

2.7 Less Frequent Types of Allergic Reactions (Types V and VI)

In addition to the four types according to Coombs and Gell, types V and VI have been suggested:

- *Type V* as "granulomatous hypersensitivity," with differing kinetics from type IV and a specific macroscopic and microscopic morphology (see Sect. 5.8)
- *Type VI* as "stimulating/neutralizing hypersensitivity," where antibodies act like hormones through specific interaction with the receptor on a target cell starting a signaling cascade without amplifying inflammation (see Sect. 5.9)

2.8 Pseudo-allergic Reactions

In concluding our comments on the different types of allergic diseases, it needs to be mentioned that activation of different cells and plasma systems with release of mediators and induction of inflammatory reactions may also take place without involvement of specific immune reactions. These cases of hypersensitivity reactions have been called "pseudo-allergic reactions" (PAR).

Clinical examples are certain hypersensitivity reactions to drugs (e.g., local anesthetics, radiographic contrast media, intravenous anesthetics, and volume substitution solutions) (see Sect. 5.7.2).

2.9 Mediators of Allergic Reactions

The clinical symptoms of allergic diseases are determined by so-called mediator substances derived from different cells (mast cells, basophils, eosinophils, and neutrophils) (Table 2.7, Figs. 2.18a,b, 2.19). Many of these substances have general physiologic or pathophysiologic significance in inflammatory diseases.

2.9.1 Histamine

Histamine is the best-known mediator substance of the immediate-type allergic reaction. It is synthesized and stored in mast cells (Fig. 2.17) and basophil leukocytes. Histamine exerts its effects via several receptors (H1: endothelium, smooth muscles; H2: gastric mucosa, acid secretion, superficial skin vessels, heart; H3: CNS, autocrine inhibition of histaminergic neurons; H4: eosinophil granulocytes) [2, 44, 45, 55, 58, 64, 70] (Table 2.8).

2.9.2 Eicosanoids

Arachidonic acid in the cell membrane is transformed via cyclooxygenase into prostaglandins, via different lipoxygenases into leukotrienes (Fig. 2.20). Prostaglandins are unsaturated C-20 fatty acids formed via cyclooxygenase (COX) and an intermediate of highly active unstable endoperoxides PGG2 and PGH2 [79].

Inhibitors of cyclooxygenase are acetylsalicylic acid, indomethacin, and non-steroidal anti-inflammatory drugs (NSAIDs) acting throughout the body (COX-1 inhibitors); in inflamed tissue, a specific cyclooxygenase (COX-2) is expressed which can be specifically inhibited.

Table 2.7. Relevant mediator substances from human mast cells and basophils. M, monocytes; EOS, eosinophils; PMN, polymorphonuclear neutrophils

Mediator substance	Structure	Function
Preformed		
Histamine	β-Imidazolyl-ethylamine	H_1 permeability increase, vasodilatation, contraction smooth muscle
		H_2 gastric mucosa: acid secretion
		Heart: arrhythmia
		Skin: flush
		H_3 CNS: regulation (?)
		H_4: eosinophils (?)
Neurophil chemotactic activity (NCA)	Protein MW 75,000	Chemotaxis
Basophil kallikrein of anaphylaxis (BK-A)	Kallikrein	Kininogenase
Proteoglycans	Heparin, chondroitin sulfate, dermatan sulfate	Anticoagulating complement inhibiting?
Enzymes	Chymase,[a] tryptase	Proteolysis
Newly formed		
Protease inhibitors	$α_1$-Chymotrypsin	Inhibition of chymase
Lipoxins	Trihydroxytrienes	Bronchoconstriction
Leukotrienes (LT-C_4, D_4, E_4)	Sulfido-LT	Contraction of smooth muscles (long-lasting), permeability increase, chemotaxis
Leukotriene B_4, 15-HETE		Mucus secretion
Prostaglandins	Prostaglandins D_2 Prostaglandins E_2	Contraction smooth muscles, vasodilatation
Platelet-activating factor (PAF)	Acyl-glyceryl-phosphoryl-choline	Chemotaxis
		Chemotaxis (particularly eosinophils), bronchospasm
Cytokines	Interleukin-4	Activation of M, EOS, PMN, fever
	TNF-α	Fibrosis
	Fibroblast growth factor	

[a] Only in mucosa mast cells

Table 2.8. Histamine effects, receptors and symptoms

Effect	Receptor	Symptoms/disease
Stimulation of nociceptive nerve fibers	H_1	Itch, urticaria, eczema, allergic rhinoconjunctivitis, pharyngitis
Increase of endothelial permeability	H_1/H_2	Wheal, urticaria, allergic rhinitis, anaphylaxis
Constriction of smooth muscles	H_1	Bronchoconstriction, allergic asthma, food anaphylaxis
Increased mucosecretion	H_1	Allergic rhinitis, asthma
Tachycardia	H_1 (probably via suprarenals)	Anaphylaxis
Blood pressure changes (hypo- and hypertension)	H_1/H_2	Anaphylaxis
Arrhythmia	H_2	Anaphylaxis
Gastric acid secretion	H_2	Peptic ulcer
Inhibition of leukocyte function	H_2	Immune deviation?
Prostaglandin formation	H_1	Allergic asthma?
Increase of intracellular cAMP	H_2	Negative feedback on mast cell activation and immune function
Increase of intracellular cGMP	H_1	Enhancement of mast cell secretion?
Autocrine inhibition of histaminergic neurons	H_3	Sleep-wake rhythm, headache (?)
Activation of eosinophils	H_4	?

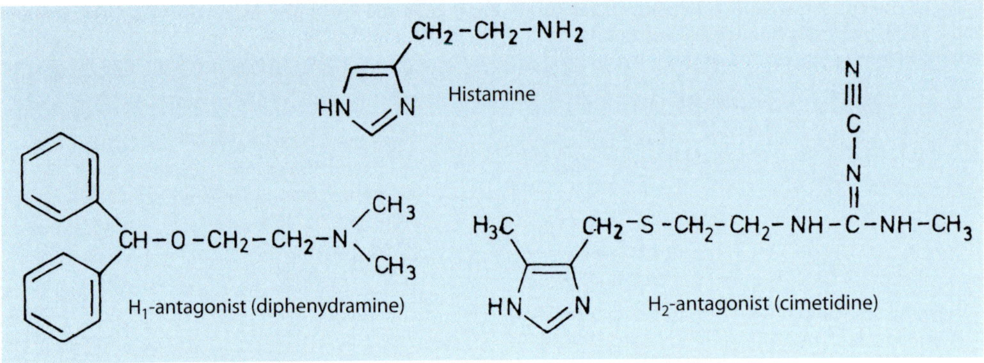

2 Pathophysiology of Allergic Reactions

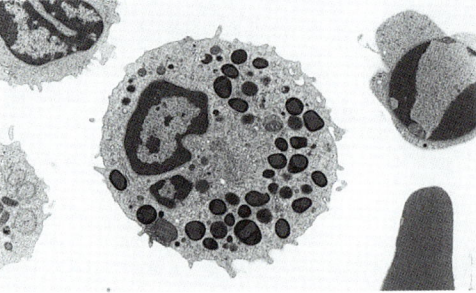

Fig. 2.17. Structural formulas of histamine and of an H_1- and an H_2-receptor antagonist

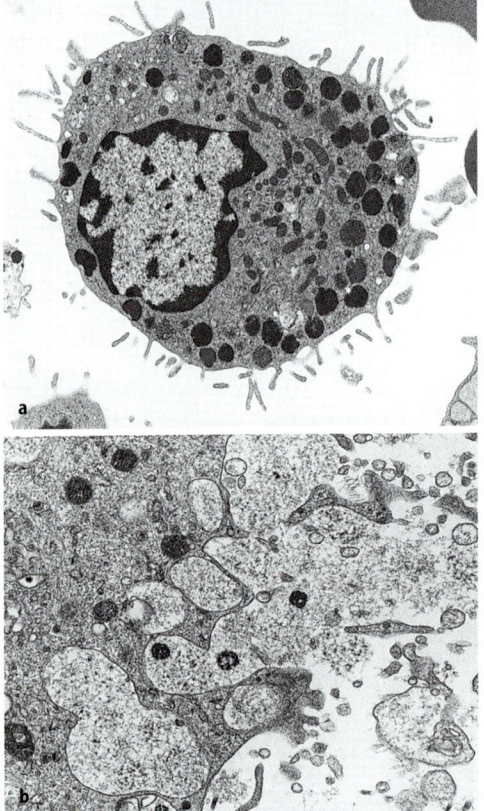

Fig. 2.19. Human eosinophilic leukocyte ($\times 15,000$) (electron microscopic photos: H. Behrendt)

Four relevant groups of prostaglandins are distinguished with different effects:

- PGE: vasodilation
- PGF and PGD (the latter produced by mast cells): vasoconstriction and bronchoconstriction
- PGI (= prostacyclin): inhibition of platelet aggregation
- Thromboxane: platelet aggregation

Prostaglandins not only act at the smooth muscle, but also at white blood cells and are involved in regulation of the immune reaction, PGE2 enhancing TH2 patterns.

Arachidonic acid is produced in a metabolic cycle between lecithin and lysolecithin from membrane phospholipids.

Fig. 2.18. a Human mast cells obtained from an asthmatic patient by bronchoalveolar lavage ($\times 18,000$). **b** Human cutaneous mast cells, degranulation ($\times 47,100$)

2.9.3 Leukotrienes

The chemical nature of the "slow-reacting substance of anaphylaxis" (SRS-A) has been elucidated since 1979, being shown to comprise leukotrienes, which were so called since they were isolated from leukocytes [23, 54, 63]. Similar to prostaglandins, they are formed from arachidonic acid, not via cyclooxygenase but via 5-lipoxygenase (Fig. 2.20). While LTB4 has chemotactic activity on neutrophils and eosinophils, the sulfido-leukotrienes LTC4, LTD4, and LTE4 have anaphylactogenic and bronchoconstricting effects.

2.9.4 Platelet-Activating Factor

Platelets are also involved in the course of the immediate-type allergic reaction. The so-called "platelet drop" has been used as a diagnostic test in food allergy provocation tests. Platelet-activating factor (PAF) is produced from mast cells and basophils and induces aggregation and degranulation of platelets. PAF is a phospholipid (2-acyl-sn-glyceryl-3-phosphorylcholine) and also has chemotactic activities (Fig. 2.21) [9].

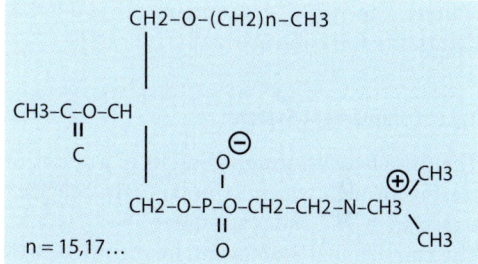

Fig. 2.21. Structural formula of the platelet-activating factor (PAF)

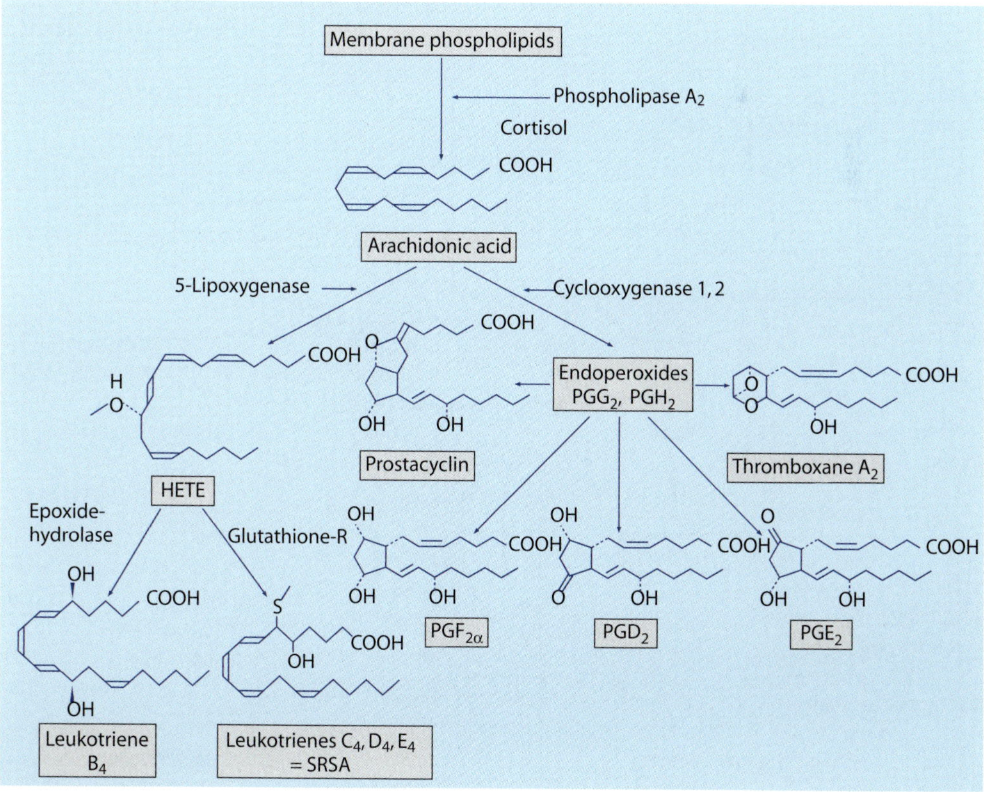

Fig. 2.20. Schematic representation of the most important products of arachidonic acid metabolism, including products of cyclooxygenase (prostaglandins) and lipoxygenase (leukotrienes)

2.9.5 Serotonin

Platelets represent the most important store for serotonin in human blood. Serotonin (5-OH tryptamine) is a biogenic amine with pronounced vasoactive properties. When increased – e.g., in carcinoid syndrome – attacks of flushing are characteristic. Similar manifestations have been observed in anaphylactic reactions. The role of serotonin in human allergic diseases is still controversial.

2.9.6 Complement System

The complement system consists of a series of plasma proteins which – similar to the coagulation system – activate each other like a cascade. The complement system can be activated with or without specific immunologic antigen recognition. Activated complement induces either cell lysis or inflammation [50]. Two pathways of complement activation, the "classical" and the "alternative," can be distinguished (Fig. 2.22). The classical pathway consists of a total of 11 different components starting with C1q-recognizing immune complexes and once activated leading to further activation of the factors C1r, C1s, C4, and C2. These components of the classical pathway are also called "recognition" (= C1) and "activation" units (C4, C2, and C3).

C3 represents the central component of the complement system which is activated through both pathways. Activated C3 leads to activation of C5 and the so-called "attack" unit (components C6–C9), leading to lysis of cells (bacteria, protozoa, but also red blood cells).

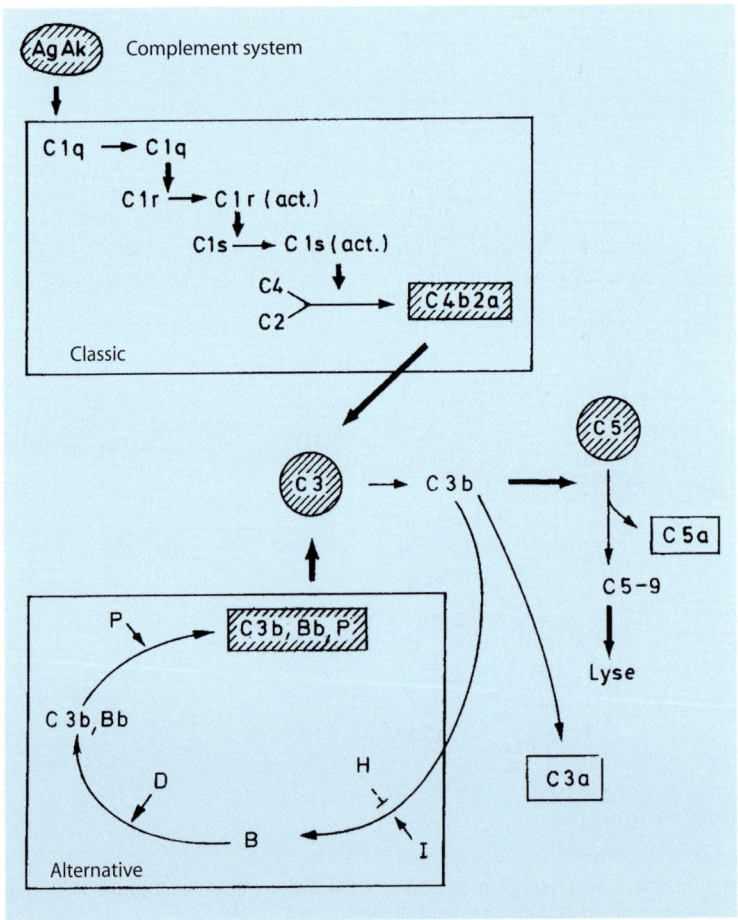

Fig. 2.22. Schematic representation of the two pathways for complement activation

Apart from the "classical" pathway, complement can be activated via the "alternative" pathway (also called bypass activation) without antigen-antibody complexes. The alternative pathway consists of three components: factor B, factor D, and properdin. The postulated initiating factor I of the alternative pathway playing a comparative role as an "antibody" on the surface of certain bacteria or cell surfaces is still controversial. Factor I may recognize common frequently repeating carbohydrate structures characteristic of bacterial surfaces. Indeed, polysaccharides or lipopolysaccharides from many bacteria are very effective in activating the alternative pathway of the complement system.

Properdin seems to have a stabilizing effect in the alternative pathway activation, conserving the activity of the enzyme complex C3bBb and allowing feedback between the classical and alternative pathways.

During complement activation, certain peptides C3a or C5a – so-called anaphylatoxins – are formed with chemotactic, histamine liberating and direct vasoactive effects [50].

The various methods of activation of the complement system are counteracted in nature by certain inhibitors; if they are defective, clinical diseases with allergy-like symptoms become manifest: C1-inactivator deficiency leads to the hereditary angioneurotic edema (see Sect. 5.1.3). In the case of deficiency of anaphylatoxin inactivator (carboxypeptidase B), which inactivates anaphylatoxins by digesting the arginine end, relapsing infectious diseases, urticaria, and eosinopenia are observed.

2.9.7 Mediators from Neutrophil Granulocytes

Both IgE-mediated mast cell reactions and complement activation lead to chemotactic factors acting on granulocytes [82], e.g., leukotriene B4 has a chemotactic action not only on eosinophil but also on neutrophil granulocytes. According to Behrendt, in a humid environment pollen grains are able to release eicosanoid-like substances which have a neutrophil chemotactic activity in the "initiation" of sensitization [5] (see Sect. 3.3).

Neutrophil granulocytes contain highly active lysosomal enzymes, stored in different granules (proteinases, hydrolases, peroxidases) [26]. Interacting with other cells as well as the complement system, these enzymes influence the amplification of inflammation (activation of mast cell, basophils, platelets, C5, formation of kinins and leukotrienes).

In many inflammatory reactions, activated oxygen species (radicals) formed via lysosomal peroxidases play a role. Superoxide dismutases (SOD) able to inactivate these radicals have inhibitory activity and are used in certain inflammatory diseases. They have also been characterized as major allergens from certain molds (e.g., *Aspergillus*) (see Sect. 3.4).

2.9.8 Mediators from Eosinophil Granulocytes

While eosinophils some decades ago were regarded as anti-inflammatory cells, clearing up the sequelae of tissue destruction ("dawn of inflammation") (Charcot-Leyden crystals contain the leukotriene-degrading enzyme phospholipase D), they are regarded today as active proinflammatory cells contributing to tissue destruction through cationic proteins such as major basic protein (MBP) or eosinophil cationic protein (ECP). Eosinophils can bind endotoxin and become activated through CD14 [56].

2.9.9 Kallikrein-Kinin System

The kallikrein-kinin system, when activated, leads to formation of potent vasoactive substances, e.g., bradykinin – with possible involvement in allergic diseases (Fig. 2.23). The close relationship with coagulation, fibrinolysis, and the complement system as well as with the enzymes of prostaglandin metabolism suggest important interactions.

These interactions are of practical importance for patients with hereditary angioneurotic edema (C1 inactivator deficiency). C1 inactivator inhibits not only C1 but also plasmin and prekallikrein. In a state of deficiency, trivial events such as minimal trauma during dental procedures lead to excessive activation of all three systems with autocatalytic processes within the kinin molecule [23].

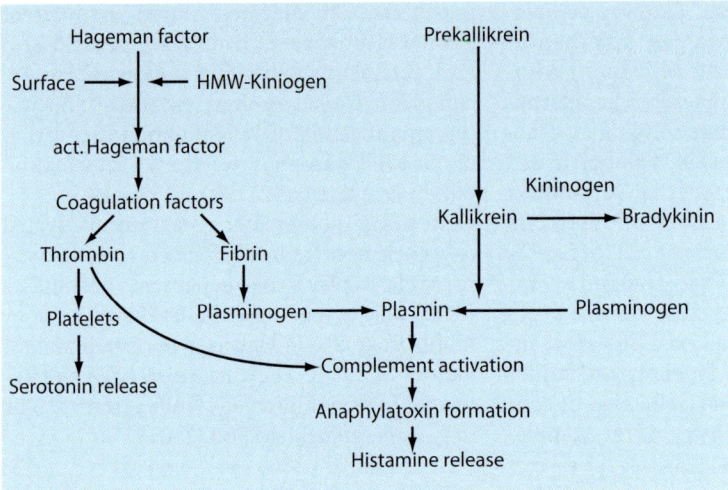

Fig. 2.23. Relationships between the complement, coagulation and kallikrein-kinin systems

The differential therapy of this hereditary disease includes:

- Epsilon-amino-caproic acid as fibrinolysis inhibitor
- The androgenic substances danazol or stanazolol lead to an increased production of C1 inactivator protein
- In acute treatment or for prophylaxis prior to surgery, highly purified C1 inactivator can be infused

2.9.10 Tachykinins

Neuropeptides (e.g., substance P, calcitonin-gene-related peptide, CGRP, vasoactive intestinal peptide, VIP) induce mast cell activation and influence the end phase of allergic reactions [12]. Tachykinins may play a role in the pathophysiology of itch (see Sect. 6.2.11).

2.10 Synopsis of Mediator Release and Inactivation

The release of mediators and cytokines during an allergic response represents a complex interaction with activating and inhibitory components. Experiments in knock-out mice have shown the redundancy of important phenomena: defects in certain cytokines, receptors, or mediators often show no clinical abnormal phenotype, while severe symptoms may be observed with overexpression of certain factors.

Some mediators released during cell activation induce (via negative feedback) inhibitory influences on the releasing cell or induce inactivation via activation of other cells and release of inhibitory enzymes. Inhibitory enzymes for relevant mediators are:

- Diaminoxidase (DAO = histaminase) for histamine
- Phospholipase D for platelet-activating factor
- Peptidases for sulfido-leukotrienes

Certain drugs have DAO inhibitory activity; especially in elderly persons on multiple pharmacotherapy, DAO blockade may occur and may be relevant for increased histaminergic reactions (see Sect. 5.7.3).

Some humoral and cellular reactions of the allergic cascade described are also under control of the nervous system through neuropeptides, autonomic transmitters and suprarenal hormones. Cytokines can act on nerve cells and neurotrophins on lymphocytes. This complex interaction might help to explain the well-known psychosomatic influence upon many allergic diseases (see Chap. 7).

References

1. Askenase PW, Geba GP, Levin J, Ratzlaff RE, Anderson GM, Ushio H, Ptak W, Matsuda H (1995) A role for platelet release of serotonin in the initiation of contact sensitivity. Int Arch Allergy Immunol 107:145–147
2. Austen KF (1979) Biologic implications of the structural and functional characteristics of the chemical mediators of immediate-type hypersensitivity. The Harvey lectures, series 73. Academic Press, New York, pp 93–161
3. Baggiolini M (1998) Chemokines and leukocyte traffic. Nature 392:565–568
4. Barnes PJ (1996) New drugs for asthma. Clin Exp Allergy 26:738–745
5. Behrendt H, Becker W-M (2001) Localization, release and bioavailability of pollen allergens: the influence of environmental factors. Curr Opin Immunol 13:709–715
6. Bergstresser PR, Takashima A (eds) (2001) Gamma-delta T cells. Chemical immunology, vol 79. Karger, Basel
7. Blaser K, Carballido JM, Faith A, Crameri R, Akdis CA (1998) Determinants and mechanisms of human immune response to bee venom phospholipase A_2. Int Arch Allergy Immunol 117:1–10
8. Bennich H, Johansson SGO (1971) Structure and function of human immunoglobulin E. Adv Immunol 13:1
9. Benveniste J, Arnoux B (eds) (1983) Platelet-activating factor and structurally related ether-lipids. INSERM Symp 23. Elsevier, Amsterdam
10. Bienenstock J, Befus AD (1980) Mucosal immunology. Immunology 41:249–270
11. Billingham RE, Brent L, Medawar PB (1953) Actively acquired tolerance of foreign cells. Nature 172:603–606
12. Capron M, Capron A (1994) Immunoglobulin E and effector cells in schistosomiasis. Science 264:1876–1877
13. Coffmann RL, von der Weid T (1997) Multiple pathways for the initiation of T helper 2 (Th2) responses. J Exp Med 185:373–375
14. Cohen D, Dausset J (1973) HLA-gene polymorphism. Progr Immunol 5:1–12
15. Coombs RRA, Gell PGH (1963) The classification of allergic reactions underlying disease. In: Gell PGH, Coombs RRA (eds) Clinical aspects of immunology. Davis, Philadelphia, p 317
16. Denburg JA, Sehmi R, Saito H, Pil-Seob J, Inman MD, O'Byrne PM (2000) Systemic aspects of allergic disease: Bone marrow responses. J Allergy Clin Immunol 106:S242–246
17. Dixon FJ, Vasquez JJ, Weigle WO, Cochrane CG (1958) Pathogenesis of serum sickness. Arch Path 65:18
18. Elsner J, Kapp A (2001) Eosinophile Granulozyten im Netzwerk der Chemokine. Allergologie 24:368–389
19. Foreman I (1987) Substance P and calcitonin gene-related peptide: effects on mast cells in human skin. Int Arch Allergy Appl Immunol 82:366–371
20. Galli SJ, Costa JJ (1995) Mast-cell-leukocyte cytokine cascades in allergic inflammation. Allergy 50:851–862
21. Gleich GJ (2000) Mechanisms of eosinophil-associated inflammation. J Allergy Clin Immunol 105:651–663
22. Goetzl EJ, Austen KF (1977) Cellular characteristics of the eosinophil compatible with a dual role in host defense in parasitic infections. Am J Trop Med Hyg 26:142
23. Grant JA, Lichtenstein LM (1974) Release of slow reacting substance of anaphylaxis from human leukocytes. J Immunol 112:897–904
24. Hemmi H, Takeuchi O, Kawai T, Kaisho T, Sato S, Hoshino K, Wagner H, Takeda K, Akira S (2000) A novel Toll-like receptor that recognizes bacterial DNA. Nature 408:740–745
25. Herz U, Schnoy N, Borelli S, Weigl L, Käsbohrer U, Daser A, Wahn U, Köttgen E, Renz H (1998) A human-SCID mouse model for allergic immune responses: bacterial superantigen enhances skin inflammation and suppresses IgE production. J Invest Dermatol 110:224–231
26. Henson P (1972) Pathologic mechanisms in neutrophil mediated injury. Am J Pathol 68:593
27. Holgate S (1999) The epidemic of allergy and asthma. Introduction. Nature 402 [Suppl 6760]:B2–B4
28. Ishizaka K, Ishizaka T (1978) Mechanisms of reaginic hypersensitivity and IgE antibody response. Immunol Rev 41:109
29. Jakob T, Udey MC (1999) Epidermal Langerhans cells: from neurons to nature's adjuvants. Adv Dermatol 14:209–258
30. Jankovic D, Sher A, Yap G (2001) Th1/Th2 effector choice in parasitic infection: decision making by committee. Curr Opin Immunol 13:403–409
31. Jerne NK (1974) Towards a network theory of the immune system. Ann Immunol 125c:373–379
32. Johansson SGO (1967) Raised levels of a new immunoglobulin (IgND) in asthma. Lancet 11:951–954
33. Intel M, Watanabe T, Klunker S, et al (2001) Histamine regulates T cell and antibody responses by differential expression of H1 and H2 receptors. Nature 413:420–425
34. Kaliner M (1977) Human lung tissue and anaphylaxis. 1. The role of cyclic GMP as a modulator of the immunologically active secretory process. J Allergy Clin Immunol 60:204
35. Kaplan AP (2001) Chemokines, chemokine receptors and allergy. Int Arch Allergy Immunol 124:423–431
36. Kapsenberg ML, Wierenga EA, Bos JD, Jansen HM (1991) Functional subsets of allergen-reactive human DC4+ T cells. Immunol Today 12:392–395

37. Kay AB, Barata L, Meng Q, Durham SR, Ying SL (1997) Eosinophil and eosinophil-associated cytokines in allergic inflammation. Int Arch Immunol 113:196–199
38. Kemeny DM, Noble A, Homes BJ, Diaz-Sanchez D, Lee TH (1995) The role of CD8+ T cells in immunoglobulin E regulation. Allergy 50 [Suppl 25]:9–14
39. Kinet JP (1999) The high-affinity IgE receptor (Fc epsilon RI): from physiology to pathology. Annu Rev Immunol 17:931–972
40. Knop J, Stremmer R, Neumann C, De Maeyer E, Macher E (1982) Interferon inhibits the suppressor T cell response of delayed-type hypersensitivity. Nature 296:775–776
41. Krammer PH, Behrmann I, Daniel P, Dhein J, Debatin K-M (1994) Regulation of apoptosis in the immune system. Curr Opin Immunol 6:279–289
42. Lanzavecchia A, Sallusto F (2000) Dynamics of T lymphocyte responses: intermediates, effectors, and memory cells. Science 290:92–97
43. Levi-Schaffer F, Garbuzenko E, Rubin A, Reich R, Pickholz D, Gillery P, Emonard H, Nagler A, Maquart FA (1999) Human eosinophils regulate human mast cells. Proc Natl Acad Sci U S A 96:9660–9665
44. Lichtenstein LM (1975) The mechanism of basophil histamine release induced by antigen and by the calcium ionophore A 23187. J Immunol 114:1692
45. Marone G, Spadaro G, Genovese A (1995) Regulation of human mast cell and basophil function. Prog Allergy Immunol 3:19–25
46. Matzinger P (1994) Memories are made of this? Nature 369:605–606
47. Messer G, Rupec RA (2001) Nuklearfaktor-kappa-B (NF-κB). Hautarzt 52:677–685
48. Metzger H, Rivnay B, Henkart M, Kanner B, Kinet J-P, Perez-Montfort R (1984) Analysis of the structure and function of the receptor for immunoglobulin E. Mol Immunol 21:1167
49. Mossmann TR, Sad S (1996) The expanding universe of T-cell subsets: Th1, Th2 and more. Immunol Today 17:138–146
50. Müller-Eberhard HJ (1969) Complement. Ann Rev Biochem 38:389
51. Nakao A (2001) Is TGF-β1 the key to suppression of human asthma? Trends Immunol 22:115–118
52. O'Reilly M, Algeit R, Jenkins S, et al (2002) Identification of a histamine H4 receptor on human eosinophils - role in eosinophil chemotaxis. J Recept Signal Transduct Res 22:431–448
53. Ovary Z (1952) Cutaneous anaphylaxis in the albino rat. Int Arch Allergy 3:293–305
54. Parker CW, Koch D, Huber MM, Falkenhein SF (1980) Formation of the cysteinyl form of slow reacting substance (leukotriene E4) in human plasma. Biochem Biophys Res Commun 97:1038
55. Pearce FL, Ali H, Barrett KE, Befus AD, Bienenstock J, Brostoff J, Ennis M, Flint KC, Hudspith B, Johnson NM, Leung KBP, Peachell PT (1985) Functional characteristics of mucosal and connective tissue mast cells of man, the rat and other animals. Int Arch Allergy Appl Immunol 77:274–276
56. Ploetz SG, Lentschat A, Behrendt H, Plötz W, Hamann L, Ring J, Rietschel ET, Flad H-D, Ulmer AJ (2001) The interaction of human peripheral blood eosinophils with bacterial lipopolysaccharide is CD14 dependent. Blood 97:235–241
57. Renz H, Enssle K, Lauffer L, Kurrle R, Gelfand EW (1995) Inhibition of allergen-induced IgE and IgG1 production by soluble IL-4 receptor. Int Arch Allergy Immunol 106:46–54
58. Ring J, Burg G (eds) (1986) New trends in allergy II. Springer, Berlin Heidelberg New York
59. Roecken M, Urban JF, Shevach EM (1994) Antigen-specific activation, silencing and reactivation of the IL-4 pathway in vivo. J Exp Med 179:1885–1893
60. Romagnani S (1994) Lymphokine production by human cells in disease states. Ann Rev Immunol 12:227–257
61. Rother KO, Till G (1987) The complement system. Springer, Berlin Heidelberg New York
62. Saloga J, Enk AH, Ross R, Reske-Kunz AB, Knop J (2001) Dendritic cells in the allergic immune response – from a key player in the pathological process to a potential therapeutic tool. ACI Int 13:107–112
63. Samuelsson B (1983) Leukotrienes: mediators of immediate hypersensitivity reactions and inflammation. Science 220:568
64. Schmutzler W, Poblete-Freundt G, Rauch K, Schoenfeld W (1979) Response to immunological or cholinergic stimulation of isolated mast cells from man, guinea pig and rat. Monogr Allergy 14:288
65. Schuler G, Steinmann RM (1985) Murine epidermal Langerhans cells mature into potent immunostimulatory dendritic cells *in vitro*. J Exp Med 161:526–546
66. Schwartz LB (1994) Mast cells: function and contents. Curr Opin Immunol 6:91–97
67. Sen R, Baltimore D (1986) Inducibility of κ immunoglobulin enhancer-binding protein NF-κB by a post-translational mechanism. Cell 47:921–928
68. Simon HU, Plötz SG, Dummer R, Blaser K (1999) Abnormal clones of T cells producing interleukin-5 in idiopathic eosinophilia. N Engl J Med 341:1112–1120
69. Springer TA (1994) Traffic signals for lymphocyte recirculation and leukocyte emigration: the multistep program. Cell 76:301–314
70. Stanworth DR (1973) Immediate hypersensitivity. North-Holland, Amsterdam
71. Stingl G, Katz SI, Clement L, Green I, Shevach EM (1978) Immunological functions of Ia bearing epidermal Langerhans cells. J Immunol 121:2005

72. Szentivanyi A (1968) The beta adrenergic theory of the atopic abnormality in asthma. J Allergy 42:203
73. Tada T, Kubo S, Nakayama T (1997) Self-tolerance: multiple strategies for peripheral unresponsiveness of T cells. In: Ring J, Behrendt H, Vieluf D (eds) New trends in allergy IV. Springer, Berlin Heidelberg New York, pp 358–364
74. Tamaki K, Nakamura K (2001) The role of lymphocytes in healthy and eczematous skin. Curr Opin Allergy Clin Immunol 1:455–460
75. Thomson AW (ed) (1998) The cytokine handbook, 3rd edn. Academic Press, San Diego
76. Thomas ML (1999) The regulation of antigen-receptor signaling by protein tyrosine phosphatases: a hole in the story. Curr Opin Immunol 11:270–276
77. Thueson D, Speck L, Lett-Brown M, Grant A (1979) Histamine-releasing activity (HRA): II. Interaction with basophils and physiochemical characterization. J Immunol 123:633–639
78. Tonegawa S (1983) Somatic generation of antibody diversity. Nature 302:575–581
79. Vane JR (1964) The use of isolated organs for detecting active substances in the circulating blood. Br J Pharmacol 23:360–373
80. Vercelli D, Geha RS (1992) Regulation of isotype switching. Curr Opin Immunol 4:794–797
81. Wagner H, Röllinghoff M (eds) (1980) Interleukin 2. Behring Inst., Mitt. 67, Marburg
82. Wasserman SJ, Soter NA, Center DM, Austen KF (1977) Cold urticaria: recognition and characterization of a neutrophil chemotactic factor which appears in serum during experimental cold challenge. J Clin Invest 60:189
83. Weck AL de (1995) What can we learn from the allergic zoo? Int Arch Allergy Immunol 107: 13–18
84. Zinkernagel RM, Doherty PC (1979) MHC-restricted cytotoxic T cells: Studies on the biological role of polymorphic major transplantation antigens determining T cell restriction-specificity, function and responsiveness. Adv Immunol 27:51–177
85. Zlotnik A, Yoshie O (2000) Chemokines: a new classification system and their role in immunity. Immunity 12:121–127
86. Ring J (1991) Atopy: condition, disease, or syndrome? In: Ruzicka T, Ring J, Przybilla B (eds) Handbook of atopic eczema. Springer, Berlin Heidelberg New York

3 Genetics and Environment in the Development of Allergy

3.1 Genetics of Allergy

3.1.1 Classical Genetics

The fact that certain allergies occur in families has already been described for the Julian-Claudian imperial family (see Sect. 1.1). A scientific description of the phenomenon was given by Wyman [32] and especially by Cooke [5], leading finally to the development of the term "atopy" for hay fever and asthma. Wise and Sulzberger [28] and Schnyder [23] have since also included atopic eczema in this group of familial allergies. Characteristic "Venn" diagrams of the age groups can be drawn showing the occurrence of predominantly eczema in childhood and rhinoconjunctivitis in adult age (Fig. 3.1) with obvious overlaps. The genetic basis of this inheritance of allergies has not yet, however, been completely established.

After the search for *an* allergy or atopy gene proved unsuccessful, we now know that the disease does not follow a monogenic pattern but that a multifactorial polygenic inheritance with partial genomic imprinting (maternal influences are stronger than paternal influences) plays a role. The classic method of twin analysis showed a concordance of approximately 80% for homozygous twins compared to 30% for heterozygous twins [2, 24, 31]. Sixty percent of patients suffering from one atopic disease are also affected by another manifestation of the disease.

Family studies with long-term follow-up in Linköping [12] have determined the atopy risk for children of atopic parents, which is highest when both parents are suffering from the same atopic manifestation (e.g., "eczema" or "asth-

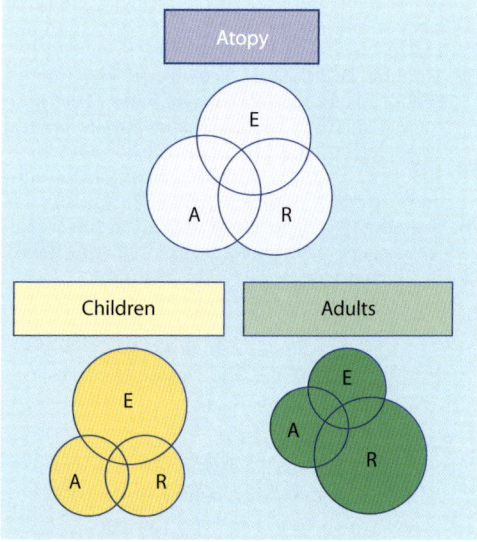

Fig. 3.1. "Venn" diagram showing overlap between atopic diseases in childhood and adult life. *A*, asthma; *E*, eczema; *R*, rhinoconjunctivitis

Table 3.1. Atopy risk for children (according to Kjellman)

Parents	Atopy risk (%) at the age of 12 years
Without atopy	Approx. 10–15
One parent atopic	20–30
Two parents atopic (different organ manifestation)	30–40
Two parents atopic (same organ manifestation)	60–80

ma") (Table 3.1). As well as the increased IgE production, the occurrence in certain organs is also genetically influenced.

As for other immunologically mediated diseases, the search for associations between certain HLA (human leukocyte antigen) characteristics and allergic phenotypes has been without success. Associations with certain HLA haplotypes [11] have been detected only for the specificity of an IgE response.

3.1.2 Molecular Genetics

The advances made in molecular genetics have allowed the definition of certain gene loci for clinical phenotypes [4, 9]. This is done using naturally occurring DNA sequences, which as polymorphic genetic markers (so-called microsatellites) are distributed over the whole genome. Studies can be performed using different methods:

Coupling analysis investigates why genetic markers and defined clinical phenotypes show cosegregation within families (e.g., "affected sib pair" studies with several affected family members). *Association studies* investigate large populations of affected and non-affected individuals for the allelic distribution pattern of polymorphic gene markers in order to determine associations between phenotypes and certain chromosomal markers.

Principally two different approaches are possible: In *candidate gene analysis* defined genetic markers in proximity to genes coding for other gene-relevant protein products (e.g., IL-4 gene on chromosome 5 [14, 16, 22]) are studied. The second approach is the *whole genome screen* method, which allows the identification of new chromosomal regions of genes possibly involved in the manifestation of phenotypes [7, 8, 20].

Another method measures mutations of DNA sequences within candidate genes and their promotors (*single nucleotide polymorphisms – SNP*). Interesting data for the β-chain of the high-affinity IgE receptor on chromosome 11 [6] as well as for the endotoxin receptor (CD14) on chromosome 5 have been found [30].

Since the description of the whole human genome with approximately 4 billion base pairs and an SNP frequency of 1:1,000, we know that there are approximately 4 million SNPs to be investigated. Molecular biological techniques need to progress in parallel with the exact clinical description of phenotypes (disease, severity, test results, functional methods, etc.) in these genetic analyses.

Associations in the human system need to be verified for the actual functional importance in experimental systems mostly in the mouse, which shows a high degree of analogy

Table 3.2. Atopy-relevant gene loci

Chromosome (region)	Candidate gene	Phenotype
3	CD80/86?	Infantile atopic eczema
5 q 31–35	"Cytokine cluster":	IgE
	IL-4	Asthma
	IL-13	BHR
	IL-5	
	IL-3	
	IL-9	
	CD14 (endotoxin receptor)	
	β-Adrenergic receptor (ADRB2)	
	Glucocorticoid receptor (GLR) on lymphocytes	
6 p 21	MHC II	Specific IgE
	TNF-α	Asthma
11 q 13	β-chain Fcε RI	IgE
12 q 14	IFNγ, STAT-6	Specific IgE
14 q 11	T-cell receptor α/δ	Specific IgE
	Mast-cell chymase	Specific IgE
16 p 11	Interleukin-4Rα	Specific IgE
17 q 25	?	Atopic eczema
20 p 31	ADAM 33	Asthma

to the human genome. There are already dictionaries of human-mouse synteny. New insights can be expected through hybridization experiments of different mouse strains with known allergy susceptibility or through selective new mutations induced with mutagens (e.g., ENU = ethylnitrosourea mutagenesis project) [10].

Table 3.2 shows the most important candidate genes or gene loci involved in the development of atopic diseases. Some still have no functional correlates. Recently, coupling of infantile atopic eczema with a gene locus on chromosome 3 has been described [20]. This locus also has been implied in psoriasis, stressing the importance of different pathways for inheritance of immunological abnormalities and organ manifestation.

The genetics of other allergic diseases (e.g., anaphylaxis, allergic contact dermatitis) are much less well established; occasional studies have shown associations of nickel allergy with certain HLA haptotypes [15].

The major difficulty of these genetic investigations is in the allergen exposure, which until now has not or has only preliminarily been considered and which is different for different family members (e.g., insect stings). It is speculated that in the manifestation of allergy, not only one or a few genes are involved; experts estimate there to be approximately 150 atopy-relevant genes.

References

1. Barnes KC, Marsh DG (1998) The genetics and complexity of allergy and asthma. Immunol Today 19:325–332
2. Daser A, Daheshia M, De Sanctis GT (2001) Genetics of allergen-induced asthma. J Allergy Clin Immunol 108:167–174
3. Blumenthal MN, Björksten M (1997) Genetics of allergy and asthma. Marcel Dekker, New York
4. Deichmann KA (2001) Asthmagenetik – der immunologische Fingerabdruck. Allergologie 24: 330–338
5. Cooke RA, Van der Veer A (1916) Human sensitization. J Immunol 1:305
6. Cookson WO, Sharp PA, Faux JA, Hopkin JM (1989) Linkage between immunoglobulin E responses underlying asthma and rhinitis and chromosome 11 q. Lancet 1:1292–1295
7. CSGA (Collaborative Study on the Genetics of Asthma) (1997) A genome-wide search for asthma susceptibility loci in ethnically diverse populations. Nat Genet 15:389–392
8. Daniels SE, Bhattacharrya S, James A, Leaves NI, Young A, Hill MR, Faux JA, Ryan GF, le Souef PN, Lathrop GM, Musk AW, Cookson WO (1996) A genome-wide search for quantitative trait loci underlying asthma. Nature 383:247–250
9. Heinzmann A, Deichmann KA (2001) Genes for atopy and asthma. Curr Opin Allergy Clin Immunol 1:387–392
10. Hrabe de Angelis M, Flaswinkel H, Fuchs H, Rathkolb B, Soewarto D, Marschall S, Heffner St, Pargent W, Wuensch K, Jung M, Reis A, Richter T, Alessandrini F, Jakob T, Fuchs E, Kolb H, Kremmer E, Schaeble K, Rollinski B, Roscher A, Peters Ch, Meitinger Th, Srom T, Steckler Th, Holsboer F, Klopfstock Th., Gekeler F, Schindewolf C, Jung Th, Avraham K, Behrendt H, Ring J, Zimmer A, Schugart K, Pfeffer K, Wolf E, Balling R (2000) Genome-wide, large-scale production of mutant mice by ENU mutagenesis. Nature Genet 25: 444–447
11. Huang SK, Zwollo P, Marsh DG (1991) Class II major histocompatibility complex restriction of human cell responses to short ragweed allergen, Amb a V. Eur J Immunol 21:1469–1473
12. Kjellman NM (1976) Immunglobulin E and atopic allergy in childhood. Linköping Univ Med Diss No 36
13. Kulig M, Bergmann R, Klettke U, Wahn V, Tacke U, Wahn U, and the Multicenter Allergy Study Group (1999) Natural course of sensitization to food and inhalant allergens during the first 6 years of life. J Allergy Clin Immunol 103: 1173–1179
14. Marsh DG, Neely JD, Breazeale DR, Ghosh B, Freidhoff LR, Ehrlich-Kautzky E, Schou C, Krishnaswamy G, Beaty TH (1994) Linkage analysis of IL-4 and other chromosome 5q31.1 markers and total serum immunoglobulin E concentrations. Science 264:1152–1156
15. Menné T, Holm NV (1986) Genetic susceptibility in human allergic contact sensitization. Semin Dermatol 5:301–306
16. Meyers DA, Postma DS, Panhuysen CIM, Xu J, Amelung PJ, Levitt RC, Bleecker ER (1994) Evidence for a locus regulating total serum IgE levels mapping to chromosome 5. Genomics 23: 464–470
17. Moffat MF, Hill MR, Cornelis F, Schou C, Faux JA, Young RP, James AL, Ryan G, le Souef P, Musk AW, et al. (1994) Genetic linkage of T-cell receptor α/β complex to specific IgE responses. Lancet 343: 1597–1600
18. Nanavaty U, Goldstein AD, Levine SJ (2001) Polymorphisms in candidate asthma genes. Am J Med Sci 321:11–16
19. Nickel R, Wahn U, Hizawa N, Maestri N, Duffy DL, Barnes KC, Beyer K, Forster J, Bergmann R, Zepp F, Wahn V, Marsh DG (1997) Evidence for linkage of chromosome 12q15-q24.1 markers to

high total serum IgE concentrations in children of the German multicenter allergy study. Genomics 46:159–162
20. Lee YA, Wahn U, Kehrt R, Tarani L, Businco L, Gustafsson D, Andersson F, Oranje AP, Wolkertstorfer A, v. Berg A, Hoffmann U, Kuster W, Wienker T, Ruschendorf F, Reis A (2000) Chromosome 3 and infantile atopic dermatitis. Nature Genet 26:470–472
21. Postma DS, Bleecker ER, Amelung PJ, Holroyd KJ, Xu J, Panhuysen C, Meyers DA, Levitt RC (1995) Genetic susceptibility to asthma – bronchial hyperresponsiveness coinherited with a major gene for atopy. N Engl J Med 333:894–900
22. Rosenwasser LJ, Klemm DJ, Dresback JK, Inamura H, Mascali JJ, Klinnert M, Borish L (1995) Promoter polymorphisms in the chromosome 5 gene cluster in asthma and atopy. Clin Exp Allergy 25:74–78
23. Schnyder UW (1960) Neurodermitis, asthma, rhinitis. Eine genetisch-allergologische Studie. Karger, Basel
24. Schulz-Larsen F, Holm NV, Henningsen K (1986) Atopic dermatitis: A genetic-epidemiologic study in a population-based twin sample. J Am Acad Dermatol 15:487–494
25. Shirakawa T, Li A, Dubowitz M, Dekker JW, Shaw AE, Faux JA, Ra C, Cookson WOCM, Hopkin JM (1994) Association between atopy and variants of the subunit of the high-affinity immunoglobulin E receptor. Nature Genet 7:125–129
26. Vom Eerdewegh P, Little RD, Dapuis J, et al. (2002) Association of the ADAM33 gene with asthma and bronchial hyperresponsiveness. Nature 418:426–430
27. Wahn U, Lau S, Bergmann R, Kulig M, Forster J, Bergmann K, Bauer CP, Guggenmoos-Holzmann I (1997) Indoor allergen exposure is a risk factor for sensitization during the first three years of life. J Allergy Clin Immunol 99:763–769
28. Wise F, Sulzberger MB (1934) Editorial remarks in: The 1933 yearbook of dermatology and syphilology. Year Book Medical, Chicago, p 38
29. Wjst M, Fischer G, Immervoll T, Jung M, Saar K, Rueschendorf F, Reis-Ulbrecht M, Gomolka M, Weiss EH, Jaeger L, Nickel R, Richter K, Kjellman NI, Griese M, von Berg A, Gappa M, Riedel F, Boehle M, van Koningsbruggen S, Schoberth P, Szczepanski R, Dorsch W, Silbermann M, Wichmann HE, et al. (1999) A genome-wide search for linkage to asthma. German Asthma Genetics Group. Genomics 58:1–8
30. Vercelli D, Baldini M, Martinez F (2001) The monocyte/IgE connection: may polymorphisms in the CD14 gene teach us about IgE regulation? Int Arch Allergy Immunol 124:20–24
31. Wüthrich B (ed) (1999) The atopy syndrome in the third millennium. Karger, Basel
32. Wyman M (1872) Autumnal catarrh (hay fever). Hurd & Houghton, Cambridge, p 82

3.2 Epidemiology of Allergic Diseases

3.2.1 Atopic Diseases

Allergies have shown a dramatic increase in prevalence worldwide during recent decades [2, 5, 7, 13, 14]. An international study with comparable methods (questionnaires) (International Study of Asthma and Allergy in Childhood ISAAC) showed marked differences around the globe. Highest prevalence rates were found for the United Kingdom, New Zealand, and Australia (asthma 30–35%, hay fever 20%, atopic eczema 15–20%). The lowest rates were found in countries such as Albania or Indonesia (asthma 2–3%, hay fever 4–5%, atopic eczema 1–2%) [5] (Fig. 3.2).

In Germany, a variety of intensive epidemiological investigations have been performed on different age groups and areas of both former East and West Germany [7, 8, 10, 11, 12, 13]. There are significant regional differences, not only between east and west but also between north and south, which can be summarized as follows:

- Ten to 20% of adult Germans are suffering from allergy.
- In children (5–6 years old), bronchial asthma occurs in 2–5%, hay fever in 1–7% (in 9–10 year olds approximately 10%), and eczema in 6–19%. East German children showed a lower prevalence than West German children for asthma and hay fever and a higher rate of eczema after reunification in the early 1990s.
- The rates of atopic sensitization (skin test or sIgE in serum) against aero-, food, or insect venom allergens are approximately twice as high.
- Not only hay fever and asthma but also sensitization against housedust mites and birch pollen was significantly rarer after reunification (1990) in East Germany than in West Germany. For grass pollen, there is an increase from north to south (up to 40% in Bavaria).

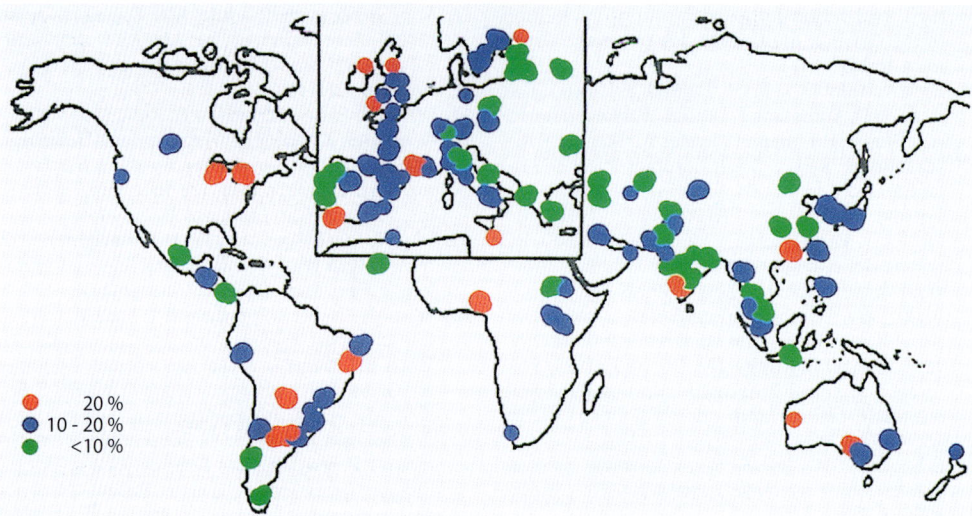

Fig. 3.2. Prevalence of allergic rhinitis among 13- and 14-year-old children (ISAAC study [4])

- The observed East-West German differences vary according to the year of birth. Apparently, influences active since the early 1960s are of importance (Fig. 3.3) [13]. In the second half of the 1990s, increasing prevalences of hay fever have been found also for East German children.
- Children growing up on farms seem to have fewer allergies than children from an urban environment [3].
- The higher the parental educational level (e.g., university degree), the higher the allergy risk for the children.
- There are diseases which are associated with a decreased atopy risk, for instance diabetes mellitus [6].

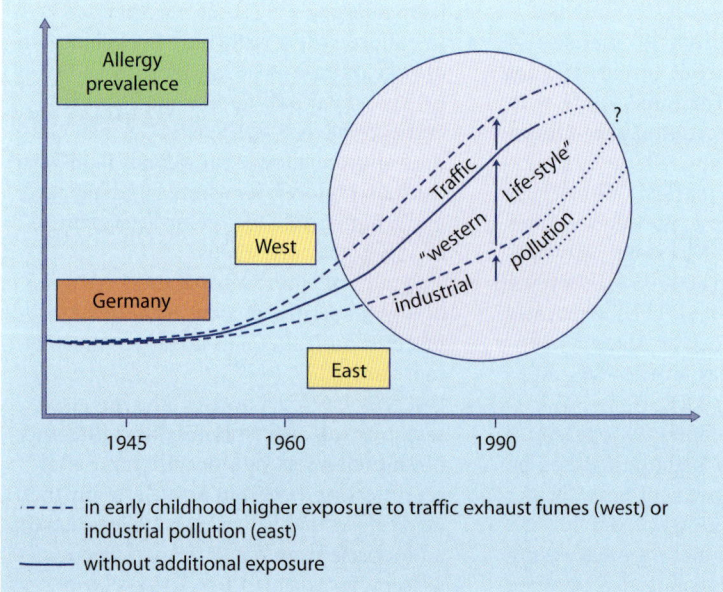

Fig. 3.3. Importance of cumulative environmental factors for the increase of allergies in Germany (according to Wichmann [14])

The causes for the increase in allergy prevalence are not yet clear; there are only hypothetical concepts (Table 3.3), which show some influence of "fashion" trends in science [1, 3, 4, 8, 12, 13]. It is likely that there is *more than one* factor responsible for the increase in allergies. However, before arriving at practical recommendations for allergy prevention, we should have some exact knowledge of the causal factors. It does not make sense – on the basis of the attractive but still not finally proven "hygiene hypothesis" (also "jungle hypothesis") – to stop vaccination programs or to recommend insufficient body hygiene for allergy protection ("dirt is healthy"!).

Table 3.3. Hypothetical concepts aiming to explain the increase in allergy prevalence

- Genetic predisposition
- Increased awareness and improved diagnostics
- Allergen exposure
- Increasing age of mothers (primiparae)
- Increasing social mobility (womens' emancipation, professional and holiday life)
- Lower number of children (smaller families)
- Decreased immune stimulation ("training of immune system") through improved hygiene, fewer infections, fewer parasite infestations, etc. ("hygiene" or "jungle" hypothesis)
- Loss of protective (tolerance-inducing) factors
- Influence of antiallergic therapy (?)
- Allergy-promoting influence of environmental pollution

3.2.2 Epidemiology of Contact Allergies

Very little information exists on the epidemiology of other allergic diseases (see Chap. 5). Exact data on population-related prevalence rates of sensitizations in the patch test exist from contact dermatitis research groups such as the "Informationsverbund Dermatologischer Kliniken" (IVDK) in Germany [11] as well as from patch tests on representative adult populations (the KORA Study in Augsburg) [10] (Table 3.4).

Table 3.4. Prevalence of contact allergy in dermatology patients (1999, 2000 [11]) and in the general population (2001 [10])

Allergen	1999 ($n=9{,}994$)	2000 ($n=88{,}868$)	2001 ($n=1{,}141$)
Nickel sulfate	17.6%	15.6%	13.1%
Fragrance mix	13.1%	10.2%	15.9%
Balsam of Peru	10.3%	8.4%	3.8%
Thimerosal	9.1%	7.3%	4.7%
Cobalt chloride	7.2%	5.3%	2.4%
Woolwax alcohols	5.1%	4.3%	1.4%
Colophony	4.4%	4.2%	1.6%
p-Phenylenediamine	4.5%	4.0%	1.5%
MDBGN/PE (Euxyl K400)	4.6%	3.8%	1.7%
Potassium dichromate	4.1%	3.4%	1.1%
Thiuram mix	2.6%	2.4%	0.7%
CMI/MI (Kathon CG)	2.0%	2.3%	1.8%
Neomycin sulfate	2.5%	2.3%	1.4%
Mercury-(II)-aminochloride	2.6%	2.2%	1.0%
Turpentine	2.9%	2.2%	2.5%
Formaldehyde	1.9%	1.8%	0.6%
Propolis	(2.5%)	1.8%	n.d.
Bufexamac	(2.3%)	1.4%	n.d.
Benzocaine	1.4%	1.3%	1.0%
Epoxy resin	1.4%	1.2%	0.6%
Cetylstearyl alcohol	1.3%	1.2%	0.8%
Parabene mix	1.2%	1.4%	0.6%

References

1. Alm JS, Swartz J, Lilja G, Scheynius A, Pershagen G (1999) Atopy in children of families with an anthroposophic lifestyle. Lancet 353:1485–1488
2. Burr M (ed) (1992) Epidemiology of clinical allergy. Karger, Basel
3. Gassner-Bachmann B, Wüthrich B (2000) Bauernkinder leiden selten an Heuschnupfen und Asthma. Dtsch med Wschr 125:924–931
4. The International Study of Asthma and Allergics in Childhood Steering Committee (ISAAC) (1998) World-wide variation of asthma, allergic rhinoconjunctivitis and atopic eczema in prevalence of symptoms. 351:1225–1232
5. Lewis SA, Weiss ST, Platts-Mills TAE, Syring M, Gold DR (2001) Association of specific allergen sensitization with socioeconomic factors and allergic disease in a population of Boston women. J Allergy Clin Immunol 107:615–622
6. Mutius E von (1999) Asthma bronchiale und atopische Erkrankungen im Kindesalter. Prävalenz und Risikofaktoren. Dustri, Munich
7. Olesen AB, Juul S, Birkebaek N, Thestrup-Pedersen K (2001) Association between atopic dermatitis and insulin-dependent diabetes mellitus: a case-control study. Lancet 357:1749–1752
8. Ring J, Krämer U, Schäfer T, Behrendt H (2001)

Why do allergies increase? Curr Opin Immunol 13:201–208
9. Ring J, Wenning J (eds) (2000) Weißbuch Allergie in Deutschland 2000. Urban und Vogel, Munich
10. Schäfer T, Ring J (1998) Epidemiologie des atopischen Ekzems. Allergologie 21:259–271
11. Schäfer T, Böhler E, Ruhdorfer S, Weigl L, Wessner D, Filipiak B, Wichmann HE, Ring J (2001) Epidemiology of contact allergy in adults. Allergy 56:582–585
12. Schnuch A, et al. (2001) Informationsverbund dermatologischer Kliniken. Prävalenz von Kontaktallergien. Hautarzt 52:582–586
13. Wahn U, Wichmann HE (eds) (2000) Spezialbericht Allergien. Statistisches Bundesamt, Metzler und Poeschel, Stuttgart
14. Wichmann HE (1995) Environment, life-style and allergy. The German answer. Allergo J 6:315–316
15. Wüthrich B (2001) Epidemiologie der Allergien in der Schweiz. Ther Umschau 58:253–258

3.3 Allergy and Environment

The reasons for the dramatic increase in allergy prevalence in the past few decades are not known; among the hypothetical concepts proposed (see Sect. 3.2), the role of environmental pollution has been the subject of particular controversy. In this debate, the term "environment" has to be defined: One has to distinguish between natural (physical, chemical, biological) influences and anthropogenic environmental pollution.

Allergies belong to the few diseases in which environmental factors (namely allergens) of both natural and anthropogenic origin have been defined as causal and characterized in their molecular structures (they are partly available as recombinant proteins). Allergy can be regarded as "the environmental disease no. 1" [32]. Allergen exposure is not only relevant for the development of sensitization but also for the severity of clinical symptoms. Allergy follows dose-response relations in the manifestation of skin and mucous membrane inflammation.

3.3.1 Environment and Health

Anthropogenic noxious agents in the environment ("environmental pollution") have been known to affect human health for a long time, especially as toxic agents (cytotoxic, mutagenic or cancerogenic effects). It is true that in the environment increasing amounts of noxious agents disturb not only the ecologic equilibrium but also endanger the life of plants, animals, and humans [4].

Apart from the causal factors from the environment (allergens), other environmental substances may modulate the development of diseases such as allergies (adjuvant effects) and may contribute to the chronification of diseases or influence the intensity and severity grade of clinical symptoms.

3.3.2 Allergotoxicology

The new research concept of "allergotoxicology" deals with the "influence of environmental factors upon the induction, elicitation, and maintenance of allergic reactions" (Behrendt 1979, cited in [2]) (Fig. 3.4). The investigation of the role of environmental pollutants in allergy development is complicated by the following factors [4]:

- There is limited knowledge on the quantitative dose-response relationships between allergen exposure and sensitization or disease.

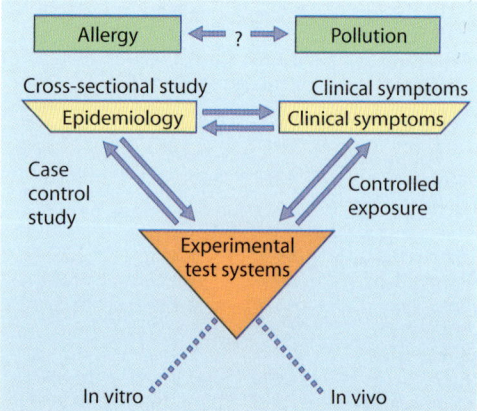

Fig. 3.4. Investigation objectives and paths in the field of allergotoxicology (according to Behrendt [2])

- Combined effects of different substances may lead to complex manifestations when acting simultaneously. Only rarely can the apparent clinical symptoms be attributed to one single substance.
- Noxious effects of environmental pollutants sometimes only become apparent after many years, making causal associations difficult.
- Environmental factors may act differently at the different levels from induction of allergy (sensitization) via development of hyperreactivity of skin and mucous membranes until the manifestation of clinical symptoms and chronification of the disease.
- It is possible that atmospheric pollutants interact with allergen carriers in the ambient air, influencing the development of allergy in humans [2].
- Phobic attitudes ("environmentophobia") can lead to psychosomatic interactions and perpetuation of subjective environmentally induced feelings of impaired health (see Sect. 5.9, "Eco-syndrome", "MCS").

Few medical problems of today are discussed with such emotional (sometimes almost ideological) intensity as the relationship between environmental pollution and allergy. It seems appropriate to summarize briefly the facts from the multitude of opinions and discuss their relevance.

The best knowledge exists on the role of air pollutants. Effects of anthropogenic constituents of food (xenobiotics such as contaminants, pesticides, and additives) have been poorly investigated. Equally, the influence of ionizing radiation of natural (e.g., radon) or anthropogenic origins (e.g., nuclear catastrophies) in the development of human allergy has not been well investigated [26].

3.3.2.1 Classification of Air Pollutants

Air pollutants may be classified as *primary* (emitted into the atmosphere as such) (e.g., SO_2 NOx, VOC, large dust particles) or *secondary*, which are only formed within the atmosphere through chemical or physical processes (e.g., ozone, fine and ultrafine particles) (Table 3.5).

Table 3.5. Anthropogenic air pollutants with possible allergy-relevant influence

Gaseous air pollutants
Sulfur dioxide (SO_2)
Nitric oxides (NO_x)
Ozone (O_3)
Particulate air pollutants
Indoor
Environmental tobacco smoke
Outdoor
Atmospheric dust (fine and ultrafine particles most prominent)
Diesel exhaust particles

Furthermore, a distinction needs to be made between outdoor and indoor pollutants, with certain overlaps. Finally, air pollution present over wide areas and regions needs to be distinguished from specific regional and mostly industrial emissions (e.g., asbestos, beryllium, mercury, arsenic or radioactive nuclides). These agents are subject to strict legal regulations. Increased exposure only occurs as a consequence of illegal actions or catastrophies and has to be regarded as the exception [4]. While the toxic effects of most substances are well known, their role in the development of allergies is poorly understood.

Air pollutants may be *gaseous* or *particulate* in nature. In the ambient air, there is always a mixture of different air pollutants, many of them chemically not yet identified. It is crucial to distinguish qualitatively between certain types of air pollution (Table 3.6):

Table 3.6. Types of air pollution (according to Behrendt)

Type I	Type II
Sulfur dioxide	Nitric oxides
	Volatile organic compounds (VOCs)
Large dust particles	Ozone
	Fine and ultrafine particles (PM 2.5 and smaller)
Airway inflammation	*Airway inflammation*
Bronchitis	Allergy
Type "East"	Type "West"

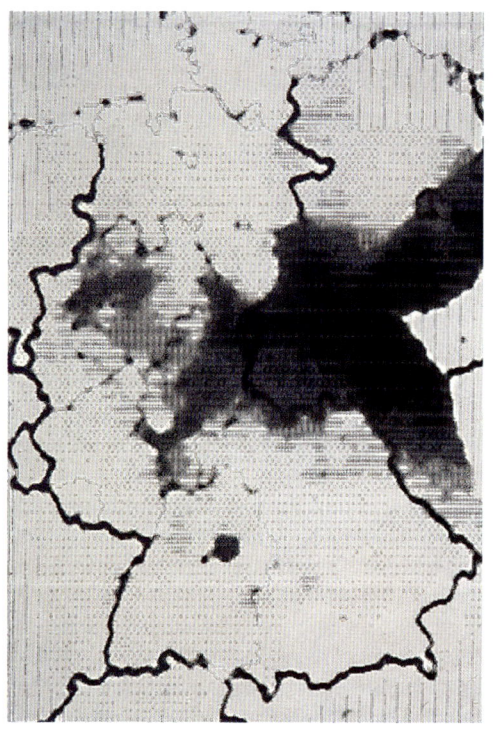

Type I air pollution was characteristic in East Germany prior to reunification in 1990 and is still present in many Eastern European countries. This type of air pollution can be associated with irritative and inflammatory reactions of the upper airways (Fig. 3.5).

Type II air pollution is present over highly populated industrialized urban regions and has been found to be associated with allergic sensitization and disease [13] (Fig. 3.6).

The sequelae of air pollution include simply an "unpleasant feeling" and range from irritation to the development of serious diseases.

The irritative effect of some air pollutants on skin and mucous membranes may possibly be increased in atopics. On the other hand, there are increased susceptibilities (e.g., for ozone) which are not connected with atopy and are not yet understood in humans. However, ozone is able to increase allergen-induced bronchial hy-

◁

Fig. 3.5. Type 1 air pollution caused by primary air pollutants (concentration of SO_2 and coarse particles in the outside air) (according to U. Krämer)

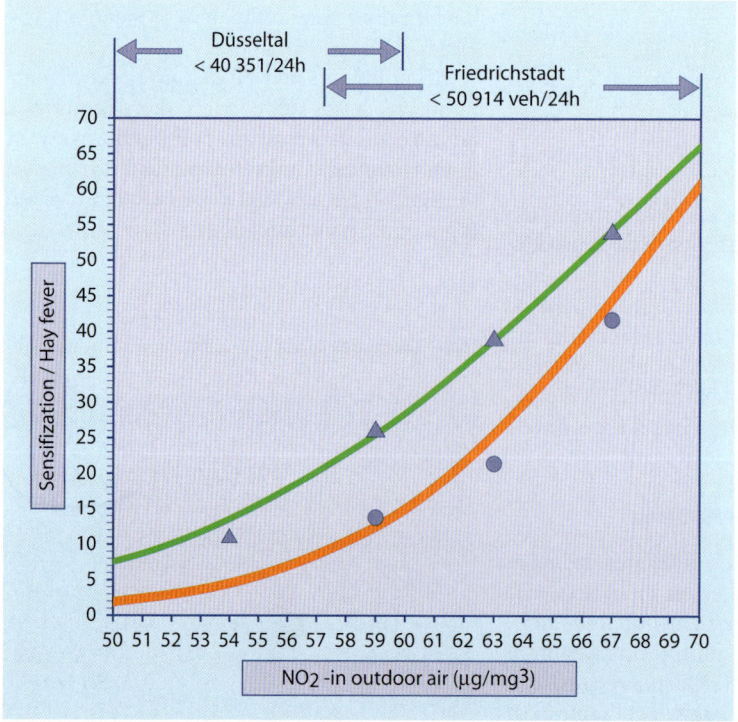

Fig. 3.6. Relationship between traffic-related NO_2 concentration of the outdoor air, atopic sensitization to aeroallergens, and hay fever symptoms in 306 nine-year-old German children (according to Krämer et al. [13]) (adjusted percentages for exposure groups with the same distance to the regression curve for urban areas; *veh*, traffic units = motor vehicle)

perreactivity – especially together with exercise [10, 16].

Asthmatics often react with increased bronchial constriction to sulfur dioxide, also to sulfites in foods (see Sect. 5.1.5). However, SO_2 does not cause an increased allergy prevalence in the phase of sensitization (as shown by the decreased rates of asthma and hay fever in East Germany before reunification).

3.3.2.2 Animal Experiments, and Epidemiologic and Clinical Studies

It has been shown in various animal experiments that air pollutants, especially fine particles from diesel exhaust fumes, increase IgE production [15]. These results were confirmed in human cell cultures by a deviation of the T-cell response towards TH2 [7]. Dust samples collected over West German cities were able to induce release of mediators from a variety of inflammatory cells (basophil leukocytes or neutrophil granulocytes in a non-toxic and dose-dependent manner). Certain pollutants show differentiated effects: Cadmium can increase leukotriene synthesis in rat mast cells, but at the same time can inhibit degranulation and histamine release (Behrendt).

The fall of the Berlin Wall in November 1989 offered the unique chance to study a genetically similar population in comparable geographic and climatic situations, which for only political reasons existed for over 40 years under quite different environmental conditions and with quite different lifestyles. It was surprising that all the groups performing East-West-German epidemiologic comparison studies found that respiratory atopies were significantly more prominent in the West compared to the East [2, 12, 24, 25]. Many people – especially politicians – falsely concluded from this finding that air pollution does not play a role in allergy. Detailed analyses of qualitative differences in air pollution patterns led to new conclusions: Air pollution type I exposure is not or is rather negatively associated with allergy, while air pollution type II has been found by a variety of studies to be associated with allergic sensitization and disease [6, 13]. These air pollutants derive mostly from traffic exhaust fumes in outdoor air and tobacco smoke in indoor air.

Irritative and infectious respiratory disease induced through classical air pollutants (type I) in East Germany decreased dramatically in the early 1990s while at the same time hay fever prevalence increased in children born after 1991 [12, 24, 25].

Taken together, risk factors which have been shown to be significantly associated with atopy in multivariate logistic regression in our own studies [2, 11, 12, 13, 20, 22, 23] are:

- Genetic predisposition (maternal influence stronger than paternal influence)
- Animal contact (dead or alive)
- Higher social status of parents
- Environmental tobacco smoke
- Traffic exhaust

Apart from allergy-enhancing factors, a decrease in protective influences may be considered. This might play a role in the improved hygiene (lack of parasitic infestations) but also in the higher social status of parents. Children growing up on a farm have fewer allergies than children from non-farmers living in the same village. The cause of this difference is not yet known (see Sect. 3.2).

3.3.2.3 Interaction Between Pollen and Air Pollutants

Both Latin-derived terms "pollen" and "pollution" are etymologically only weakly related (*pollen* = flour, *pollutio* = impurity); however, research into the interaction between pollen and pollutants has thrown fresh light on our understanding of allergy [2, 3, 18].

Pollen grains are altered by air pollutants in a polluted atmosphere. Pollen agglomerations have been found over West German cities together with air pollutant particles (Figs. 3.7, 3.8). In vitro exposure of pollen with air pollutant particles led to changes in the surface structure and allergen liberation. This was especially marked for pollutants of type II, while pollutants of type I showed a greater tendency toward inhibitory influences on pollen activation [3]. Possibly the lower hay fever prevalence in East German children may be explained as a sequel of the tremendously high outdoor SO_2 exposure.

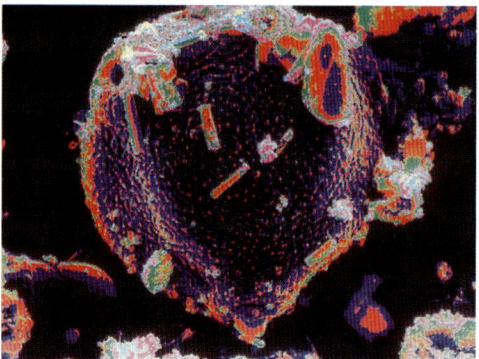

Fig. 3.7. Scanning electron microscopic photo of a pollutant-laden grain of birch pollen (H. Behrendt)

Table 3.7. Indoor air and health

Elicitors	Possible clinical conditions
Physicochemical irritants	Irritation (dyspnea, headache, conjunctival problems with contact lenses)
Pathogenic microbes	Infectious diseases (e.g., legionellosis)
Allergens	IgE-mediated: allergic rhinitis, conjunctivitis, asthma, atopic eczema (?), urticaria (?)
	IgG/cellular-mediated: hypersensitivity pneumonitis (e.g., humidifier lung)

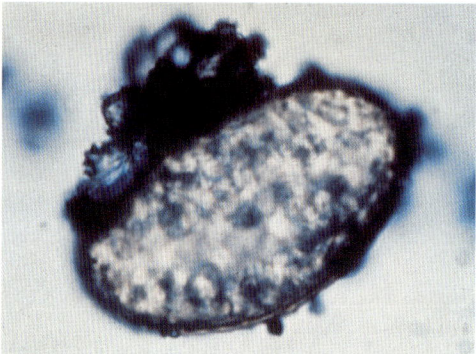

Fig. 3.8. Photo taken under a light microscope of a pine pollen sac with particulate deposits (H. Behrendt)

In regions with high air pollution, allergens are released into the humid atmosphere and allergen aerosols occur outside the pollen fraction. The simple pollen count therefore does not necessarily reflect the actual allergen exposure in a certain region.

Recently, Behrendt et al. have shown that in a humid milieu pollen grains themselves release proinflammatory eicosanoid-like substances able to attract neutrophil and eosinophil granulocytes ("pollotrienes" or "PALMs" = pollen-associated lipid mediators) [3]. The formation of these substances was significantly enhanced after exposure of pollen to type II pollutants (e.g., VOCs).

3.3.2.4 Indoor Air Pollution

Most people spend 80–90% of their time indoors. Almost always indoor air is worse than outdoor air. Particularly since the oil crisis and the introduction of energy-saving measures with increased insulation, people have forgotten the need for proper ventilation [previously houses were first ventilated over weeks or possibly preliminarily inhabited until dry (poor people were invited to live there until the apartment was dry)]. Many diseases are due to indoors air pollution (Table 3.7).

Apart from natural factors such as molds and animal allergens, the biggest producer of air pollution indoors is the smoking human. Environmental tobacco smoke is the classical type II pollutant leading to increased IgE formation [22, 38] and allergic disease.

The first and major practical recommendation is "improved ventilation"! (see Sect. 3.4.).

3.3.3 Conclusions

From clinical, epidemiological, and experimental investigations there can be no doubt that certain air pollutants or pollutant mixtures play a role in the development of allergy. Causal factors (allergens) and allergy-modulating factors (e.g., pollutants) need to be differentiated. There are distinct differences in pollutant effects at the different levels of allergy development in sensitization and disease (Fig. 3.9). Genetic susceptibility, allergic sensitization, skin and mucous membrane hyperreactivity, and manifest allergic disease are different parameters and may be influenced in different ways.

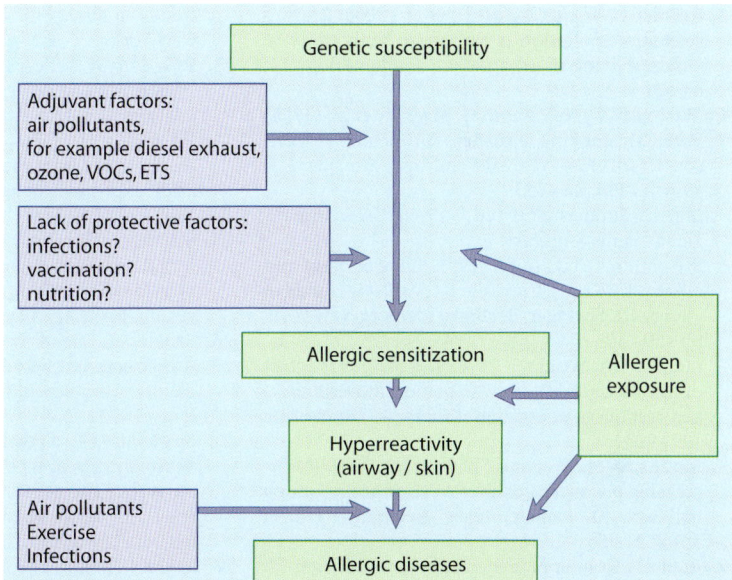

Fig. 3.9. Factors contributing to the development of allergic disorders (according to Behrendt et al. [4])

References

1. Behrendt H, Nolte D, Ring J (1993) Allergie und Umwelt. In: Vademecum für die Praxis. Bayr. Staatsmin. Landesentwicklung und Umweltfragen, Munich
2. Behrendt H, Krämer U, Schäfer T, Kasche A, Eberlein-König B, Darsow U, Ring J (2001) Allergotoxicology – a research concept to study the role of environmental pollutants in allergy. Allergy Clin Immunol Int 13:122–128
3. Behrendt H, Kasche A, Ebner von Eschenbach C, Risse U, Huss-Marp J, Ring J (2001) Secretion of proinflammatory eicosanoid-like substances precedes allergen release from pollen grains in the initiation of allergic sensitization. Int Arch Allergy Immunol 124:121–125
4. Behrendt H, Ewers HJ, Hüttl RF, Jänicke M, Plaßmann E, Rehbinder E, Sukopp H (1999) (Der Rat der Sachverständigen für Umweltfragen). Umwelt und Gesundheit. Risiken richtig einschätzen. Sondergutachten. Metzler-Poeschel, Stuttgart
5. Börkstén B (1995) Genetic and environmental interaction in the development of allergy in children. Prog Allergy Immunol 3:184–189
6. Braun-Fahrländer C, Vuille JC, Sennhauser FH, et al. (1997) Respiratory health and long-term exposure to air pollutant in Swiss schoolchildren. SCAR-POL Team. Swiss Study in childhood allergy and respiratory symptoms with respect to air pollution, climate and pollen. Am J Respir Crit Care Med 155:1042–1049
7. Diaz-Sanchez D, Tsiwn A, Fleming J, Saxon A (1997) Combined diesel exhaust particulate and ragweed allergen challenge markedly enhances human in vivo nasal ragweed-specific IgE and skews cytokine production to a helper cell 2-type pattern. J Immunol 158:2406–2413
8. Eberlein-König B, Przybilla B, Kühnl P, et al. (1998) Influence of airborne nitrogen dioxide or formaldehyde on parameters of skin function and cellular activation in patients with atopic eczema and control subjects. J Allergy Clin Immunol 101:141–143
9. Hirsch T, Weiland SK, von Mutius E, et al. (1999) Inner city air pollution and respiratory health and atopy in children. Eur Respir J 14:669–677
10. Jörres R, Nowak D, Magnussen H (1996) The effect of ozone exposure on allergen responsiveness in subjects with asthma or rhinitis. Am J Respir Crit Care Med 153:56–64
11. Krämer U, Altmann L, Behrendt H, Dolgner R, Islam MS, Kayers HG, Ring J, Stiller-Winkler R, Turfeld M, Weishoff-Houben M, Willer H, Winneke G (1997) Comparison of the influence of socioeconomic factors on air pollution health effects in West and East Germany. In: Jantunen H (ed) Socioeconomic and cultural factors in air pollution epidemiology. Air pollution epidemiology report series, No. 8. Brussels, EU, pp 41–49
12. Krämer U, Behrendt H, Dolgner R, et al. (1999) Airway diseases and allergies in East and West Germany children during the first 5 years after reunification: Time trends and the impact of sulphur dioxide and total suspended particles. Int J Epidemiol 28:865–873

13. Krämer U, Koch T, Ranft U, et al. (2000) Traffic-related air pollution is associated with atopy in children living in urban areas. Epidemiology 11: 64–70
14. Martinez FD, Antognoni G, Macri F, et al. (1998) Parental smoking enhances bronchial responsiveness in nine-year-old children. Am Rev Respir Dis 138:518–523
15. Mersch-Sundermann (ed) (1999) Umweltmedizin. Thieme, Stuttgart
16. Miyamoto T, Takafuji S (1991) Environment and allergy. In: Ring J, Przybilla B (eds) New trends in allergy III. Springer, Berlin Heidelberg New York, pp 459–468
17. Molfino NA, Wright SC, Katz I, et al. (1991) Effect of low concentrations of ozone on inhaled allergen responses in asthmatic subjects. Lancet 338: 199–203
18. Mutius E von, Weiland SK, Fritzsch C (1998) Increasing prevalence of hay fever and atopy among children in Leipzig, East Germany. Lancet 351:862–866
19. Riedel F, Kramer M, Scheibenbogen C, Rieger Ch (1984) Effects of SO_2 exposure on allergic sensitization in the guinea pig. J Allergy Clin Immunol 82:527–534
20. Riedler J, Edler W, Oberfeld G, Schreuer M (2000) Austrian children living on a farm have less hay fever, asthma and allergic sensitization. Clin Exp Allergy 30:94–200
21. Ring J, Krämer U, Schäfer T, et al. (1999) Environmental risk factors for respiratory and skin atopy: Results from epidemiologic studies in former East and West Germany. Int Arch Allergy Immunol 118:403–407
22. Ring J, Behrendt H, Vieluf D (eds) (1997) New trends in allergy IV. Springer, Berlin Heidelberg New York
23. Ring J (1997) Allergy and modern society: Does "western life style" promote the development of allergies? Int Arch Allergy Immunol 113:7–10
24. Rusznak C, Devalia JL, Davies RJ (1996) Airway response of asthmatic subjects to inhaled allergen after exposure to pollutants. Thorax 51:1105–1108
25. Schäfer T, Dirschedl B, Kunz B, et al. (1997) Maternal smoking during pregnancy and lactation increases the risk for atopic eczema in the offspring. J Am Acad Dermatol 36:550–556
26. Schäfer T, Vieluf D, Behrendt H, et al. (1996) Atopic eczema and other manifestations of atopy: results of a study in East and West Germany. Allergy 51:532–539
27. Spieksma FT, Nikkels BH, Dijkman JH (1995) Seasonal appearance of grass pollen allergen in natural, paucimicronic aerosol of various size fractions. Relationship with airborne grass pollen concentration. Clin Exp Allergy 25:234–239
28. Vialuf D, Beil D, Beauregard K, et al. (1997) Xenobiotics and food allergy: In vivo and in vitro studies in patients with apple allergy. Int Arch Allergy Immunol 113:352–354
29. Wichmann H (1995) Environment, life-style and allergy: The German answer. Allergo J 6:315–316
30. Wüthrich B (1989) Epidemiology of the allergic diseases; are they really on the increase? Int Arch Allergy Appl Immunol 90:3–10
31. Zetterström O, Osterman K, Machedo L, Johannson SGO (1981) Another smoking hazard: Raised IgE concentration and increased risk of occupational allergy. Br Med J 283:1215–1217
32. Ring J (1988) Interview with *Natur*.

3.4 Allergens

Allergens are antigens able to start an allergy (induction of sensitization and elicitation of symptoms). They thus differ from other antigens able to induce specific immunologic reactions without disease characteristics. In this definition, allergens are not restricted to IgE-mediated reactions. According to the type of allergy elicited, allergens differ in nature, e.g., small chemicals for contact allergy, proteins and carbohydrates for immune complex reactions, proteins and glycoproteins for IgE-mediated allergies.

Allergens can be classified according to different criteria:

- Origin or allergen source (e.g., plant, animal, etc.)
- Route of contact [e.g., aeroallergens – often incorrectly called "inhalation" allergens, but skin and eye do not inhale!, through food (ingestion) or through injection (naturally by insect stings or iatrogenic)]
- Pathomechanism of allergy elicited (e.g., immediate-type allergens, IgE-inducing allergens, type IV allergens)
- Elicitation of certain diseases (e.g., so-called atopens in asthma, rhinoconjunctivitis, or atopic eczema)
- Situation of the affected individual (e.g., occupational allergens)

Terminology is critical: pollen grains themselves are not allergens but allergen carriers from which up to 30 different allergens can be released under certain conditions. Table 3.8 il-

Table 3.8. From the allergen source to the allergen (e.g., birch pollen)

Allergen source	Plant (e.g., birch)
Allergen contact route	Air ("inhalation")
Allergen carrier	Pollen (e.g., birch pollen)
Allergen extract	Extract from purified birch pollen
Allergen	e.g., major allergen Bet v 1

lustrates the different levels of allergen formation using the example of birch pollen grain.

3.4.1 "Allergenic Potency"

In spite of the great progress made in the elucidation of the molecular nature of many allergens, it is not known so far what makes an allergen an allergen. The best knowledge available is in the area of contact allergy, where certain aromatic ring structures with a special tendency for nucleophilic substitution and a high binding capacity to proteins represent very potent allergens and elicitors of type IV contact allergy (see Sect. 5.2). Allergens eliciting type III allergies such as hypersensitivity pneumonitis derive from allergen carriers of < 2 µm, can pass into the alveolar space and induce an IgG, IgA, and IgM response. Here – similar to serum sickness – high allergen doses are required for elicitation of symptoms.

In the following, IgE-inducing allergens will be discussed in particular: They are proteins, sometimes glycoproteins, with a molecular weight of between 5,000 and 70,000. Many allergens are known in molecular structure and are available either as recombinant or chemically synthesized "pure" allergens [1, 9, 10, 18, 22, 29, 31, 32, 41, 45, 46, 58].

Contrary to earlier simplifications, according to which allergic reactions – in contrast to toxic phenomena – do not follow dose response relations, we now know that the allergic process – like any natural phenomenon – underlies a dose response principle. However, the quantitative relationships often take place in very low and almost undetectable concentrations below so-called threshold values. Several micrograms of an allergen may kill a sensitized person (e.g., in insect venom allergy).

In the induction of IgE-mediated reactions, rather low concentrations seem to favor sensitization especially when applied together with certain adjuvants (e.g., aluminum hydroxide in animals). Higher doses can induce tolerance. Unfortunately, knowledge of dose response relationships in humans is so limited that practical recommendations cannot be given at the moment for prevention (e.g., "let the children keep their cat"). Allergen avoidance remains the only rational preventive principle (see Sect. 6.5).

Often the term "allergenic potency" is used by scientists and doctors without critical reflection. There is no doubt that the phenomenon exists: There are marked differences between different pollens in their capacity to induce allergies. The term has to be considered at different levels (Table 3.9) describing either the prevalence, the intensity, or the speed of reaction or induction of sensitization. Poppy seeds contain allergens which, except for the affected individual, rarely induce allergy very "potently."

One interesting hypothesis claims that potent allergens are enzymes, which holds true for some major allergens (e.g., proteases as major allergens of housedust mites, phospholipase of bee venom). However, most of the structurally known proteins are enzymes. Furthermore, many "potent" allergens do not have enzyme properties. Many plant allergens belong to so-called "pathogenesis-related proteins" or "stress proteins," which are formed by the plant in the defense of danger [45]. An interesting and almost philosophical speculation is that man by creating increasing environmental pollution or through financial greed is himself contributing to the increasing development of allergies (e.g., latex allergens as defense proteins in the milk of the hevea tree).

Table 3.9. Aspects of "allergenic potency"

- Frequency of sensitization
- Intensity of sensitization
- Speed of sensitization
- Frequency of allergy
- Intensity (severity) of allergy
- Speed of elicitation of allergy (e.g., anaphylaxis)

3.4.2 Standardization of Allergen Extracts

A committee of the International Association of Allergology and Clinical Immunology (IAACI)/World Allergy Organization (WAO) and the "International Union of Immunological Societies (IUIS)" has been working on the standardization of allergens for many years. Standard extracts are prepared which contain 100,000 IU (international units) per vial. With these standardized extracts, further comparisons can be performed. There are different methods of measuring allergen content:

In vitro allergen extracts can be standardized using RAST inhibition with positive sera from at least 20 specifically allergic patients.

In vivo extracts can be standardized using skin tests – compared to the histamine reaction (measured as wheal size) – as histamine equivalent potency (HEP) or as "biological units" (BU).

In the United States, intradermal tests are preferred to the prick test, and the diameter of the flare is measured and expressed as "biological activity units" (BAU). Furthermore, allergen concentrations can be determined which induce 50% of the intradermal test reaction obtainable with histamine (ID_{50}-EAC) (equivalent allergen concentration).

3.4.3 Terminology of Allergens

The above-mentioned WHO committee has published a nomenclature of allergens, which is being revised continuously [29] and contains all the molecularly characterized IgE-inducing allergens (Table 3.10). The first three letters of the name (genus) are followed after a space by the first letter of the species and after another space by an Arabic number, mostly according to the chronology of identification, but frequently also according to the homology with other known allergens (e.g., first described allergen of *Betula verrucosa* = Bet v 1). If necessary, four letters or suffixes can be used (e.g., to avoid confusion between dog [can] and candida [cand] allergens).

Within allergens of one species, related molecules with high degrees of homology (more than 67% of the amino acid sequence is identical) are often called iso-allergens [37]. These are characterized by the further addition of a four-digit Arabic number (e.g., ragweed iso-allergens amb a 2.0101 or 2.0102). Recombinant allergens contain a prefix "r," synthetic allergens an "s." While earlier allergens were printed in italics, names in the new nomenclature are in normal type and also identify the respective genes. The major cat allergen Fel d 1 consists of two polypeptide chains coded via two different genes (Fel d 1A and Fel d 1B).

The importance of allergens is evaluated according to the frequency of sensitized individuals. Major allergens are those against which more than 50% of tested patients have developed specific IgE antibodies.

The most important aeroallergens are discussed briefly below. Elicitors of contact, food and drug allergies are considered in the respective chapters.

3.4.4 Aeroallergens

The most important aeroallergens of natural and anthropogenic origin are listed in Table 3.11. The molecular characterization of many allergens has helped us to understand a clinical phenomenon known for 30 years, namely "cross-sensitization" ("celery-mugwort-spice syndrome") [54, 67]. Homologous allergen structures sometimes do not correspond to taxonomic classifications and can give rise to unexpected symptoms after contact with unsuspicious substances (apple allergy in birch pollen allergic patients) (Table 3.12).

The most important cross-sensitizations occur between pollen and foods derived from plants, but also between animal epithelia and milk constituents as well as latex and certain fruits.

3.4.4.1 Allergen Detection

Pollen and Mold Counts. The most important aeroallergens in the outdoor air are pollen and mold spores with a diameter of 2–60 µm, which are transferred through the air over large distances [3, 12, 20, 26, 27, 42, 44, 49, 51, 65].

The identification and quantification of defined and specifically relevant particular air

Table 3.10. Terminology of a selection of natural allergens

Allergen source (species)	Allergen	Function	Molecular weight
A. Pollen			
Alnus glutinosa (alder)	Aln g 1	Pathogenesis-associated (PR-) protein	17
Betula verrucosa (birch)	Bet v 1	PR protein	17
	Bet v 2	Profilin	14
	Bet v 3	Ca-binding protein	24
Corylus avellana (hazel)	Cor a 1	Stress protein	17
Castanea sativa (sweet chestnut)	Cas s 1	Stress protein	17
Dactylis glomerata (cocksfoot)	Dac g 1	–	32
	Dac g 2	–	11
	Dac g 3	–	
	Dac g 5	–	31
Lolium perenne (perennial ryegrass)	Lol p 1	Group I	27
	Lol p 2	Group II	11
	Lol p 3	Group III	11
	Lol p 5		31
	Lol p 9	Group IX	31/35
Phleum pratense (timothy grass)	Phl p 1	Protease	27
	Phl p 4	–	50–60
	Phl p 5	Ribonuclease	32/38
	Phl p 6	–	11
	Phl p 11	Profilin	14
Triticum aestivum (wheat)	Tri a 2.1	Profilin	14
	Tri a 2.2	Profilin	14
	Tri a 2.3	Profilin	14
Zea mays (corn)	Zea m 1	Lol p I homolog	27
Ambrosia artemisiifolia (ragweed)	Amb a 1	–	38
	Amb a 5	–	5
Artemisia vulgaris (mugwort)	Art v 1	–	47
	Art v 2		30.35
B. Mites			
Dermatophagoides pteronyssinus (house dust mite)	Der p 1	Cysteine protease	25
	Der p 2	Profilin	14
	Der p 3	Serine protease	28/30
	Der p 4	Amylase	60
	Der p 5	–	14
	Der p 6	Chymotrypsin	25
	Der p 7	–	22–28
C. Insects			
Apis mellifera (honey bee)	Api m 1	Phospholipase A2	19
	Api m 2	Hyaluronidase	45
	Api m 3	Melittin	2.8
	Api m 4	Acid phosphatase	49
Vespa crabro (hornet)	Ves c 1	Phospholipase	34
	Ves c 5	–	23
Vespula germanica (wasp)	Ves g 1	Phospholipase A1/B	35
	Ves g 2	Hyaluronidase	45
	Ves g 5	–	23
Blatella germanica (cockroach)	Bla g 2	–	20

Table 3.10. *(Cont.)*

Allergen source (species)	Allergen	Function	Molecular weight
D. Mammals			
Felis domesticus (cat)	Fel d 1	–	35
Canis familiaris (dog)	Can f 1	–	25
	Can f 2	–	27
Mus musculus (mouse)	Mus m 1	–	19
Rattus norvegicus (rat)	Rat n 1	α-2a-globulin	17
E. Molds			
Alternaria alternata	Alt a 1	–	30
	Alt a 2	–	28
	Alt a 10	Aldehyde dehydrogenase	53
Aspergillus fumigatus	Asp f 1	Mitogillin	18
Cladosporium herbarum	Cla h 1	–	30
	Cla h 6	Enolase	48
F. Foods			
Arachis hypogaea (peanut)	Ara h 1	Vicilin	63.5
	Lektin	Agglutinin	17
Glycine max (soy)		Glycinin	
		β-Conglycinin	
		Soy lectin	
		Kunitz trypsin inhibitor	
Malus domestica (apple)	Mal d 1	PR protein	17
Triticum aestivum (flour)	Gluten	α/β-Gliadin	
Bos domesticus (cattle)	Bos d 4	α-Lactalbumin	14
	Bos d 5	β-Lactoglobulin	18
	Bos d 6	Serum albumin	67
	Bos d 8	Casein	25–35
Gadis callarias (cod)	Gad c 1	β-Parvalbumin	
		Allergen M	
Gallus domesticus (hen)	Gal d 1	Ovomucoid	28
	Gal d 2	Ovalbumin	44
	Gal d 3	Ovotransferrin	78
	Gal d 4	Lysozyme	14
Metapenaeus ensis (shrimp)	Met e 1	Tropomyosin	36
G. Other			
Hevea brasiliensis (latex)	Hev b 1	Rubber elongation factor	14.5
	Hev b 2	β-1,3-glucanase	35
	Hev b 3	Hev b 1-homolog	23–27
	Hev b 4	Micro helix component	50–57
	Hev b 5	Major allergen	16
	Hev b 6.01	Prohevein	21.8
	Hev b 6.02	Hevein	4.7
	Hev b 6.03	Prohevein C terminal	14
	Hev b 7	Patatin-like protein	42.9
	Hev b 8	Profilin	14.2

3.4 Allergens

Table 3.11. Origin of common airborne allergens

Plants	Pollen, grain dust, flour, fibers, mold spores, housedust, natural rubber latex, etheric oils, enzymes
Animals	Mammalian epithelia (dander, hair), feathers, insects (e.g., bee, wasp), arthropods (e.g., housedust mites)
Bacteria[a]	Enzymes
Chemicals[a]	Isocyanates, formaldehyde, epoxide resins, acid anhydrides, hexachloroplatinate, azo-dyes

[a] Predominantly occupational

Table 3.12. Common "cross-sensitizations"

Tree pollen Birch, alder, hazel	• Foods (fruit, vegetables) Stone fruit, hazelnut, kiwifruit, carrot, celery
Grass pollen Grass pollen	• Cereals, vegetables, fruits Flour, peanut, soy, tomato, potato
Weed pollen Mugwort, ragweed	• Vegetables, spices, fruits • Celery, carrot, spices, melon, banana, cucumber
Latex constituents Natural rubber latex	• Exotic fruits Avocado, banana, buckwheat, kiwifruit, mango
Feathers Bird feathers	• Egg Poultry, meat, eggs
Arthropods Housedust mite	• Crustacea Lobster, crab, shrimp
Mammalian epithelia Cattle epithelia Horse epithelia	• Meat, milk Cow's milk, beef Mare's milk

constituents is not only of scientific importance. Over the years, exposure calendars (pollen calendars) with concentration curves over the season have been prepared [4, 20, 28, 34, 53] (Fig. 3.10). In the media (radio, TV), pollen counts together with metereologic and field observations ("phenology") enable a pollen forecast to be given and thus preventive action can be taken [4, 28, 34, 53, 62].

In the selection of allergens for the formulation of an allergen extract for specific immunotherapy, the clinical relevance is of crucial importance and can be determined in comparing symptom diaries with pollen counts. A common mistake is the selection of allergens according

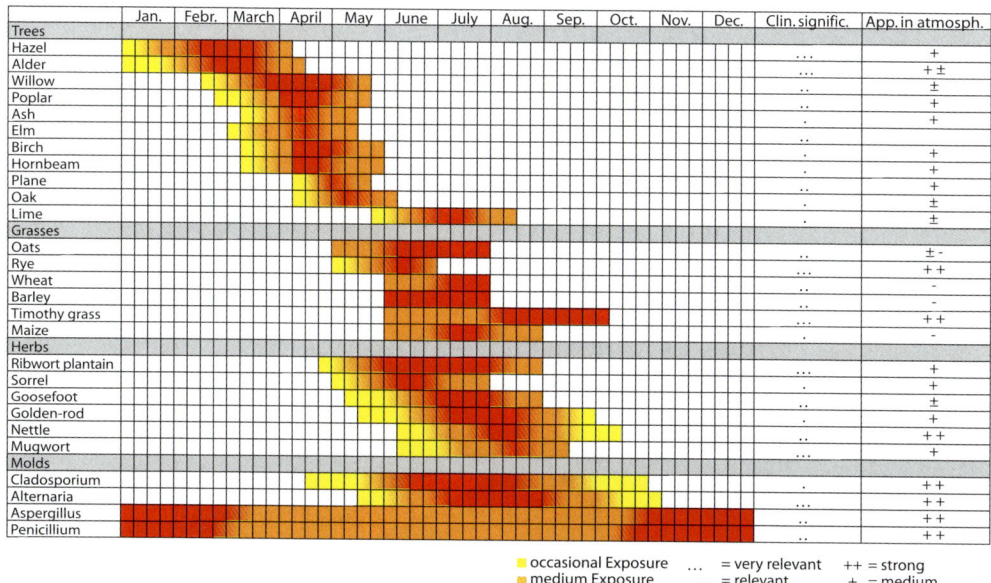

Fig. 3.10. Pollen and spore flight calendar for Germany (Stiftung Deutscher Pollen-Informationsdienst, German Pollen Information Service Foundation)

to the intensity of skin test or RAST results without consideration of history and pollen counts.

In order to collect particular air constituents, various methods are used. The most simple one is the so-called gravimetric collection (Durham) whereby the sedimentation of certain pollen or molds per square unit (mostly cm²) is measured. Equally, mold spores can be collected in indoor environments on agar plates in Petri dishes and cultured. Rotor samplers (Rotorod) are mainly used in the United States [48]. Here the number of pollen or mold spores is determined on a surface of a rotating device.

The best and scientifically most acceptable results are obtained by Burkard traps (Fig. 3.11a), which suck air with constant speed and can be positioned according to the wind direction; the airstream passes over Scotch tape on which the particles stick and can be quantified exactly according to intervals of time per m³ air. The "Anderson sampler" also works with airstreams and different cascades (cascade impactor) where the air passes over several agar-coated plates.

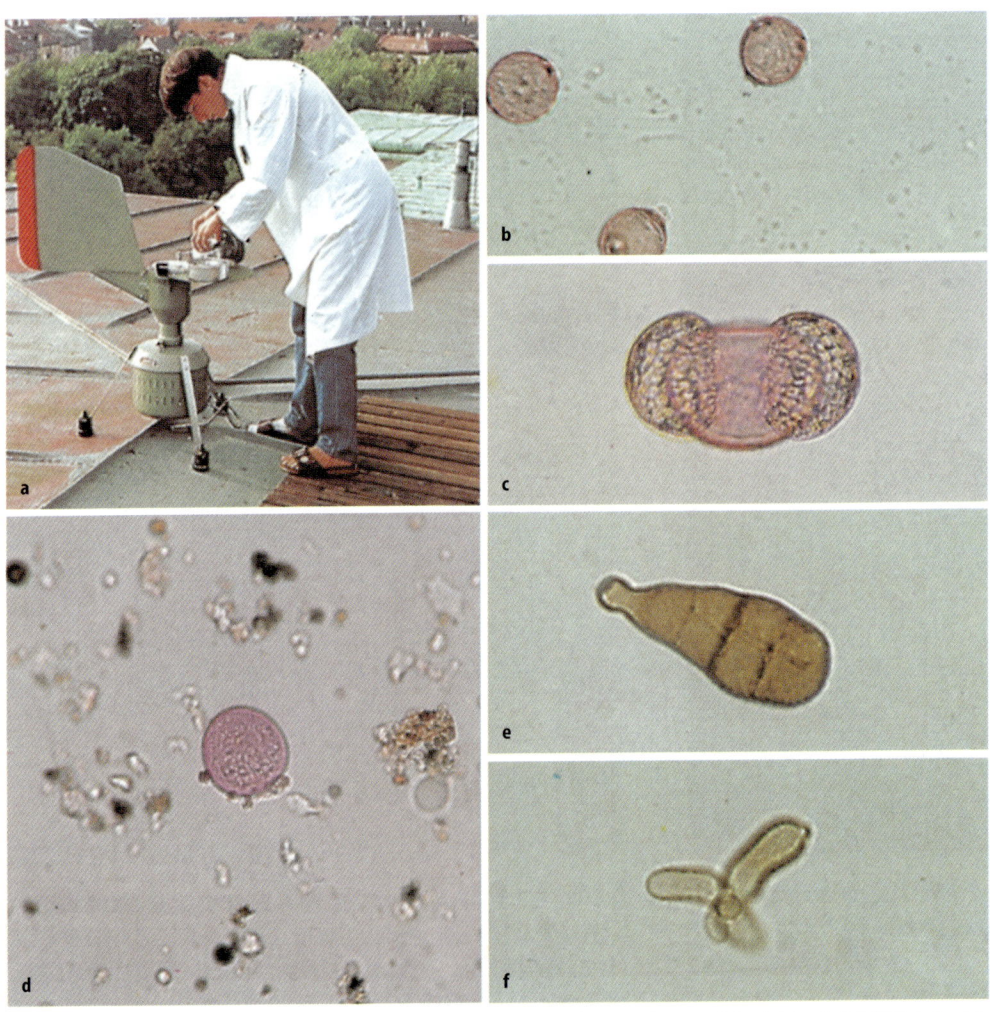

Fig. 3.11. a Burkard traps on the roof of the Division of Dermatology at the Municipal Hospital (affiliated with University Hospital) in Thalkirchnerstr. in Munich. **b–f** Light microscopic preparations of pollen and fungus spores; **b** birch pollen (*Betula*); **c** pine (*Pinus*); **d** rye pollen (*Secale cereale*); **e** *Alternaria alternata*; **f** *Cladosporium herbarum*

Crucial for all types of pollen counts is the correct localization of the device. It should be positioned at least 5 m above ground in an area with free air circulation in order to avoid walls, trees, or house ventilation devices. The immediate environment should be known and botanically characterized.

The collected particles are transferred to a microscopic slide and for better contrast stained with safranil or fuchsin. Then they are differentiated under the microscope using a water immersion objective (Fig. 3.11b–f). Slides can be stored under airproof conditions (e.g., nail polish).

3.4.4.2 Pollen

The pollen is the carrier of the male genes in higher plants ("gametophyte"). Pollen grains have a very resistant wall consisting of two layers, the external exine and the internal intine [51] (Fig. 3.12). The intine consists of the cell wall materials cellulose and pectin overlaid by the exine consisting of carotinoid complexes. The pollen wall covers the cytoplasm and the nucleus. Allergenic substances are derived from cytoplasm and released under humid conditions when pollen is activated in a similar way as for germination. Water intake and swelling occur either on a moist flower or on the surface of a mucous membrane. During this process other constituents of the cytoplasm (fat, carbohydrates, and proteins such as allergens) are also mobilized. According to D. Marsh the inhalation of 10 ng pollen allergen is enough to elicit symptoms of hay fever (personal communication).

Pollen grains vary in size between 5 and 60 μm (it is commonly assumed that large particles of more than 10 μm do not reach the bronchi).

Allergists interested in pollinosis should have some botanical and specifically palynological knowledge. The taxonomy of the different pollen carriers (Table 3.13) is of major importance for the formulation of allergen extracts. Pollen of different species but the same order may be used as allergen mixtures while that from different orders should be used as single allergen sources in one extract [19]. Table 3.14 lists the international (Latin) names of important allergy-relevant plants.

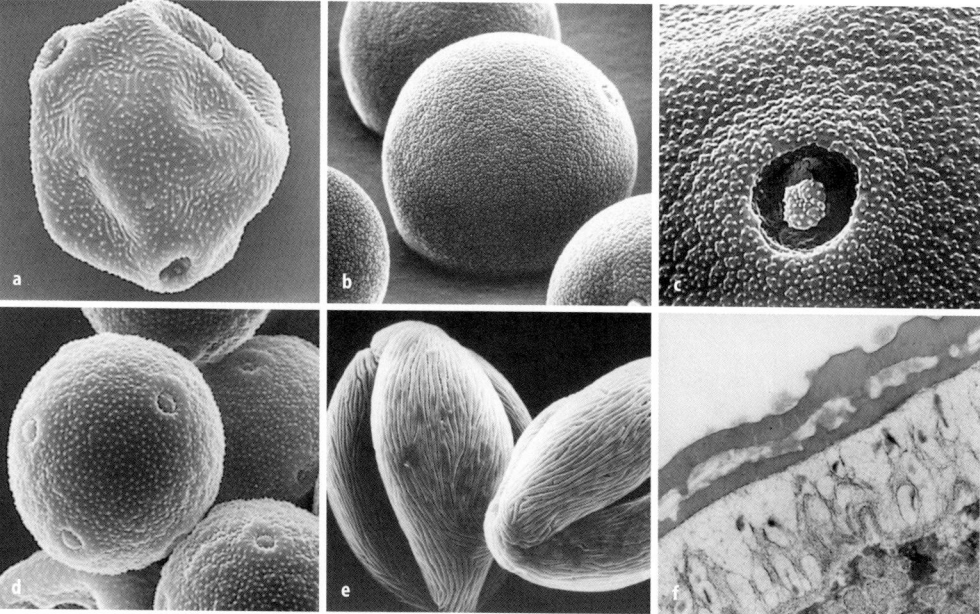

Fig. 3.12a–f. Pollen grains seen under the electron microscope. **a** Birch (*Betula*); **b** timothy grass; **c** timothy grass, pore (*Phleum pratense*); **d** narrow-leaved plantain or ribwort (*Plantago lanceolata*); **e** mugwort pollen (*Artemisia vulgaris*); **f** transmission electron microscopic photo pollen wall with intine and extine (H. Behrendt)

Table 3.13. Taxonomy

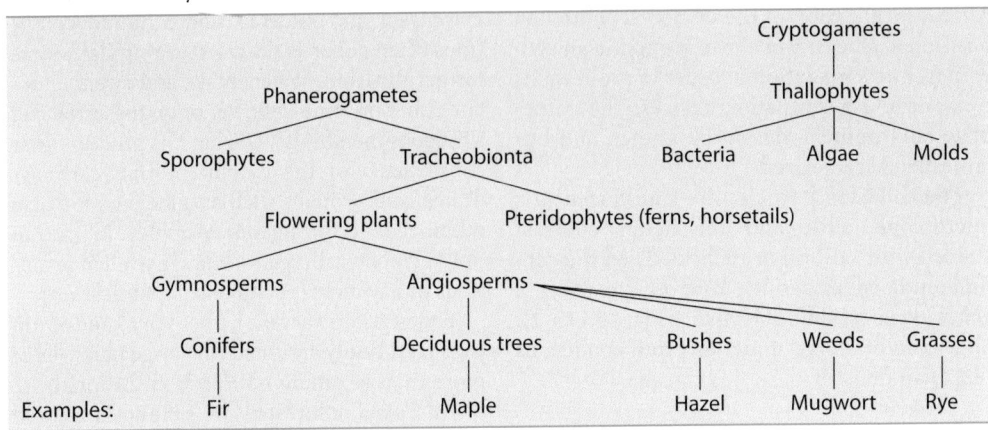

Table 3.14. Index of allergy-relevant plant names

Alder – *Alnus*	Maize – *Zea mays*
Ash – *Fraxinus excelsior*	Male fern – *Dryopteris*
Barley – *Hordeum vulgare*	Maple – *Acer*
Beech – *Fagus sylvatica*	Meadow-rue – *Thalictrum*
Birch – *Betula verrucosa*	Meadow foxtail – *Alopecurus pratensis*
Bird cherry – *Prunus padus*	Mugwort – *Artemisia*
Bog myrtle – *Myrica gale*	Nettle – *Urtica*
Bulrush – *Typha*	Norway maple – *Acer platanoides*
Clover – *Trifolium*	Oak – *Quercus*
Common chickweed – *Stellaria media*	Oats – *Avena sativa*
Common oak – *Quercus robur*	Ox-eye daisy – *Chrysanthemum leucanthemum*
Common polypody – *Polypodium vulgare*	Perennial ryegrass – *Lolium perenne*
Clubmoss – *Lycopodium*	Pondweed – *Potamogeton*
Cocksfoot – *Dactylis glomerata*	Pine – *Pinus*
Cotton-grass – *Eriophorum*	Plane – *Platanus*
Cow parsley – *Anthriscus sylvestris*	Poplar – *Populus*
Cornflower – *Centaurea cyanus*	Ragweed – *Ambrosia*
Dandelion – *Taraxacum*	Red-berried elder – *Sambucus racemosa*
Dropwort – *Filipendula vulgaris*	Reed – *Phragmites communis*
Dwarf birch – *Betula nana*	Ribwort plantain – *Plantago lanceolata*
Elder – *Sambucus nigra*	Rock-rose – *Helianthemum*
Elm – *Ulmus*	Rye – *Secale cereale*
Field mustard – *Brassica campestris*	Sea buckthorn – *Hippophae rhamnoides*
Fir – *Abies*	Sea club-rush – *Scirpus maritimus*
Golden-rod – *Solidago virgaurea*	Sedge – *Carex*
Goosefoot – *Chenopodium album*	Sorrel – *Rumex*
Grasses – *Poaceae*	Spruce – *Picea abies*
Greater plantain – *Plantago major*	Sweet chestnut – *Castanea*
Hazel – *Corylus avellana*	Sweet vernal grass – *Anthoxanthum odoratum*
Heather – *Calluna vulgaris*	Timothy – *Phleum pratense*
Hops – *Humulus lupulus*	Walnut – *Juglans*
Hornbeam – *Carpinus betulus*	Water milfoil – *Myriophyllum*
Horse chestnut – *Aesculus hippocastanum*	Wheat – *Triticum*
Horsetail – *Equisetum*	Willow – *Salix*
Ivy – *Hedera helix*	White birch – *Betula pubescens*
Juniper – *Juniperus communis*	Woodrush – *Luzula*
Larch – *Larix*	Yarrow – *Achillea millefolium*
Lime – *Tilia*	Yew – *Taxus*

Obviously, in allergy, wind-activated pollinated (anemophilous) plants are of major importance. There are, however, allergies against insect-activated orders when there is close contact as in agriculture or floristics [22, 26]. A less widely known but in some areas of the world very important allergy through aeroallergens should be mentioned, namely "airborne contact dermatitis," where allergens induce eczematous skin lesions after skin contact on uncovered skin surface areas. Often these reactions are mixed with photoallergy (see Sect. 5.6). An epidemic occurrence of these diseases has been reported in India with parthenium plants (composite family).

Table 3.15. Morphological criteria for pollen differentiation

- Number of pores (mono-, di-, triporate)
- Number of colpi (e.g., mono-, di-, tricolpate)
- Pores and colpi (colporate)
- Distribution of pores on the surface (periporate, stefanoporate)

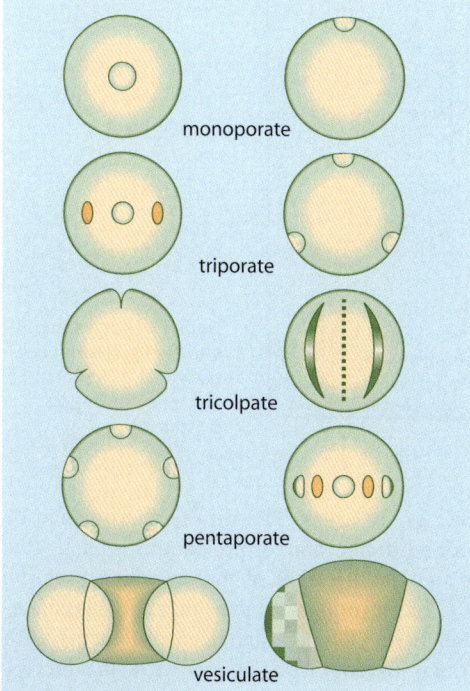

Fig. 3.13. Pollen forms

The differentiation of pollen grains has been performed according to different criteria, the most important of which are size, form, kind, and number of spores and grooves as well as surface characteristics (Table 3.15) (Fig. 3.13).

Apart from the quantitative measurement of pollen, allergologic expertise is important for interpretation considering regional aspects. Interestingly, much very commonly found pollen in the air in rather high concentrations, such as pine or fir pollen, is of only marginal allergological relevance. Certain pollen species are difficult to differentiate so that they are taken together in some pollen counts.

The most important allergen carriers in Central Europe in the spring (often as early as February) are hazel, alder, birch, then other trees, from May to July the different grasses and then up to September and October weeds such as *Plantago*, mugwort and others, in the United States especially ragweed.

Circadian rhythms of pollen counts have to be considered. In the countryside, the highest pollen counts can be measured during the day, especially over meadows. In cities, pollen maxima often occur only in the evening (9 p.m.) due to smog conditions (Figs. 3.14, 3.15).

For illustration of quantitative relations, one may imagine that one rye ear contains over 4 million pollen grains, one hazel bush approximately 600 million pollen. The pollen can rise up to 5,000 m. In Central Europe, on average 27,000 pollen grains/cm^2 are deposited [26].

Of course geographic differences are reflected in pollen counts. In the United States, in autumn ragweed (*Ambrosia artemisiifolia*) is the major allergen carrier. Recently, ragweed has also been observed in Germany and Austria along the big river valleys [4]. While in Central Europe pollinosis patients are sensitized mostly against a spectrum of various pollen species (grasses, weeds, trees), monovalent allergy against ragweed is typical.

Between pollen of different species and also orders, cross-reactivities exist (see above) [32, 40, 54, 67] which are of practical importance for diagnosis and therapy. Almost all known grass pollen shows common allergens, which also holds true for reed [40], with individual

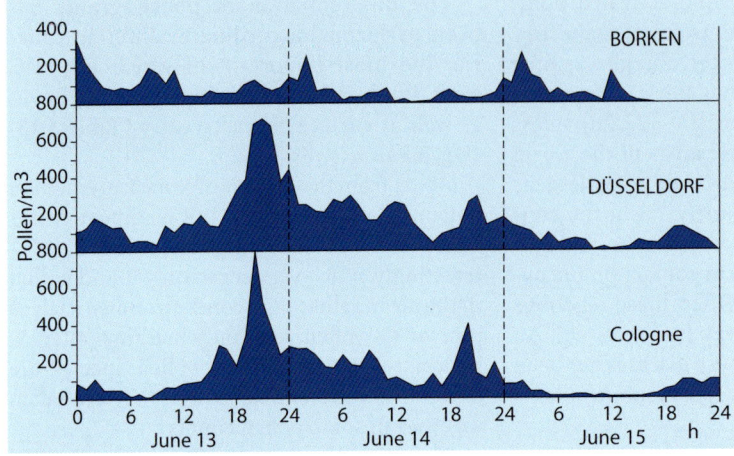

Fig. 3.14. Diurnal fluctuations in grass pollen concentration measured in a rural area (Borken, Westphalia) and two large cities (Düsseldorf and Cologne) in Germany with different degrees of air pollution (according to Behrendt)

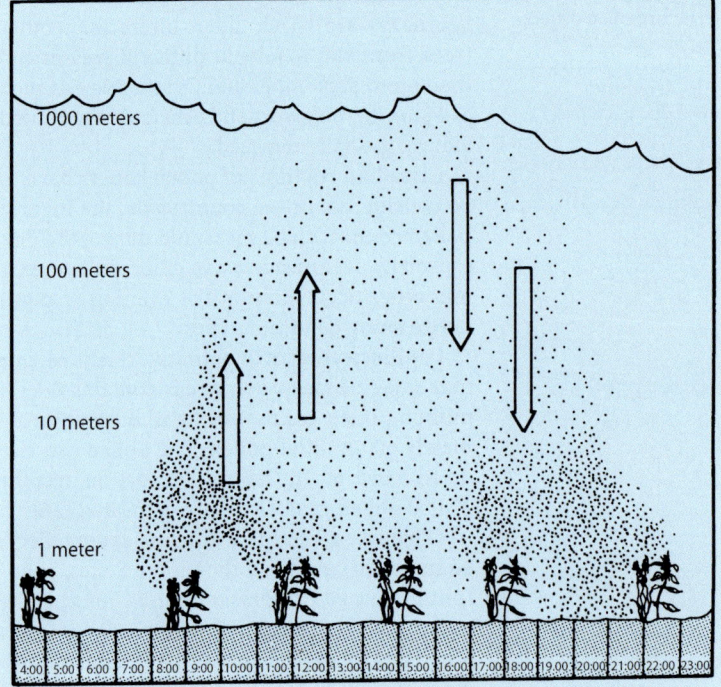

Fig. 3.15. Diurnal fluctuations in pollen concentration at different altitudes (according to Behrendt)

characteristics in single allergens. For routine treatment of allergy, grass pollen can be used as allergen mixture.

3.4.4.3 Mold Spores

Mold spores – rarely mycel fragments – form the major part of biological particles in the air over green areas. The differentiation may be more difficult than for pollen; this is partly due to the classification of molds, which uses the type of reproduction as the means of classification, with divisions between organisms with sexual (teleomorph, spores as a product of combining nuclei and meiotic division) and asexual spores (anamorph, simple mitotic division) [33, 42, 44, 49, 65]. Most molds form both sexual and asexual spores, which however differ in morphology and therefore also terminology (e.g., teleomorph: *Leptosphaeria* species, *Mycosphaerella* species, *Eurotinum* species; anamorph: *Alternaria* species, *Cladosporium* species, *Aspergillus* species). Fungi imperfecti have no sexual reproduction.

The most common airborne fungi are listed in Table 3.16. Mold spores in the air are especially enhanced by high humidity (fog, smog, rain), e.g., for *Ascospora*, *Basidiospora* (*Fusarium*, *Phoma*, etc.). In dry air, spores from *Cladosporium herbarum*, *Alternaria*, *Epicoccum*, and *Helminthosporium* are predominant. With certain activities like collecting of leaves, but also simple sports exercise, spore clouds can be formed. Also basidiomycete spores may be present in the air and elicit allergies [23]. Molds need oxygen, carbohydrates, as well as high humidity (over 65%) for growth. Hyphae grow best at a temperature between 18 and 32 °C. Temperatures over 71 °C are lethal.

Actinomycetes are often classified under molds. They represent, however, filiform bacteria with dry spores. In allergy, they predominantly play a role in hypersensitivity pneumonitis (farmer's lung due to thermophilic actinomycetes) (see Sect. 5.4).

Certain mold species have active mechanisms for spore release, for instance basidiomycetes and ascomycetes needing humidity. That is why these spores are especially prevalent at high air humidity. There are also circadian rhythms for mold spore concentrations. Dry spores (*Cladosporium*, *Alternaria*, *Epicoccum*) have their maximum around noon. Basidiospores are especially prevalent in the early evening hours.

Identification of mold spores is performed according to the following criteria:

- Size (ranging between 1 µm and 100 µm, average 7–12 µm)
- Color: while many spores are colorless, i.e., transparent, some may be yellowish brown to black (Demiataceae = black fungi)
- Morphology (spherical, oval, elliptic, cylindric, filiform, with or without dendrites)
- Septal structure (with septa or without, only transverse and longitudinal = muriform) (Fig. 3.11)
- Surface characteristics (smooth, rough, punctated, wartiform, etc.)

A major problem for practical allergology is the production of mold allergen extracts, which mostly consist of vegetative mycel and few spores [21, 32, 65]. Recently, the major allergen of *Aspergillus fumigatus* was characterized as superoxide dismutase with a strong homology to the human enzyme. Possible autoimmune phenomena in chronic disease have been discussed [9]. In practical allergy, intramural and extramural molds are distinguished (Table 3.17).

Intramural molds play a role in perennial diseases, while extramural molds follow the patterns of pollinosis.

In the indoor environment, humid walls, old humidifiers, window frames with condensation water, air conditioners, foam mattresses, waste baskets with old food, and indoor plants represent the most favorable environments for mold growth.

Other mold products (enzymes) play a role in the food industry (amylase in bakery). Food allergies against edible fungi (basidiomycetes) such as champignons or shiitake are rare but can occur [23, 47].

Table 3.16. Taxonomy of fungi

Fungi Myxomycetes	Eumycetes			
1	2	3	4	5
Mastigomycetes	Zygomycetes (e.g., *Mucor*, *Rhizopus*)	Ascomycetes (e.g., *Chaetomium*)	Basidiomycetes (e.g., *Rhodotorula*, *Sporobolo-myces*, smuts – Ustilaginomyctes)	Deuteromycetes (e.g., *Aspergillus*, *Alternaria*, *Cladosporium*, *Botrytis*, *Curvularia*, *Penicillium*)

1, mobile, flagellated spores; *2, 3, 4, 5*, immobile spores

Extramural	Intra- and extramural	Intramural
Alternaria tenuis	Aspergillus	Chaetomium globosum
Phoma betae	Botrytis cinerea	Mucor racemosus
Ustilago	Trichothecium roseum	Penicillium notatum nigricans
Fusarium	Pullularia pullulans	Neurospora sitophila
Cladosporium		Merulius lacrimans
Epicoccum purpurescens		
Helminthosporium		

Table 3.17. Selection of allergy-relevant molds

3.4.4.4 Mammalian Epithelia

Allergies against animal epithelia are increasing in prevalence in parallel with the increasing tendency for pet-keeping. Rudolph et al. found among 2,638 animal-exposed patients with suspected respiratory allergies 45% with sensitization against animal epithelia, among them 30% with sensitization against several species. Especially dangerous with regard to sensitization are cats and rodents (55% sensitized of exposed), guinea pigs (60%), while dogs (17%) and birds (10%) showed lower rates [43]. The chemical nature of cross-reactivities between different animal orders or species has not yet been fully elucidated. In rodents, a major allergen from epithelia has been shown to be serum albumin [63, 64]. In standard allergen extracts, up to 20 different allergens of doubtful relevance have been demonstrated in some animal epithelia extracts.

Cat allergen represents a major problem since it only slowly sediments and stays present in aerosols of indoor air for many weeks, which can be noticed by affected individuals by their immediate symptoms (red eyes, itchy nose, etc.), while housedust mite allergen mostly stays sedimented in the dust. Cat allergen mostly comes from saliva (androgen-dependent, male cats form less allergen when castrated) [68]. According to recent investigations, cat allergen can be regarded as ubiquitous; it has been demonstrated in apartments where cats have never been kept [25]. Animal allergens are transferred through the clothing of pet keepers. Allergic individuals may suffer severe attacks in the subway, in school, or in restaurants when meeting pet keepers. The problem of "passive allergy" ("derivative" allergy according to E. Fuchs) should be taken as seriously as the problem of "passive smoking"!

Recent studies showing the protective effects of cat keeping have induced controversial debates [7] (see Sect. 6.5). Increasing sensitization rates are reported against horse epithelia (also commonly transferred through clothes in public rooms). The dramatic increase in small rodents (rats, mice) kept as pets in childrens' bedrooms seems alarming from an allergy point of view. The allergen in mouse urine corresponding to a prealbumin fraction is extremely "potent" and until now has mostly been relevant as an occupational allergen in laboratory workers.

Animal allergic individuals are mostly allergic against the whole order although there are differences in sensitization prevalence between different species. Rarely allergies are reported against individual animals of one species. The mechanism of such MHC-dependent allergies is not clear; possibly psychological aspects (e.g., particularly close contact with a favorite horse) might play a role (F. Wortmann, personal communication).

More exotic are the occasional press reports of allergy against human hair. This phenomenon is known in allergic dogs. I myself have seen three patients with a clear-cut history of allergy against human hair (from the partner or from a child); however, in spite of very extensive investigations and double-blind provocation tests including psychosomatic consultation, I did not find convincing explanations. IgE antibodies against human HLA determinants have so far not been described. However, IgE antibodies against epidermal proteins (Hom s1-s4) have been observed in severe atopic eczema (see Valenta, Sect. 5.5.3).

3.4.4.5 Sperm Allergy

A special case of mammalian allergy against human proteins is the rare sperm allergy, more precisely allergy against seminal plasma proteins, which occurs predominantly in atopic females, sometimes after the first contact with sperma (e.g., contact urticaria on the skin, anaphylaxis on the wedding night). This suggests the possibility of cross-reactions with another as yet unknown allergen. Successful hyposensitization has been reported [31]. Rare cases of noninfectious vaginitis with IgE antibodies against spermicide substances or *Candida* have to be considered in the differential diagnosis [66].

3.4.4.6 Bird Allergens

The previously common "feather" allergy most likely corresponds to a housedust mite allergy. There are, however, allergies against bird proteins present in feathers but also in bird droppings, especially for budgerigars, pigeons, and parrots. These diseases have to be differentiated from hypersensitivity pneumonitis in birdkeeper's lung (see Sect. 5.4).

3.4.4.7 Arthropods: Housedust and Storage Mites

Housedust is an ill-defined mixture of sedimented particles differing according to the localization of collection, the major constituents being animal and human epithelia, mites, fibers and molds. Since 1964, it has been known that certain mites induce housedust allergy [61]. The species *Dermatophagoides pteronyssinus* (Fig. 3.16) and *D. farinae* of the Pyroglyphidae family are the major housedust mites of the world; in tropical climates, *Bloomia* species are also important. Only in Arctic and Alpine climates are mites rarely found [7, 21]. In Germany, an especially high mite exposure is found in Freiburg [13, 15], while in Davos, Switzerland, and other high-altitude (above 1,500 m) regions, housedust mites are rare. There are more than 30,000 mite species. Housedust mites are present predominantly in bed, mattress, and upholstery dust. In Birmingham, 4,241 mites per gram bed dust and 1,088 per gram floor dust in the bedroom were counted, but only 80 mites per gram dust in kitchen floors [7].

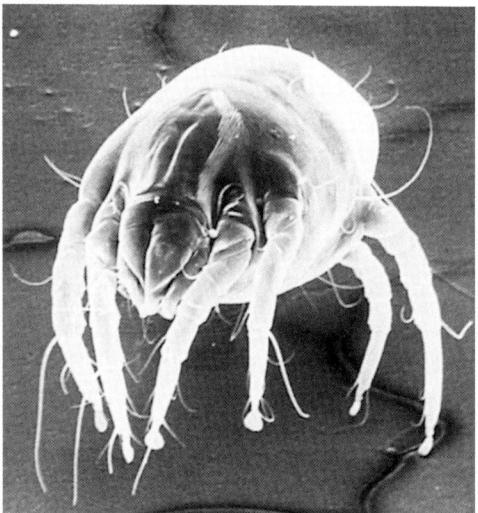

Fig. 3.16. House dust mite (*Dermatophagoides pteronyssinus*) seen under the scanning electron microscope (JEMH von Bronswijk)

Housedust mites are also found in furs and grain stores. The living conditions of housedust mites follow a complex ecosystem with enhancing factors such as high humidity, mold growth, high temperature, and quantity of organic or fiber material (Fig. 3.17). Acaricides used comprise benzylbenzoate, tannin, and hypertonic saline [5, 11, 57].

The relevant allergen of housedust mite is present in 95% of the 10- to 40-µm-diameter feces balls [55]. It is a glycoprotein P1 (molecular weight 24,000).

Mites can be measured by different methods (e.g., counted in the microscope view of a dust sample). Using a color reaction a metabolic product of mites, guanine, can be measured [5]. Progress is achieved through the use of monoclonal antibodies against the major allergen Der p1 with enzyme immunoassays (ELISA) [13, 15, 35]. With the measurement of mites in different samples from, for instance, couch, carpet, furniture, and clothes, very specific avoidance recommendations can be given.

Apart from housedust mites, also storage mites occurring in grain stores and in households (*Lepidoglyphus destructor, Euroglyphus maynei, Acarus siro*) are relevant especially in farmers but also persons engaged in other oc-

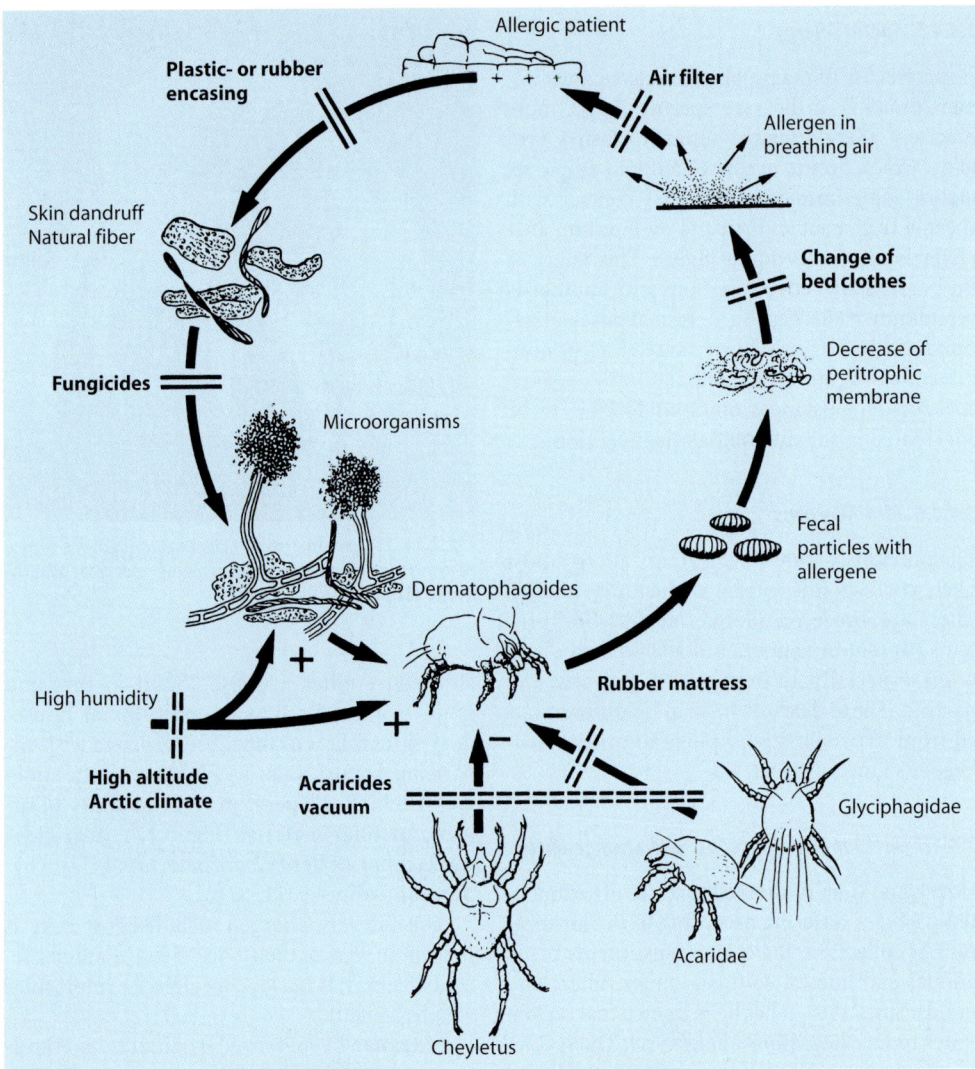

Fig. 3.17. "Ecosystem" of house dust and house dust mites (according to JEMH von Bronswijk)

cupations with contact with hay and straw (e.g., thatchers) [16, 59, 60].

Storage mites show little cross-reactivity to housedust mites, but clear cross-reactions to the scabies mite *Sarcoptes scabiei*, leading to positive skin test reactions in scabies patients [35].

3.4.4.8 Insect Allergens

Apart from the well-known allergens in Hymenoptera venoms, which will be covered in the section on insect venom allergy (Sect. 5.1.6), there are IgE-mediated allergies against airborne allergens from insect dander (beekeeper's asthma). Also allergies against the red midge larvae in aquarium owners (*Chironomus thummi*) are very common in northern Africa, where they also represent an outdoor air problem. The allergen corresponds to the *Chironomus* hemoglobin and its molecular structure is known [2]. Other sources of indoor aeroallergens are cockroaches, mostly reported in the United States, against *Blatella germanica*.

Allergies against products of silkworms (natural silk) are easily overlooked [14]. Rare cases of allergies against other insects such as dust lice, bread beetle, museum beetle, and silverfish (*Daphia*) have been reported; however, they have not been well investigated due to the limited allergen extract amounts. If there is a specific history together with objective complaints in certain rooms, sampling and site visits are recommended.

3.4.4.9 Allergy Against Parasites

During evolution, IgE was functional as a carrier of defense against large organisms such as helminths. Indeed, intestinal parasite infestation occurs with high IgE and sometimes allergic symptoms such as urticaria or anaphylaxis (see Sect. 5.1.3). The complication of anaphylaxis after rupturing of an echinococcal cyst in the liver is also IgE mediated; the condition of acute anisakiasis is similarly IgE mediated.

It is not known what role IgE-mediated allergy plays in cutaneous parasitosis such as that by nematode larvae of *Larva migrans* or persistent ictus reactions in scabies. Ascariasis in the dog and *Nippostrongylus brasiliensis* in the rat are the best-established animal models for IgE reactions.

Sheep when infested with ticks develop a special form of cutaneous basophil inflammation with IgE against saliva proteins of ticks.

3.4.4.10 Occupational Aeroallergens

Apart from the ubiquitous and common aeroallergens, certain occupations are characterized by IgE-mediated diseases against occupational substances such as low-molecular-weight chemicals; these diseases manifest mainly as asthma (see Sect. 5.1.2), but also as rhinoconjunctivitis, urticaria, and eczema. Particular consideration should be given to natural rubber latex allergy, which has increased in prevalence dramatically since the 1980s, especially in the health professions (20% of the employees of a large hospital in Munich are sensitized!). Risk factors for latex allergy are atopic diathesis, history of frequent surgical interventions, especially in the urogenital tract, spina bifida, and also other professions with increased rubber contact [39].

The latex milk from *Hevea brasiliensis* contains more than 12 molecularly characterized allergens, some of them involved in the typical property of elasticity of the product (rubber elongation factor). Attempts to produce allergen-free latex gloves of equal hygienic and surgical quality are continuing. Especially dangerous is the transport of the latex allergen from the glove into powder, which then is transported through the air (e.g., in operation theaters) and has led to fatal anaphylaxis in patients with previously undiagnosed latex allergy. Natural rubber-latex-free operation theaters and materials (intubation tubes, etc.) should be available [39].

References

1. Aalbersee RC (2000) Structural biology of allergens. J Allergy Clin Immunol 106:228–238
2. Baur X, Aschauer H, Dewair M, et al. (1982) Relationship between primary structures and allergenicity of asthma-inducing insect proteins (chironomid hemoglobins). Chest 82:254
3. Behrendt H, Becker WM (2001) Localization, release and bioavailability of pollen allergens: the influence of environmental factors. Curr Opin Immunol 13:709–715
4. Bergmann KC/Stiftung Deutscher Polleninformationsdienst (ed) (2001) Pollenbestimmungsbuch der Stiftung Deutscher Polleninformationsdienst. Takt, Paderborn
5. Bischoff E, Krause-Michel B, Nolte D (1986) Zur Bekämpfung der Hausstaubmilben in Haushalten von Patienten mit Milbenasthma. Allergologie 9:448–457
6. Breiteneder H, Ferreira F, Reikerstorfer A, et al. (1992) Complementary DNA cloning and expression in *Escherichia coli* of Aln g I, the major allergen in pollen of alder (*Alnus glutinosa*). J Allergy Clin Immunol 90:909–917
7. Celedon JC, Litonjua AA, Ryan L, Platts-Mills T, Weiss ST, Gold DR (2002) Exposure to cat allergen, maternal history of asthma and wheezing in first 5 years of life. Lancet 360:781–782
8. Bronswijk JEMH van (1972) Hausstaub-Ökosystem und Hausstaub-Allergen(e). Acta Allerg 27:219
9. Chapman MD, Smith AM, Vailes LD, Arruda LK (1997) Recombinant mite allergens. Allergy 52:374–379
10. Crameri R (1998) Recombinant *Aspergillus fumigatus* allergens: from the nucleotide sequences to

clinical applications. Int Arch Allergy Immunol 115:99–114
11. Custovic A, Simpson A, Chapman MD, Woodcock A (1998) Allergen avoidance in the treatment of asthma and atopic disorders. Thorax 53: 63–72
12. D'Amato G, Spieksma FTHM (1995) Aerobiologie and clinical aspects of mould allergy in Europe (position paper). Allergy 50:870–877
13. Ehnert B, Lau-Schadendorf S, Weber A, Buettner P, Schou C, Wahn U (1992) Reducing domestic exposure to dust mite allergen reduces bronchial hyperreactivity in sensitive children with asthma. J Allergy Clin Immunol 90:135–138
14. Eng PA, Wüthrich B (1994) Silkwaste – a further allergen in the bedroom. Schweiz Rundsch Med Prax 83:402–406
15. Fahlbusch B, Heinrich J, Gross I, Jäger L, Richter K, Wichmann HE (1999) Allergens in house-dust samples in Germany: results of an East-West German comparison. Allergy 54:1215–1222
16. Franz JT, et al. (1998) Domestic-Mite-Fauna auf Bauernhöfen in Deutschland. Allergologie 21: 371–380
17. Franz JT, Masuch G, Bergmann KC, Müsken H (2000) Entwicklung und Entwicklungsstadien der Milbe Glycyphagus domesticus (De Geer 1778). Allergologie 23:219–225
18. Grobe K, Becker WM, Schlaak M, Petersen A (1999) Grass group I allergens (beta-expansins) are novel, papain-related proteinases. Eur J Biochem 263:33–40
19. Fuchs E (1979) Allergische Atemwegsobstruktion (Allergisches Extrinsic Asthma bronchiale). In: Ulmer WT (ed) Bronchitis, Asthma, Emphysem. Springer, Berlin Heidelberg New York, p 543
20. Fuckerieder K (1976) Der Graspollengehalt der Luft in Mitteleuropa. Umweltbundesamt Berichte 9:1–85
21. Hart BJ (1998) Life cycle and reproduction of house-dust mites: environmental factors influencing mite population. Allergy 53 [Suppl 48]: 13–17
22. Hausen BM, Vieluf IK (1997) Allergiepflanzen – Pflanzenallergene. Ecomed, Landsberg
23. Helbing A, Gayer F, Pichler WJ, Brander KA (1998) Mushroom (Basidiomycete) allergy: diagnosis established by skin test and nasal challenge. J Allergy Clin Immunol 102:853–858
24. Hinze S, Bergmann KC, Lowenstein H, Hansen GN (1996) Differente Schwellenwertkonzentrationen durch das Rinderhaarallergen Bos d 2 bei atopischen und nichtatopischen Landwirten. Pneumologie 50:177–181
25. Hoppe A, Müsken H, Bergmann KC (1994) Häufigkeit allergischer Atemwegserkrankungen durch Katzenallergene bei Patienten mit und ohne Katzenhaltung. Allergo J 3:96–100
26. Horak F, Jäger S (1979) Die Erreger des Heufiebers. Urban & Schwarzenberg, Munich
27. Jorde W (1998) Schimmelpilzallergie. Dustri, Munich
28. Kersten W, Puls KE (1984) Pollenflugvorhersage. Allergologie 7:84–114
29. King TP, et al. (1999) Allergen nomenclature. IUIS/WHO Allergen Nomenclature Subcommittee. In: Turner MW, Natrig JB (eds) Immunology Nomenclature. Hogrefe & Huber, Seattle, pp 125–138
30. Knox RB (1993) Grass pollen, thunderstorms and asthma. Clin Exp Allergy 23:354–359
31. Köhn FM, Ollert M, Schuppe HC, Rakoski J, Schill WB, Ring J (2000) Spermaallergien. Reproduktionsmedizin 16:183–188
32. Kraft D, Sehon A (eds) (1993) Molecular biology and immunology of allergens. CRC Press, Boca Raton
33. Krempl-Lamprecht L (1981) Mykoallergosen durch spezielle Schimmelpilze. In: Borelli S, Düngemann H (eds) Fortschritte der Allergologie und Dermatologie. IMP, Basel, pp 344
34. Leuschner RM (1983) Pollenzählungen und Informationsdienst über Pollen und Pilzsporen der Luft. Schweiz Ärzteztg 64:1799–1804
35. Lind P (1985) Purification and partial characterization of two major allergens from the house dust mite Dermatophagoides pteronyssinus. J Allergy Clin Immunol 76:753–761
36. Partti-Pellinen K, Marttila O, Mäkinen-Kiljunen S, Haahtela T (2000) Occurrence of dog, cat, and mite allergens in public transport vehicles. Allergy 55:65–68
37. Petersen A, Grobe K, Lindner B, Schlaak M, Bekker WM (1997) Comparison of natural and recombinant isoforms of grass pollen allergens. Electrophoresis 18:819–825
38. Platt-Mills TA, Vaughan JW, Blumenthal K, Pollart Squillace S, Sporik RB (2001) Serum IgG and IgG4 antibodies to Fel d 1 among children exposed to 20 microg Fel d 1 at home: relevance of a nonallergic modified Th2 response. Int Arch Allergy Immunol 124:126–129
39. Przybilla B, et al. (1996) Zur gesundheitlichen Gefährdung durch die Allergie vom Soforttyp gegenüber Naturlatex. Positionspapier der Deutschen Gesellschaft für Allergologie und Klinische Immunologie. Allergo J 5:185–192
40. Rakoski J, Düngemann H (1981) Kreuzsensibilisierung durch Pollen. In: Borelli S, Düngemann H (eds) Fortschritte der Allergologie und Dermatologie. IMP Verlag, Neu-Isenburg, p 116
41. Reese G, Jeoung BJ, Daul CB, et al. (1997) Characterization of recombinant shrimp allergen Pen a 1 (tropomyosin). Int Arch Allergy Immunol 113: 240–242
42. Ring J, Krempl-Lamprecht L (1987) Aerogene Allergene. Erfassung und Identifizierung. MMW Münch Med Wochenschr 129:145–147
43. Rudolph R, Kunkel G, Blome B, et al. (1981) Zur Häufigkeit und klinischen Bedeutung von Allergien gegen Tierepithelien. Allergologie 4:230

44. Salvaggio J, Aukrust L (1981) Mould-induced asthma. J Allergy Clin Immunol 68:327–346
45. Scheiner O, Kraft D (1995) Basic and practical aspects of recombinant allergens. Allergy 50: 384–391
46. Schramm G, Petersen A, Bufe A, Schlaak M, Bekker WM (1996) Identification and characterization of the major allergens of velvet grass (*Holcus lanatus*), Hol l 1 and Hol l 5. Int Arch Allergy Immunol 110:354–363
47. Senti G, Leser C, Lundberg M, Wüthrich B (2000) Allergie asthma to shiitake and oyster mushroom. Allergy 55:975–976
48. Smith EG (1984) Sampling and identifying allergenic pollens and moulds. Blewstone, San Antonio
49. Solomon R, Mathews KP (1978) Aerobiology and inhalant allergens. In: Middleton E, et al. (eds) Allergy: Principles and practice. Mosby, St. Louis, pp 1143–1202
50. Sporik R, Holgate S, Platts-Mills TAE, Cogswell J (1990) Exposure to house-dust mite allergen (Der p 1) and the development of asthma in childhood. N Engl J Med 323:502–507
51. Stanley RG, Linskens HF (1985) Pollen. Biologie, Biochemie, Gewinnung und Verwendung. Urs Freund, Greifenberg
52. Stewart GA, McWilliam AS (2001) Endogenous function and biological significance of aeroallergens: an update. Curr Opin Allergy Clin Immunol 1:95–103
53. Stix E (1981) Pollenkalender: Regionale und jahreszeitliche Verbreitung von Pollen. Wissenschaftliche Verlagsgesellschaft, Stuttgart
54. Thiel C, Fuchs E (1981) Über korrelative Beziehungen bei Kräuterpollen- und Gewürzallergenen. RAST 3 Berichtsband. Grosse, Berlin, p 178
55. Tovey ER, Chapman MD, Platts-Mills TA (1981) Mite faeces are a major source of house dust allergens. Nature 289:592
56. Tovey ER, Johanson MC, Roche AL, Cobon GS, Baldo BA (1989) Cloning and sequencing of a cDNA expressing a recombinant house dust mite protein that binds human IgE and corresponds to an important low molecular weight allergen. J Exp Med 170:1457–1462
57. Tovey E, Marks G (1999) Methods and effectiveness of environmental control. J Allergy Clin Immunol 103:179–191
58. Valenta R, Ball T, Vrtala S, Duchene M, Kraft D, Scheiner O (1994) cDNA cloning and expression of timothy grass (*Phleum pratense*) pollen profilin in *Escherichia coli*: comparison with birch pollen profilin. Biochem Biophys Res Commun 199:106–118
59. van Hage-Hamsten M, Johansson E (1998) Clinical and immunological aspects of storage mite allergy. Allergy 53 [Suppl 48]:49–53
60. Vieluf D, Przybilla B, Baur X, Ring J (1993) Respiratory allergy and atopic eczema in a thatcher due to storage and house dust mite allergy. Allergy 48:212–214
61. Voorhorst R, Spieksma-Boezeman MIA, Spieksma FTM (1964) Is a mite (*Dermatophagoides* sp.) the producer of the housedust allergen? Allergie Asthma 10:329
62. Wachter R (1982) Pollen- und Sporenflug über der Bundesrepublik Deutschland. Allergopharma Joachim Ganzer, Reinbek, Schriftenreihe 14:147
63. Wahn U, Peters TP, Siraganian RP (1980) Studies on the allergenic significance and structure of rat serum albumin. J Immunol 125:2544
64. Weißenbach T, Wüthrich B, Weiher WH (1988) Labortier-Allergien. Eine epidemiologische, allergologische Studie bei Labortier-exponierten Personen. Schweiz Med Wschr 118:930–938
65. Wilken-Jensen K, Gravensen S (eds) (1984) Atlas of moulds in Europe causing respiratory allergy. ASK, Copenhagen
66. Witkin SS, Jeremias J, Ledger JA (1988) Localized vaginal allergic response in women with recurrent vaginitis. J Allergy Clin Immunol 81:412–416
67. Wüthrich B, Schmid-Grendelmeier P (1995) Nahrungsmittelallergien. Internist 36:1052–1062
68. Zielonka TM, Charpin D, Berbis P, Luciani P, Casanova D, Vervloet D (1994) Effects of castration and testosterone on Fel d 1 production by sebaceous glands of male cats: I – Immunological assessment. Clin Exp Allergy 24:1169–1173

4 Allergy Diagnosis

The diagnosis of allergy comprises four steps which supplement each other:

- History
- Skin tests
- In vitro allergy tests
- Provocation tests

History is the major basic requirement of allergy diagnosis and customarily yields – if done carefully – half of the diagnosis. Any test – this holds true for skin, in vitro and provocation tests – should only be performed after a careful history is taken. *Blind screening does not make sense!*

4.1 History

In many offices, questionnaires are used for allergy history; if correctly answered they can be helpful, but they can never replace a physician talking to the patient. Table 4.1 shows some rough criteria for a general "allergic versus non-allergic" classification. Of special importance in the allergy history is information on the circumstances of the complaint regarding locality and time (indoors, outdoors, spring, autumn, etc.). In pollinosis the period of complaints is important, and needs to be compared with the pollen count calendar. Perennial complaints may indicate indoor allergens (house-dust mites, molds, animal epithelia). The question regarding pets – including those kept by relatives – is obligatory as is family history and possible drug therapy. The taking of an allergy history requires great experience (Table 4.2). Often several visits are necessary (e.g., a young man with nickel allergy and eczema on the left thumb: the elicitor was his bicycle bell). A good allergist has to be like Sherlock Holmes – nothing is unimportant!

Allergen avoidance has a diagnostic and a therapeutic relevance at the same time. For the general and physical examination, we refer the reader to the special disease-related sections (Sects. 5.1–5.10).

Table 4.1. History parameters for and against the appearance of allergy

	Parameter	
	Allergy probable	Allergy unlikely
Onset	Youth	Elderly age
Family history	Positive	Negative
Specific elicitors	Detectable	Unknown
Fever	No	Yes
Improvement after change of milieu	Yes	No
Symptoms	Objective, reproducible	Only subjective, not reproducible

Table 4.2. Relevant questions for allergy history

Symptoms
- Onset (first occurrence, acute complaints)
- Duration
- Timely course (circadian, yearly rhythm)
- Intensity (severity)
- Frequency of relapses
- Response to therapy
- Deterioration through therapy
- Necessity of hospital admission

Other diseases
- Personal history (atopy)
- Family history (atopy)
- Other conditions (gastroesophageal reflux, skin or airway diseases, drug or food reactions)

Elicitors and situations
- Season of the year
- Local conditions (indoor, outdoor)
- Occupation
- Holiday, leisure
- Hobby
- Drugs
- Foods
- Exercise
- Stress, emotional burden
- Infectious disease
- UV radiation
- Hormonal situation (menstruation, pregnancy)

Living conditions
- Animal contact (also passive, "derivative")
- Tobacco smoke (active, passive)
- Housedust mite, mold exposure
- Chemicals
- Plants
- Cosmetics
- Sleeping dyspnea, snoring, mouth breathing

4.2 Skin Tests

Skin tests include epidermal (patch test, friction test) and percutaneous (prick, scratch, intradermal) test procedures.

4.2.1 Patch Test

Since the first description of a patch test by J. Jadassohn (1895) [29], the patch test has been used for the diagnosis of type IV reactions, mostly allergic contact dermatitis or exanthematous drug eruptions. It will be described in detail in Sect. 5.5 on "Eczema." But also for immediate-type reactions such as contact urticaria, the so-called open patch test has gained importance, which is read after 20 min [4, 35, 43]. The "atopy patch test" (APT) with IgE-inducing allergens allows the evaluation of the relevance of a sensitization (by the prick or RAST methods) for atopic eczema [15].

4.2.2 Friction Test

In highly sensitized individuals, the friction test can be recommended (e.g., with animal hair or drugs) [22, 27]. In the friction test, the native allergen is rubbed ten times over the skin of the volar forearm (controls with pads). After tape stripping (friction test with stripping), the reaction can be enhanced.

4.2.3 Prick Test

A drop of the allergen extract is applied to the skin, which then is briefly pricked using a lancet or a needle (there should be no bleeding!). After 15 min the test solution is wiped off and the reaction is read. New standardized needles allow a defined depth of penetration [18, 40].

4.2.4 Scratch Test

Here the skin is superficially scratched under allergenic material (in the case of powder together with some drops of physiological saline). The scratches are approximately 5 mm, and there should be no bleeding.

4.2.5 Intradermal Test

In this test, 0.02–0.05 ml of the allergen solution; commonly 1/100 of the prick test solution's concentration (though this does not hold for individual allergens!) – is injected strictly intradermally using a small syringe and needle. A small wheal (approx. 3 mm) will be observed. The interpretation of intradermal test reactions is difficult. Especially for mold, food, and drugs, false-positive reactions are common.

In the diagnosis of immunodeficiency (e.g., HIV and AIDS), the intradermal test with recall antigens has practical importance. The cellular immune reaction to neoantigens can be measured with DNCB (dinitrochlorbenzene) contact sensitization and the DNCB CAT (contact

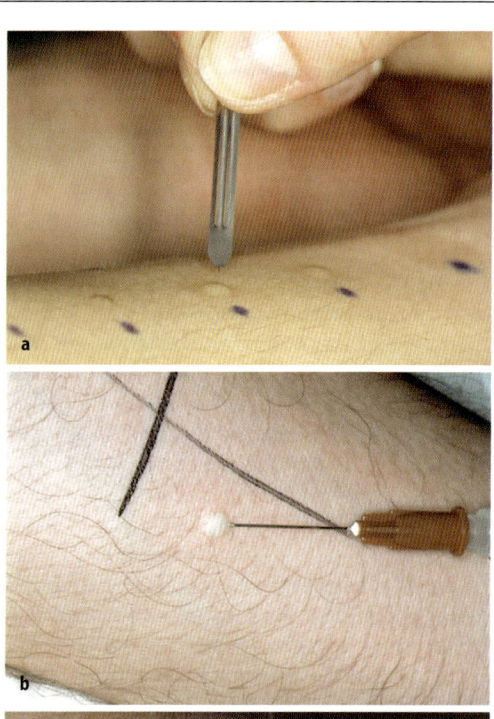
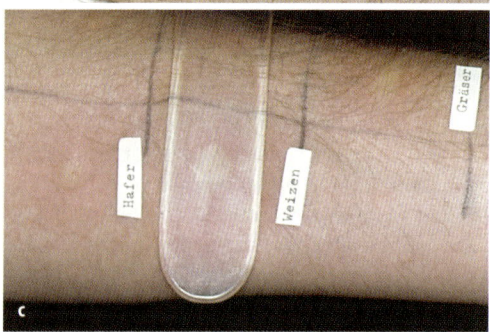
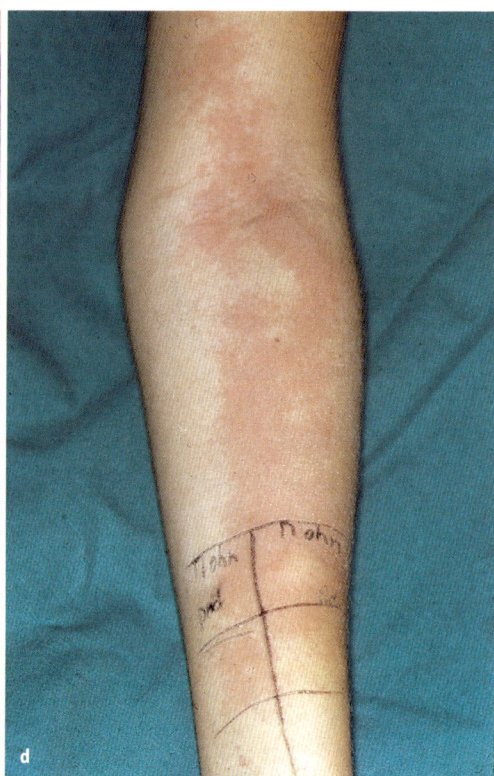

Fig. 4.1. a Prick test; **b** intradermal test; **c** positive prick test (expressible hive); **d** strongly positive intradermal test accompanied by allergic lymphangiitis in a patient with pollinosis

allergy time) determined [10]. Granulomatous reactions (type V) need up to 3 weeks to develop fully. While the Kveim (sarcoidosis) and Mitsuda tests (tuberculoid lepra) have a historical significance, this type of reaction is important prior to treatment with soluble bovine collagen (see Sect. 5.7).

In all the above-mentioned skin test procedures, adequate controls (positive with histamine or codeine, negative with saline or solvent) need to be performed. Figure 4.1 shows a positive skin prick test. The quantitative interpretation of skin test results uses a comparison with the histamine-induced wheal and flare reaction.

4.2.6 Complications

Complications can occur even in skin testing, either as hyperergic local reactions or as systemic reactions such as anaphylaxis or exacerbation of the underlying disease (asthma, eczema). Therefore, allergy tests should only be performed by experienced physicians trained for possible emergencies. Special caution has to be taken in patients with a history of anaphylaxis; we perform skin tests only under inpatient conditions when there is a history of grade III or IV anaphylaxis (see Sect. 5.1.4). Patients using beta-blockers – possibly also angiotensin-converting enzyme inhibitors – show an increased risk of anaphylaxis.

4.2.7 Reading of Skin Tests

The test reaction of percutaneous tests is evaluated using the diameter of the wheal and flare either according to an arbitrary scale from 0 to ++++ [18, 32] or in millimeters. For quantification of skin test results, the titration with different concentrations has given better results than the measurement of wheal and flare areas (Table 4.3). Flares under 3 mm in diameter as well as all reactions not significantly exceeding the negative control (saline) are negative. Wheals without flare under 3 mm diameter as well as flares without wheals under 5 mm are questionably positive and are not considered in allergy passports or for forensic questions. A repeat test at a later date can be considered.

In evaluation of immediate-type reactions, an additional reading after 6 and 24 h can give information on so-called "late cutaneous reactions" [17] (not to be confused with delayed-type reactions after 48 or 72 h = type IV), which are IgE mediated and occur after very intense immediate-type reactions, which sometimes show a biphasic course ("dual reactions"), reaching a maximum after 6–8 h. Arthus-type reactions (type III) caused by circulating immune complexes reach a maximum after 12–36 h.

Problems in test reading occur through false-positive or false-negative test reactions, e.g., through the use of irritating preparations, in patients with urticaria factitia (false positive) or when antigens are diluted too much, under the influence of drugs, in certain neurologic diseases or within too short an interval from an anaphylactic reaction (false negative) (Table 4.3).

At the time of allergy testing, there should be allergen avoidance if possible. During the pollen season or intense contact with pets, skin tests can induce an exacerbation of symptoms.

Skin reactions are subject to fluctuations in intensity according to age, sex, body surface area, season, and allergen exposure. This, however, does not play a major role in allergy practice if the test is otherwise well standardized.

4.2.8 Pharmacologic Influence

Drugs influencing immediate-type reactions comprise antihistamines, psychotropic drugs, and high-dose glucocorticosteroids. Theophylline, cyclooxygenase inhibitors and topical mast cell blockers (DNCG) do not influence immediate-type reactions (Table 4.4). In steroid-dependent asthmatics, cortisone should be reduced very slowly! In doubtful cases, one can perform a histamine prick test prior to a possible allergy skin test.

4.2.9 Special Skin Test Procedures

On the skin, physical tests are also performed, e.g., the diagnosis of physical urticaria using cold, warmth, pressure, or UV radiation (solar urticaria). UV tests are not only used in photoallergic diseases (photo patch test, photo prick test) but also in the diagnosis of certain UV-provoked dermatoses (see Sect. 5.6). Furthermore, skin tests not only give information about a specific sensitization, but also about unspecific parameters of skin function (barrier, irritability, delayed blanching reaction after acetylcholine, etc.); this is used in dermographism, nitrazine yellow test, determination of UV sensitivity (minimal erythema dosis), etc. Special problems of the patch test will be discussed in Sect. 5.5.2 on "Contact Dermatitis."

Table 4.3. Reasons for false-negative and false-positive skin test reactions

False-negative reactions
- Extract (too diluted, too weak, not soluble, wrong vehicle)
- Test procedure (depth of puncture, reading time)
- Test area (premedication, neuropathy)
- Systemic medication (antihistamines, etc.)
- Underlying disease (e.g., nervous disease)

False-positive reactions
- Extract (irritative, direct histamine release)
- Test procedure (irritative, no controls)
- Test area (inflamed skin, "angry back" patch test)
- Underlying disease (e.g., urticaria factitia)
- Artificial reaction (Munchhausen syndrome)

Medication	Application	Immediate reaction	Delayed reaction	Free interval necessary
Antihistamines	Systemic	+	–	5 days
	Topical	+	–	1 day
Antidepressives	Systemic	+	–	5 days
Beta-adrenergics	Systemic	+	–	1 day
	Topical	+	–	–
Theophylline	Systemic	–	–	–
Glucocorticosteroids				
Long-term high-dose	Systemic	+	+	3 weeks
Long-term <20 mg pred.	Systemic	±	+	3 weeks
Short-term high-dose	Systemic	±	+	1 week
Short-term <50 mg pred.	Systemic	±	–	3 days
Corticoids	Topical	±	±[a]	1 week
Cromoglycate	Topical	–	–	–
Cyclooxygenase inhibitors	Topical/systemic	–	–	–

Table 4.4. Inhibitory effect of certain drugs upon skin test results

[a] In the test site

4.3 In Vitro Allergy Tests

In vitro allergy diagnosis has an independent and equal place besides the three other pillars of allergy diagnosis [48]. In in vitro allergy investigations, there are separate tests for serologic and cellular diagnosis as well as for allergen-specific and non-specific parameters (markers of allergy or inflammation) (Table 4.5).

4.3.1 Serologic Methods

4.3.1.1 Total Serum IgE and Specific IgE Antibodies

The measurement of specific IgE antibodies can be regarded as the major advance achieved in allergy diagnosis in the last 50 years. Since the introduction of the radioallergosorbent test (RAST) [56], a multitude of procedures have

Table 4.5. In vitro allergy tests (LTT = lymphocyte transformation test)

Non-allergen-specific (general markers of allergy and inflammation)	
Serologic	**Cellular**
Total IgE	Blood count
Total Ig + subclasses	Lymphocyte subpopulations
Complement factors	Lymphocyte stimulation test (LTT) (mitogens)
Complement activity (CH50)	
Immune complexes	
Mediators in blood, tissue, and urine (histamine, methylhistamine, ECP, EPX, tryptase)	
Allergen-specific	
Serologic	**Cellular**
Specific IgE (e.g., RAST)	Histamine release
• Qualitatively (allergen mixtures, strip tests)	Basophil degranulation
• Semiquantitatively (e.g., RAST)	Basophil activation (CD63)
	Sulfido-leukotriene release (CAST)
	LTT (allergen)
Specific antibodies of other classes (type III)	
• Precipitation/immunodiffusion	
• Passive hemagglutination	
• RIA/EIA	
• Antibodies against specific proteins (immunoblot)	

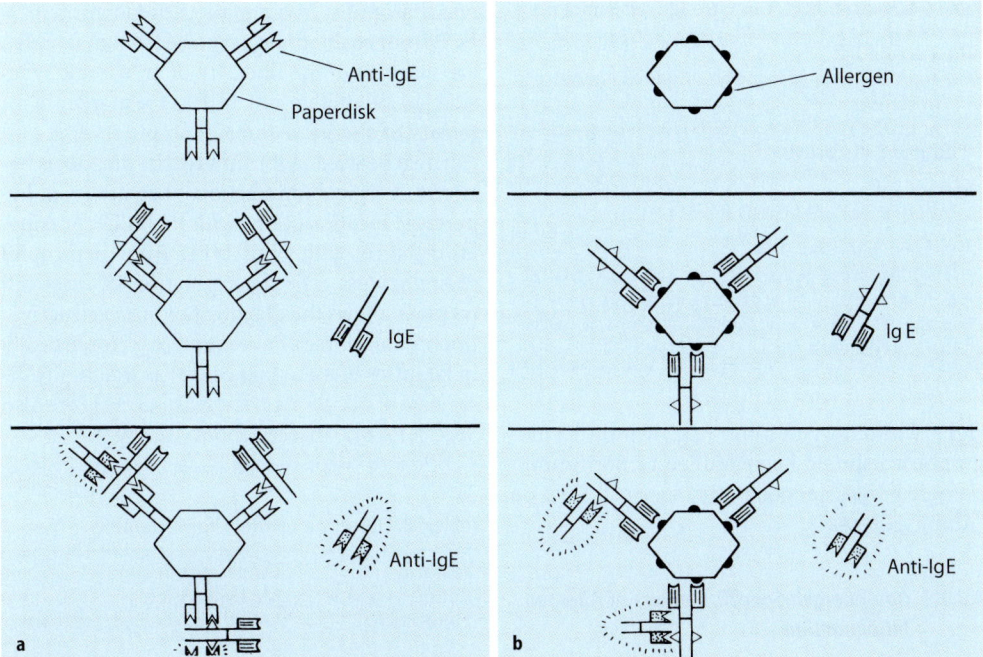

Fig. 4.2. a Schematic representation of the classic paper radioimmunosorbent test (PRIST). In this test anti-IgE is bound covalently to a paper disk (insoluble phase); **b** Schematic representation of the radioallergosorbent test (RAST)

been developed with the common principle that a bound allergen or an allergen-specific IgE antibody is recognized by a specific anti-IgE antibody. The differences consist of the separation of bound and free antibodies. Allergens are either coupled to an insoluble phase or separated in solution (e.g., after biotinylation). In the classic paper-radioimmunosorbent test (PRIST), anti-IgE is coupled covalently to a paper disk (Fig. 4.2a). IgE in the serum sample will bind and after careful washing will be recognized with a labeled (radioactive or enzyme) anti-IgE. The binding of labeled anti-IgE corresponds directly to the concentration of IgE in the serum [12, 20].

RAST differs from PRIST in that instead of anti-IgE a specific allergen is coupled to the solid phase (Fig. 4.2b).

Total serum IgE concentrations are measured in units (kU/l); 1 kU/l corresponds to the WHO standard of 2.47 ng/ml. Using standard curves with known IgE content, the IgE concentrations of samples can be measured in units (originally Phadebas-RAST-Units PRU). RAST results are commonly given semiquantitatively in classes: 0 = negative, 1 = weakly positive, 2–6 = positive in increasing intensity.

A negative RAST result does not necessarily rule out IgE-mediated sensitization. Specific IgE antibodies may be bound to mast cells in the skin or basophils in the blood (see "Skin Test," "Cellular Tests"). False-positive RAST results occur in patients with very high total serum IgE levels.

4.3.1.2 Identification of "Atopic Diathesis"

The determination of total serum IgE is indicated in certain diseases (Table 4.6). However, an "elevated IgE" does not necessarily mean "atopic diathesis"; it is also found in a variety of skin diseases (Table 4.7). Values above 400 kU/l, however, are characteristic of atopic or parasitic diseases. In the identification of "atopic diathesis," the determination of specific IgE antibodies against common environmental allergens (cat, mite, grass) in the RAST or the prick test is useful as are multiallergen disks (Phadiatop or sx1). Apart from IgE, the so-called "stigmata" of atopy representing characteristic dermatologic

Table 4.6. Indications for in vitro IgE determination

Total serum IgE
- Atopic diseases (prognosis, atopic diathesis)
- Parasitoses
- Parameters of TH2 reaction (lymphoma, autoimmune diseases)

Specific IgE
- Allergic (IgE-mediated) disease

Absolutely indicated in
- High degree of sensitization
- Life-threatening allergy (e.g., anaphylaxis)
- Impossibility of skin tests (skin lesions, medication, irritating agents)

signs without symptoms (e.g., white dermographism) should be examined as non-immunologic parameters of atopy (see Sect. 5.5.3 on "Atopic Eczema").

4.3.1.3 Non-allergen-Specific Markers of Allergen Inflammation

Apart from total serum IgE, mediators of allergy-relevant cells (histamine from mast cells and basophils, eosinophil cationic protein = ECP from eosinophils, tryptase from mast cells) are markers of the intensity of an allergic reaction [14, 30] (Table 4.8). ECP as the marker of intensity of allergic asthma or atopic eczema [30] can also be used in the differential diagnosis between allergic and infectious diseases (e.g., hyperergic local reactions with high ECP, erysipelas/cellulitis with high MPO from neutrophil granulocytes). The determination of mast cell tryptase allows the diagnosis of mast cell activation in the course of a reaction (e.g., forensically in fatalities of uncertain cause) as well as the diagnosis of occult mastocytosis [43, 51] (see also Sect. 5.1.6 on "Insect Venom Allergy").

Table 4.8. Detection methods for histamine

Bioassay	Guinea-pig ileum
Radioenzymatic	Methyltransferase
Fluorometric	O-Phthaldialdehyde, autoanalyzer
Immunoassay (RIA, EIA)	Methylhistamine, histamine

Table 4.7. Total serum IgE concentrations in various skin diseases (Xgeo = geometric mean, from [19])

Diagnosis	n	Total serum IgE (kU/l) X_{geo}	>100 kU/l (% of patients)
Atopic eczema	786	141.2	52
Bronchial asthma	72	138.7	56
Scabies	26	124.7	50
Allergic rhinitis	178	104.0	47
Ichthyosis vulgaris	11	100.7	27
Prurigo	24	100.5	46
Acute urticaria	78	95.5	47
Various immediate-type allergies	87	76.0	28
Dermatitis (not specified)	57	75.5	40
Insect venom allergy	281	74.8	39
Chronic urticaria	116	74.1	40
Allergic contact dermatitis	87	71.9	41
Physical urticaria	28	71.8	43
Nummular dermatitis	39	65.3	49
Atopic diathesis	667	57.4	34
Psoriasis	27	55.6	33
Scleroderma	11	49.5	36
Pyoderma	57	49.3	26
Mycosis fungoides, parapsoriasis	19	45.1	21
Conjunctivitis	28	40.4	21
Alopecia areata	61	38.1	20
Mollusca contagiosa	14	37.3	21
Mycosis	17	34.7	18
Melanocytic nevus	20	30.1	15
Malignant melanoma	60	27.4	13

Due to the short half-life, measurement of histamine only is useful during acute provocations; it can be supplemented by measuring metabolites (e.g., methylhistamine or EPX eosinophil protein X in the urine). EPX can also be measured in feces for diagnosis of intestinal allergy [36].

In the case of immune complex (type III) reactions, the detection of circulating immune complexes or complement activation (consumption of single components, split products, functional hemolytic activity CH50) needs to be performed.

4.3.1.4 Specific IgE Antibodies

The classic method of measuring specific antibodies is the radioallergosorbent test (RAST) [56]; this term is a brand name and at the same time represents a general term for the detection of specific IgE antibodies independent of the procedure. Most producers use cyanobromide-activated paper disks or polystyrene beads or sponges (CAP-RAST = capacity-RAST, Pharmacia) for the solid phase. The "Magic Lite" (ALK-Chiron, Bayer) and alaStat (DPC Biermann) systems use liquid allergens. Besides radioactive labeling, enzyme labeling using alkaline phosphatase, peroxidase, and β-galactosidase with and without biotinylation is common. The anti-IgE antibodies are mostly polyclonal from different species, but are also available as monoclonal (mouse).

Many manufacturers offer so-called multiallergen strips with several allergens coupled either to nitrocellulose giving a semiquantitative allergen-specific antibody pattern, e.g., Top-Screen (Biorad), Allergodip (Allergopharma), or to CLA (chemiluminescence allergy test) (Hitachi).

4.3.1.5 Immunoblot

While the above-mentioned procedures use allergen mixtures in soluble or coupled form, the specific reactivity of serum against single proteins within an allergen extract can be visualized after electrophoretic separation on nitrocellulose (Western blotting). In insect venom allergy, there is hope that in patients with a negative skin test and RAST, immunoblotting may be of diagnostic and prognostic relevance [39].

4.3.1.6 Detection of Other Antibody Classes

Allergen-specific antibodies of other immunoglobulin classes (IgM, IgG, and subclasses) may be measured with different techniques (e.g., precipitating antibodies, passive hemagglutination, RIA, EIA), but also with similar techniques as for IgE detection; because of the high background concentrations of unspecific antibodies, the main problem is finding the correct dilution.

IgG and IgM antibodies play a role in type III reactions (serum sickness, immune complex anaphylaxis, hypersensitivity pneumonitis); measuring specific IgG or IgG subclasses in food allergy has not yet shown convincing results [43]. Possibly, specific antibodies of the IgG4 class have relevance as markers during specific immunotherapy (e.g., in the ratio IgG4/IgE) [39]. Immunoblot procedures may prove more valuable here than classic RIA or EIA.

4.3.2 Cellular Tests

RAST can be negative in spite of a clear-cut history, especially when the allergic event has taken place some time previously. Then in vitro tests using cell suspensions are helpful for IgE-mediated reactions, especially the basophil leukocyte reaction.

The *in vitro histamine release* test has been proven valuable; it is, however, expensive in terms of laboratory requirements. Reactions can be performed with washed peripheral leukocytes, but also whole blood. The histamine release is measured in the supernatant using different methods (see Table 4.8) and expressed in relation to a 100% control (cell lysis by perchloric acid) as well as to the blank (spontaneous histamine release) as percentage histamine release. As positive control, cells are stimulated with anti-IgE, giving information on the non-immunologic parameter of "releasability" [13, 54].

Previously, the *basophil degranulation* test was performed using toluidine-blue staining, giving semiquantitative test results. A new procedure is the *basophil leukocyte activation* test, where the expression of surface markers CD63 or CD203c in flow cytometry is measured [19, 33, 49].

Besides the preformed mediator histamine, the newly synthesized sulfido-leukotrienes can be measured after allergen stimulation and adequate "priming" with interleukin-3 in the *cellular allergen stimulation test* (CAST) [16]. One problem is the lack of normal values for most allergens. Possibly, with CAST in vitro diagnosis of pseudo-allergic reactions (e.g., ASS idiosyncrasy) can be performed [16].

In the diagnosis of delayed-type reactions for scientific questions, the *lymphocyte transformation test* (LTT) may be used, and also as a lymphocyte stimulation test with the measurement of cytokines secreted (e.g., IL-5). In drug allergy, for certain questions the incubation of antigens with liver microsomes in order to produce relevant metabolites has been used successfully [37].

The high variability of the LTT and the lack of control values for most allergens need to be considered. In Germany, many patients come to the allergist with positive LTT results performed in laboratories of doubtful competence documenting an "allergy" against pollutants, chemicals or heavy metals. It should be known for instance that mercury itself is mitogenic leading to a positive LTT; therefore the LTT is not a suitable method for measuring mercury amalgam allergy.

4.3.3 In Vitro Detection of Allergens

With the principle of RAST, not only antibodies in the serum may be measured, but also allergens in a sample when defined antibodies are used. With the RAST inhibition assay, the potency of allergen extracts can be quantified. Using an ELISA procedure, one can directly measure allergens in dust samples (e.g., house-dust mite Der. p 1, cat, dog, cockroach allergens) [24]. This is a new dimension for allergy diagnosis. The detection of specific antibodies in humans against environmental agents is now supplemented by the specific detection of environmental allergy elicitors (allergens) through antibodies. Less specific but practical for patients to use themselves is the detection of the fecal mite product guanine (Acarex test) [9].

4.4 Provocation Tests

Strictly speaking, skin tests are also "provocation tests," namely provocation of the skin as the manifesting organ. In modern terminology, however, provocation test means the exposure of an organ involved with the respective allergen. The most important provocation tests in practice are [32, 43]:

- Conjunctival
- Nasal
- Bronchial
- Oral
- Parenteral (e.g., subcutaneous with local anesthetics) provocation.

Any provocation test should be performed under controlled and emergency conditions. Provocation tests involve a certain degree of risk for the patient!

Naturally occurring allergic reactions are imitated under control. Therefore, provocation tests should only be performed when indicated, in remission, and when other diagnostic parameters (history, skin test, in vitro test) have not given a clear-cut diagnosis.

In allergic bronchial asthma, the performance of bronchial provocation tests with acetylcholine or histamine belongs to the obligatory evaluation of lung function. Allergen provocation tests can only be done as confirmation tests; no large "test series" are possible [50].

4.4.1 Conjunctival Provocation Test

A drop of allergen solution (prick extract 1:10 or 1:100 diluted, according to degree of sensitization) is applied to the lateral conjunctiva. After 5–15 min, the reaction occurs as redness, itching, foreign body sensation, or massive edema (chemosis). When reactions develop very rapidly, the eye should be washed with saline and vasoconstrictive drops should be applied to stop the reaction [1, 7].

It is crucial that at the start a control test with a solvent solution is performed prior to the actual provocation, which is done with increasing allergen concentrations, changing from one eye to the other.

4.4.2 Nasal Provocation Test

For nasal provocation, after adaptation of the patients in the room and adequate controls, allergen solutions (or sprays or paper disks) [28] are applied under vision on the lower concha [2, 27]. The reaction is either evaluated by clinical inspection (rhinoscopy) or as sneezing, rhinorrhea, nasal obstruction, lacrimation, or in severe cases asthmoid complaints. In the nasal secretion, eosinophil leukocytes can be counted before and after provocation. The nasal provocation test should be quantified using rhinomanometry [3, 38, 46]. Using a pressure-volume diagram, the nasal obstruction can be measured as a decrease in air flow (Fig. 4.3). A decrease by more than 40% in comparison to the control is regarded as positive, whereas values of between 15% and 40% are questionable.

4.4.3 Bronchial Provocation Test

Lung function should be measured prior to any bronchial provocation. If lung function is decreased, bronchial provocation is contraindicated as in other severe diseases. See Sect. 5.1.2 for diagnosis of general asthma. Bronchial provocation tests should only be performed in patients under remission [25].

Allergen solutions are inhaled as aerosol (nebulization with a compressor, droplet size 1–4 µm, nebulization only during inspiration) after determination of the basic values. Allergen solutions commonly have a concentration similar to intradermal extracts (differences between manufacturers!). The concentration and the method of dose increase should be selected according to history and skin test reactivity.

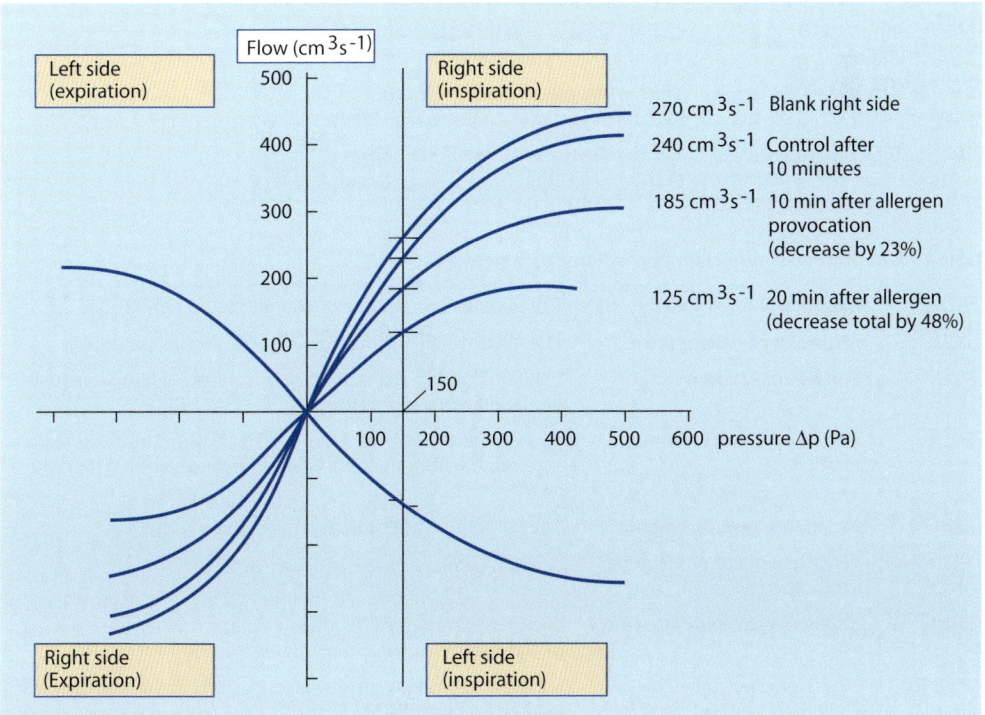

Fig. 4.3. Measurement protocol of a positive intranasal provocation test (standard representation) (from [2])

For measurement of bronchial reactivity, several methods are used [5, 20, 21, 50]:

- Pneumometry
- Spirometry
- Oscillatory airway resistance
- Flow volume diagrams
- Body plethysmography

The following parameters of airway function (Tables 4.9, 4.10) are important in the evaluation of provocation tests:

Peak expiratory flow (= PEF) can be measured by the patient regularly over certain periods.

Forced expiratory volume in the first second (FEV 1) (= Tiffeneau test) requires active cooperation from the patient. Sometimes forced breathing triggers bronchial constriction.

Modern techniques measure the *airway resistance* with body plethysmography or oscillatory methods [25]. These procedures can be performed under normal breathing conditions and also in children. Figure 4.4 shows typical curves distinguishing between obstructive and restrictive ventilation disturbance. The bronchial provocation test is regarded as positive if FEV1 drops by 15% or specific airway resistance increases by 50% and above 2 kPa s/l [25].

Table 4.9. Definition of relevant parameters in body plethysmography

RAW	Airway resistance	Defined as pressure necessary to reach a certain ventilatory flow (kPa/[l/s]). The airway resistance is a parameter for the diameter of airways
GAW	Airway conductance (*Gleitwert* airways)	
sRAW	Specific airway resistance	Product of airway resistance and intrathoracic gas volume (RAW × ITGV)
ITGV	Intrathoracic gas volume	The air volume present in the thorax at the end of a normal expiration
RV	Residual volume	The air volume present in the thorax after maximal expiration (RV = ITGV−ERV)
TCL	Total lung capacity	The maximal air volume in the thorax (TLC = VC + RV)

Table 4.10. Definition of important flow-volume parameters

VCEX	Expiratory vital capacity	The maximal air volume of complete slow expiration
VCIN	Inspiratory vital capacity	The maximal air volume of complete slow inspiration
FVC	Forced vital capacity	The most rapidly expired air volume after maximal inspiration and forced expiration
FEV1	Forced expiratory volume after 1 s	The air volume expired after maximal inspiration and forced expiration within the first second (also called the Tiffeneau test)
ERV	Expiratory reserve volume	The air volume after maximal slow expiration
FEV1%VC	FEV1 in percent of maximal vital capacity	Relative FEV1
PEF	Maximal peak expiratory flow	Maximal expiratory flow rate or the maximal airflow during forced expiration after maximal inspiration
MEF 75, 50, 25	Maximal expiratory flow at 75%, 50%, 25% of VCMAX or FVC	Maximal expiratory airflow at 75%, 50% or 25% of the expired volume (VCMAX or FVC)

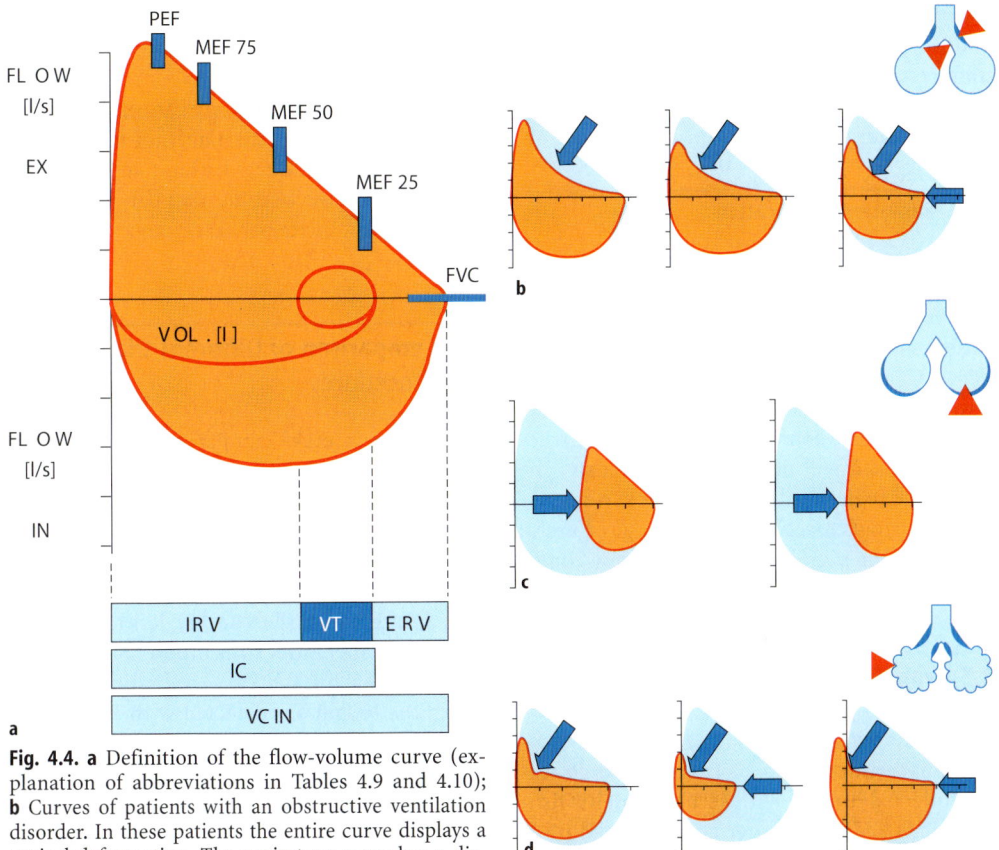

Fig. 4.4. a Definition of the flow-volume curve (explanation of abbreviations in Tables 4.9 and 4.10); **b** Curves of patients with an obstructive ventilation disorder. In these patients the entire curve displays a typical deformation. The expiratory curve has a distinctly concave form representing the decrease in expiratory flow over the entire expiration range. The degree of deformation is a measure of the severity of the disease; **c** Curves of patients with a restrictive ventilation disorder. In these patients the form of the curve is intact for the most part; however, the vital capacities (VC) and maximum expiratory flows (MEF) are distinctly reduced; **d** Curves in patients with pulmonary emphysema. These curves are similar to those obtained from patients with a respiratory tract obstruction; however, the changes are usually even more pronounced. The "emphysema kink" is typical here. In unclear cases a secure diagnosis cannot be made without body plethysmographic measurements. Residual volume (RV), intrathoracic gas volume (ITGV) and total lung capacity (TLQ) are elevated (distended lung)

4.4.4 Oral Provocation Test

Oral provocation tests [8, 47] are used in the diagnosis of food and drug reactions, urticaria, as well as pseudo-allergic reactions against additives. The suspected agent is swallowed by the patient with water. The dose depends on the severity of the allergic condition in the history (in anaphylaxis 1/100 to 1/1,000 of the eliciting dose) and increased at 2-h intervals. The patient is observed carefully. Pulse and blood pressure are regularly checked. In strongly positive reactions (blood pressure change, tachycardia, urticaria, or other signs of anaphylaxis), immediate therapy should be started (see Sect. 5.1.5 on "Anaphylaxis").

Oral provocation tests should be blinded, at least single blind, in order to rule out psychological influences. As a placebo, talcum, mannitol in capsules or blinding of food with colored substances [8] is recommended.

For scientific questions and in special cases, double-blind placebo-controlled food challenge (DBPCFC) is the method of choice. In specific cases, the reaction of the gastric or intestinal mucosa can be evaluated by X-ray or endoscopically using intragastral provocation under endoscopic control (IPEC) [45] or colonic allergen provocation (COLAP) after intramucosal allergen injection.

4.4.5 Parenteral Provocation

In the diagnosis of local anesthetics reactions, subcutaneous provocation testing is used (see Sect. 5.7). Intramuscular or intravenous provocation should only be used for scientific purposes. Controlled insect sting challenge is discussed in Sect. 5.1.6. Oral and parenteral provocations involve some risk. Normally, the reaction provoked will not exceed in intensity the reaction experienced in the history. However, anaphylactoid reactions may occur. Careful control of the patient under emergency conditions is required.

4.5 Transfer Tests

In 1921, Carl Prausnitz showed that the allergy-relevant serum factor was transferable: Prausnitz injected himself with serum from his fish-allergic colleague Küstner and observed positive skin reactions after local allergen application. This procedure, the "Prausnitz-Küstner test," corresponds to passive cutaneous anaphylaxis (PCA) in contrast to the active reaction in the classic skin test (see Sect. 2). For decades, this test was the only possible method of detecting reaginic (IgE) antibodies. Because of the risk of infectious diseases, the Prausnitz-Küstner test is no longer used as a routine method. The PCA in primates is possible but only in certain centers (for a description of the method, see Stanworth [52]).

4.6 Unconventional Methods in Allergy Diagnosis

Unfortunately, in allergology not only in therapy but also in diagnosis a multitude of so-called "alternative" procedures without any scientific background have become popular, which are confusing for patients and physicians (see Sect. 6.4).

4.7 Comparison of Different Diagnostic Procedures

Attempting to make comparisons between the different test procedures (skin test, provocation, RAST, or histamine release) and judging them as "better" or "worse" will be a fruitless task: It should be remembered that different parameters of the allergic reactions are measured with different tests (Table 4.11). It is logical that the correlation between the different test results can never reach 100% [5]. Antibodies circulating in the serum are detected with RAST. The reactivity of the mediator-secreting cell is best reflected by cellular tests such as the in vitro histamine release tests or CAST. At the affected organ, provocation tests are most useful. IgE bound to mast cells in the skin is detected by skin tests. Provocation tests are also not the absolute "gold standard"; both false-positive and false-negative provocation tests occur!

The critical evaluation of history, skin test, and in vitro tests can often save the patient from having to undergo a provocation test (Table 4.12). Out of all the diagnostic procedures used, skin tests represent the most practical method. Compared to RAST, skin test reactions stay positive over a longer period of time after allergen contact. In an overview of all the procedures, the predominant place of history is evident (Fig. 4.5).

Table 4.11. Comparison of different allergy test procedures

Information on	Skin test	Provocation	RAST	Cellular test (e.g., histamine release)
Serum antibodies	0	0	+	0
Mediator-secreting cells	±	±	0	+
Affected organ	±	+	0	0

Table 4.12. Allergy diagnosis (scoring system for indication of allergen provocation) (example) (according to Foucard et al. [20]). If score >5 points, provocation tests are usually not necessary (example)

Score (points)	History + symptoms	Skin test	RAST (class)	Total
0	0[a]	0	0	0
1	Possible	+	1	
2	Probable	+/++	2	
3	Clear-cut	+++/++++	3–6	
Sum	1	2	3	6

[a] No information or unlikely

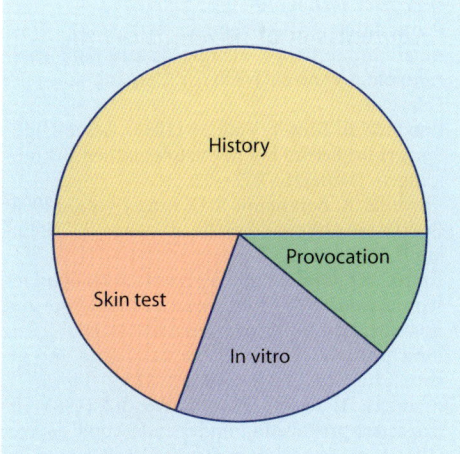

Fig. 4.5. Importance of the various methods used for allergy diagnostics

References

1. Abelson MB, Chambers WA, Smith LM (1990) Conjunctival allergen challenge. A clinical approach to studying allergic conjunctivitis. Arch Ophthalmol 108:84–88
2. Bachert C, Berdel D, Enzmann H, Fuchs E, Gonsior E, Hofmann D, et al. (1990) Richtlinien für die Durchführung von nasalen Provokationstests mit Allergenen bei Erkrankungen der oberen Luftwege. Allergologie 2:53–55
3. Bachmann W (1982) Die Funktionsdiagnostik der behinderten Nasenatmung. Einführung in die Rhinomanometrie. Springer, Berlin Heidelberg New York
4. Bandmann H-J, Fregert S (1982) Epikutantestung, 2nd edn. Springer, Berlin Heidelberg New York
5. Baur X, Fruhmann G, Liebe V v (1978) Allergologische Untersuchungsmethoden (inhalativer Provokationstest, Hauttest, RAST) für die Diagnose des Asthma bronchiale. Klin Wochenschr 56:1205
6. Becker WM, et al. (2004) In vitro Allergie-Diagnostik. DGAI-Positionspapier. Allergo J (in press)
7. Bergmann K-C, Müsken H (1993) Durchführung und Bewertung des konjunktivalen Allergentests. Allergo J 3:274–276
8. Bindslev-Jensen C (2001) Standardization of double-blind, placebo-controlled food challenges. Allergy 56 Suppl 67:75–77
9. Bischoff E, Schirmacher W (1984) Farbnachweis für allergenhaltigen Hausstaub. 1. Mitteilung. Allergologie 7:446–449
10. Burg G, Przybilla B, Bogner J (1986) Contact-allergy time. In: Ring J, Burg G (eds) New trends in allergy II. Springer, Berlin Heidelberg New York, pp 230–239
11. Brockow K, Vieluf D, Pitschel K, Grosch J, Ring J (1999) Increased postmortem serum mast cell tryptase in a fatal anaphylactoid reaction to nonionic radiocontrast medium. J Allergy Clin Immunol 104:237–238
12. Ceska M, Lundkvist U (1972) A new and simple radioimmunoassay method for the determination of IgE. Immunochemistry 9:1021–1030
13. Conroy MC (1981) Releasability – a new dimension in basophil and mast cell reactivity. In: Ring J, Burg G (eds) New trends in allergy. Springer, Berlin Heidelberg New York, p 40
14. Czech W, Krutmann J, Schöpf E, Kapp A (1992) Serum eosinophil cationic protein (ECP) is a sensitive measure for disease activity in atopic dermatitis. Br J Dermatol 126:351–355
15. Darsow U, Vieluf D, Ring J (1995) Atopy patch test with different vehicles and allergen concentrations: An approach to standardization. J Allergy Clin Immunol 95:677–684
16. De Weck AL (1993) Cellular allergen stimulation test (CAST): A new dimension in allergy diagnosis. ACI News 1/5:9–14
17. Dorsch W, Ring J (1981) Induction of late cutaneous reactions (LCR) by skin blister fluid (SBF) from allergen-tested and normal skin. J Allergy Clin Immunol 67:117–125
18. Dreborg S, Frew A (eds) (1993) Allergen standardization and skin tests. Position Papers Allergy 48 [Suppl]:48–82
19. Eberlein-König B, Rakoski J, Behrendt H, Ring J (2004) Usefulness of CD63 expression as marker of basophil activation in difficult cases of insect venom allergy. Allergy (in press)
20. Foucard T, Johansson SGO, Bennich H, Berg T (1972) In vitro estimation of allergens by RAST

using human IgE antibodies. Int Arch Allergy Appl Immunol 43:360
21. Fuchs E, Thiel Cl (1979) Zur Durchführung von inhalativen Provokationsproben mit Allergenen. Allergologie 2:38
22. Fuchs E, Gronemeyer W, Bandilla K (1981) Reibtest und Tierhaarallergie, zugleich ein klinischer Beitrag "Zum Problem der Rasse-Spezifität". Allergologie 4:241–248
23. Fuchs T, Gutsgesell C (2000) Epikutantest. In: Praktische Allergologische Diagnostik. Steinkopff, Darmstadt, pp 23–39
24. Gleich GJ, Yunginger JW (1981) Variations of the radioallergosorbent test for measurement of IgE antibody levels, allergens and blocking antibody activity. In: Ring J, Burg G (eds) New trends in allergy. Springer, Berlin Heidelberg New York, p 98
25. Gonsior E, Henzgen M, Jörres RF, Kroidl RF, Merget R, Riffelmann FW, Wallenstein GW (2001) Leitlinie für die Durchführung bronchialer Provokationstests mit Allergenen. Deutsche Ges. für Allergologie und klinische Immunologie. Allergo J 10:193–199, 257–264
26. Gronemeyer W, Fuchs E (1959) Der inhalative Antigen-Pneumometrie-Test als Standard-Methode in der Diagnose allergischer Krankheiten. Int Arch Allergy 14:217–240
27. Gronemeyer W, Debelic M (1967) Der sog. Reibtest, seine Anwendung und klinische Bedeutung. Dermatologica (Basel) 134:208
28. Hauswald B, Langbein A, Neumeister V, Hüttenbrink KB (1998) Der Nasale Applikator-Test (NAPT) – ein neues Verfahren zur Allergiediagnostik. Allergo J 7:143–147
29. Jadassohn J (1896) Zur Kenntnisse der Arzneiexantheme. Arch Derm Syph 34:103 Bericht V. Kongreß D. derm. Ges., Graz, 23–25 September 1895
30. Jakob T, Hermann K, Ring J (1990) Eosinophil cationic protein in atopic exzema. Arch Dermatol Res 283:5–6
31. Lichtenstein LM, Osler AG (1964) Studies on the mechanism of hypersensitivity phenomena. IX. Histamine release from human leukocytes by ragweed pollen allergen. J Exp Med 120:507
32. Kemp SF, Lockey R (eds) (1999) Diagnostic methods in allergy. CRC Press, Boca Raton
33. Knol EF, Mul FPJ, Jansen H, Calafat J, Roos D (1991) Monitoring human basophil activation via CD63 monoclonal antibody 435. J Allergy Clin Immunol:328–338
34. Lockey RF, Benedict LM, Turkeltaub PC, Bukantz SC (1987) Fatalities from immunotherapy and skin testing. J Allergy Clin Immunol 79:660–677
35. Maibach HI, Johnson H (1975) Contact urticaria syndrome. Arch Dermatol 111:726
36. Majamaa H, Laine S, Miettinen A (1999) Eosinophil protein X and eosinophil cationic protein as indicators of intestinal inflammation in infants with atopic eczema and food allergy. Clin Exp Allergy 29:1502–1506
37. Merk H (1989) Arzneimittelallergie: Einfluß des Fremdstoffmetabolismus. Allergologie 12:171–173
38. Ohnsorge P, Schmid W (1980) Ein neues Rhinomanometer zur rhinomanometrisch kontrollierten intranasalen Provokationstestung mit Allergenen. Allergologie 3:113
39. Ollert M, Ring J (1999) Prognostische Bedeutung von Immunoblot-Untersuchungen bei Hymenopterengift-Allergie. Allergologia 22 (Suppl 2): 78–79
40. Østerballe O, Weeke B (1979) A new lancet for skin prick testing. Allergy 34:209–212
41. Platts Mills TAE, Chapman MD (1987) Dust mites: Immunology, allergic disease, and environmental control. J Allergy Clin Immunol 80: 755–774
42. Przybilla B, Ring J, Völk M (1986) Gesamt-IgE-Spiegel im Serum bei dermatologischen Erkrankungen. Hautarzt 37:77–82
43. Przybilla B, Bergmann K-C, Ring J (eds) (2000) Praktische Allergologische Diagnostik. Steinkopff, Darmstadt
44. Rasp G, Thomas PA, Bujia J (1994) Eosinophil inflammation of the nasal mucosa in allergic and non-allergic rhinitis measured by eosinophil cationic protein levels in native nasal fluid and serum. Clin Exp Allergy 24:1151–1156
45. Reimann HJ, Ring J, Ultsch B, Wendt P (1985) Intragastral provocation under endoscopic control (IPEC) in food allergy: mast cell and histamine changes in gastric mucosa. Clin Allergy 15: 195–202
46. Riechelmann H, Klimek L, Mann W (1995) Objective measures of nasal function. Curr Opin Otolaryngol Head Neck Surg 3:207–213
47. Ring J (1987) Diagnostik von Arzneimittel-bedingten Unverträglichkeitsreaktionen. Hautarzt 38:516–522
48. Ring J (1981) Diagnostic methods in allergy. Behring Inst Mitt 68:141–152
49. Sanz ML, Maselli JP, Gamboa PM, Oehling A, Dieguez I, de Weck AL (2002) Flow cytometric basophil activation test: a review. J Invest Allergol Clin Immunol 12:143–154
50. Schultze-Werninghaus G, Merget R (2000) Asthma bronchiale. In: Praktische Allergologische Diagnostik. Steinkopff, Darmstadt, pp 165–182
51. Schwartz LB, Sakai K, Bradford TR, Ren SL, Zweiman B, Worobec AS, Metcalfe DD (1995) The alpha form of human tryptase is the predominant type present in blood at baseline in normal subjects and is elevated in those with systemic mastocytosis. J Clin Invest 96:2702–2710
52. Stanworth DR (1973) Immediate hypersensitivity. The molecular basis of the allergic response. North Holland, Amsterdam
53. Tovey ER, Chapman MD, Platts-Mills TAE (1981) Mite feces are a major source of house dust allergens. Nature 290:592–593

54. Wahn U (1980) Möglichkeiten und Grenzen der allergeninduzierten Histaminfreisetzung aus Leukozyten als in-vitro-Technik für die Allergologie. Allergologie 3:364
55. Wheeler AW, Jessberger B, Drachenberg KJ, Rakoski J (1996) Design of an optimally-diagnostic skin test solution for diagnosis of sensitivity to timothy grass (*Phleum pratense*) pollen. Clin Exp Allergy 26:897–902
56. Wide L, Bennich H, Johansson SGO (1967) Diagnosis of allergy by an in vitro test for allergen antibodies. Lancet 2:1105–1109
57. Wüthrich B, Wyss S (1979) IgE-Serumspiegel-Bestimmung: RIST oder PRIST? Ergebnisse eines Ring-Versuchs in der Schweiz. Schweiz Med Wochenschr 109:315

5 Allergic Diseases (and Differential Diagnoses)

5.1 Diseases with Possible IgE Involvement ("Immediate-Type Allergies")

There are many allergic diseases manifesting in different organs and on the basis of different pathomechanisms (see Sect. 1.3). The most common allergies develop via IgE antibodies and manifest within minutes to hours after allergen contact ("immediate-type reactions"). Not infrequently, there are biphasic (dual) reaction patterns when after a strong immediate reaction in the course of 6–12 h a renewed hypersensitivity reaction (late-phase reaction, LPR) occurs which is triggered by IgE, but amplified by recruitment of additional cells and mediators. These LPRs have to be distinguished from classic delayed-type hypersensitivity (DTH) reactions (type IV reactions) (see Sect. 5.5).

What may be confusing for the inexperienced physician is familiar to the allergist: The same symptoms of immediate-type reactions are observed without immune phenomena (skin tests or IgE antibodies) being detectable. These reactions are called "pseudo-allergic reactions" (PARs), the term "pseudo" only reflecting the not detectable participation of the immune system and not implying "psychological" phenomena. People can die from pseudo-allergic reactions! The term is negatively defined; with better techniques allowing the detection of antibodies or sensitized cells, PAR may turn into true allergy. IgE-mediated drug allergies will be covered together with other adverse drug reactions (see Sect. 5.7).

In atopic eczema, IgE antibodies play a role in many patients in the eliciting phase, albeit in close connection with T-cell-mediated reactions (combination of type I and type IV b reactions). Atopic eczema will be discussed in a separate section (see Sect. 5.5.3).

The maximal manifestation of IgE-mediated immediate-type allergic reaction is anaphylaxis. In the development of clinical symptoms, different organs may be involved and symptoms of well-known allergic diseases of skin and mucous membranes [also called "shock fragments" (Karl Hansen)] may occur according to the severity (see Sect. 5.1.4).

5.1.1 Allergic Rhinitis

5.1.1.1 Introduction

Apart from being an aesthetic organ, the nose has several very interesting functions (Table 5.1). It is true that people can live without breathing through the nose, but disturbance of this function can lead to disease. Here we are interested mostly in defense functions against particles and irritants (physical or chemical) with clinical symptoms occurring physiologically under certain conditions (e.g., secretion, sneezing, obstruction) and which can take on the characteristics of disease in intense or chronic expression [10, 12]. For these complaints, the term "rhinitis" has been accepted internationally, although the demonstration of

Table 5.1. Functions of the nose

• Airway	• Warming of air
• Olfactory sensory organ	• Air-conditioner
• Filter organ	• Body of voice resonance
• Humidifier	• Killing of microbes

inflammation cannot be done in each case. Therefore, "rhinopathy" would be a more logical term, although it is not often used [3, 4, 10]. Normal findings and disease conditions overlap in rhinitis much more often than in asthma. Often the conjunctiva is also affected ("rhinoconjunctivitis") (see Sect. 5.1.7 on "Allergy and Eye").

The most common form of allergic rhinitis and the most frequent atopic disease is pollinosis (pollen rhinitis, pollen conjunctivitis, pollen asthma, hay fever, hay asthma, hay rhinitis) [19].

The disease was known in Arabic medicine and in the late middle ages it was known as rose fever. The first scientific description dates back to 1819 when John Bostock described his own symptoms. He saw the high summer temperature as being the cause although many people called the disease "hay fever." It was not until 1873 that Charles Blackley, using a skin and provocation test, proved the disease was caused by pollen. Wolff-Eisner classified the disease in 1906 as being hypersensitivity against pollen protein (the term "allergy" had only just been introduced) (for literature see Chap. 1).

5.1.1.2 Symptoms and Pathophysiology

In industrialized countries, 10–20% of the population suffer from pollinosis [21]. As first symptoms of allergic rhinitis, sneezing (1–2 min after allergen contact) and early secretion (5 min) develop triggered by a reflex mechanism. In parallel, edema (obstruction) of the mucosa occurs, reaching a maximum after 30 min with itch, a "nasal voice," disturbance of olfactory and gustatory sensation, sinus complaints, and formation of polyps in the chronic course as products of hyperplastic rhinosinusitis [4, 7, 10, 12].

Aqueous rhinorrhea is due to a cholinergic reflex (possibly via tachykinins) while the symptom of a "blocked nose" is due to vascular dilatation and edema formation.

Among the numerous mediators of allergic reactions, histamine plays the most important role in nasal symptoms, but also other mediators have been found in nasal secretions after allergen provocation such as kinins, eicosanoids, and proteases [1].

The following mechanisms contribute to the development of nasal hyperreactivity:

- Increase in permeability
- Increase in sensitivity of irritant receptors
- Increase in number of receptors per cell surface
- Change of nerval impulses in the CNS
- Increase in number of inflammatory cells
- Increase in function of effector cells (increased releasability)
- Hormonal influences (estrogens?)

Increased mast cells and basophil leukocytes (especially during late phase reactions) have been found in the nasal smear in allergic rhinitis [9].

Clinical stigmata of patients with allergic rhinitis comprise:

- "Adenoid face"
- Permanent mouth breathing
- Periorbital halo ("allergic shiners")
- Lower lid edema
- "Allergic greeting" (frequent wiping of the nose tip) (Fig. 5.1)
- Lateral fold in the lower nasal part

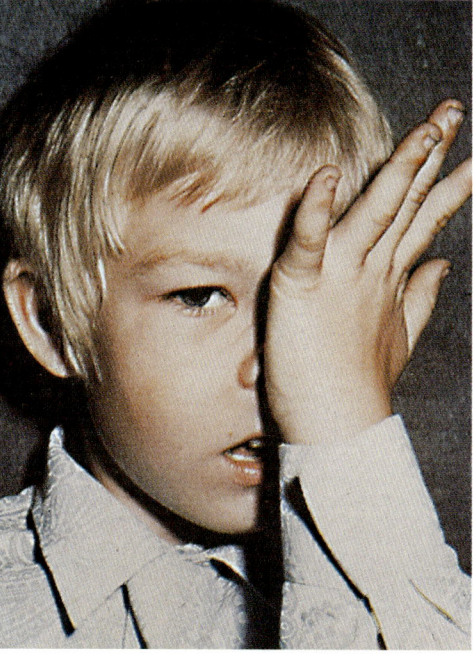

Fig. 5.1. "Allergic salutation" seen typically in children with allergic rhinitis (H. Behrendt)

5.1.1.3 Classification of Different Forms of Rhinitis

In patients with symptoms of rhinitis (itch, sneezing, secretion, obstruction), other causes of impaired nasal ventilation have to be excluded such as mechanical obstruction, structural abnormalities, septum deviation, tumors, foreign bodies, atresia, as well as other severe organ diseases (cystic fibrosis, Wegener's granulomatosis, lepra, or infectious diseases) [6, 19] (Table 5.2).

For the diagnosis of "infectious rhinitis," usually no detection of an infectious agent is required. Normally, the diagnosis is done according to the type of secretion (putrid, milky) and the rhinoscopic finding. With unilateral symptoms, hemorrhagic secretion and painfulness, rhinoscopy is obligatory. If the secretion is clear or aqueous, further classification into "allergic" and "non-allergic" (also called "vasomotor") rhinitis is done (Fig. 5.2).

While previously allergic rhinitis was classified into seasonal (hay fever) in the spring and summer months and perennial (all year), the new WHO classification in the document *Allergic Rhinitis and Its Impact on Asthma (ARIA)* recommends a new classification into "intermittent" (duration of symptoms of less than 4 weeks) and "persistent" (symptoms longer than 4 weeks). This new classification, however, does not replace the practically important distinction between seasonal and perennial.

Furthermore, the classification of the severity of allergic rhinitis into "mild," "moderate," and "severe" is important. Symptoms like "sleep disturbance," "impairment of daily activities," "impairment in school or working place," as well as other impairments in the quality of life are important.

Regarding therapy of allergic rhinitis, it is important to know that some symptoms such as itching, secretion, and sneezing respond quite well to antihistamines, while nasal obstruction is best treated with corticosteroids. This is reflected in the guidelines for therapy of allergic rhinitis [6].

While seasonal allergic rhinitis can mostly be diagnosed with classical allergy diagnosis, in perennial rhinitis sometimes overlaps between allergic (housedust mite allergy) and

Table 5.2. Classification of rhinitis (according to WHO)

Infectious
- Viral
- Bacterial
- Others

Allergic
- Intermittent
- Persistent

Occupational (allergic, non-allergic)
- Intermittent
- Persistent

Drug-induced
- Acetylsalicylic acid
- Others

Hormonal

Others
- NARES (non-allergic rhinitis eosinophilia syndrome)
- Irritants
- Gustatorial rhinitis
- Emotional factors
- Atrophic rhinitis
- Gastrointestinal reflux
- Idiopathic

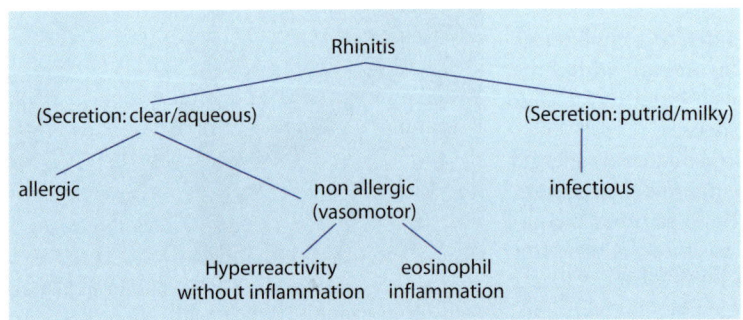

Fig. 5.2. Breakdown of rhinitis into its various forms

non-allergic mechanisms are observed. All forms of rhinitis have in common a hyperreactivity of the nasal mucosa similar to bronchial hyperreactivity in asthma.

In the group of non-allergic vasomotor rhinitis, two forms may be distinguished according to nasal cytology: an inflammatory form with increased eosinophil granulocytes and the non-inflammatory form. The form of vasomotor rhinitis with increased eosinophils is often characterized by strong swelling, formation of polyps and concomitant acetylsalicylic acid [10]. It responds better to antihistamines and glucocorticosteroids than the non-inflammatory form, which is very resistant to therapy and may respond to anticholinergics (ipratropium bromide).

Patients with vasomotor rhinitis show an increased reactivity to unspecific irritants (Table 5.3) with a pathophysiologic correlate of "autonomic nervous system dysregulation" corresponding possibly to an extreme variant of physiologic reactivity [2, 10, 14]. Dryness (draughts of air, cold air, dust) is a common triggering factor.

The relationship between allergic rhinitis and otitis media has been discussed. It seems that with atopics there is an increased risk of serous otitis media, although the latter cannot be regarded as allergic disease.

The simple hypothesis that particle size determines deposit and organ manifestation (pollen grains with diameters of around 25 μm cause rhinitis in the nose, mold spores 5 μm in diameter in the bronchi cause asthma and small actinomycete particles below 2 μm in diameter in the alveoli lead to alveolitis) is surely too mechanistic, although of didactic value [10]. We know that pollen fragments may also reach the bronchi.

5.1.1.4 Therapy

The general therapy of allergic rhinitis is covered in the sections on "Immunotherapy" (Sect. 6.3.1) and "Pharmacotherapy" (Sects. 6.2, 6.3) [6]. A characteristic of rhinitis therapy is the use of α-adrenergics as vasoconstrictors (orally as pseudoephedrine or norephedrine or topically as naphthazoline, xylometazoline, or oxymetazoline). The possible adverse reaction of rhinitis medicamentosa after long-term use of topical vasoconstrictors with mucosal damage should be mentioned!

When selecting pharmacotherapy, the clinical symptoms should be considered. If obstruction is prominent, a combination of antihistamines, vasoconstrictors, and steroids is recommended while patients with predominant rhinorrhea usually respond well to antihistamines and anticholinergics. Mucosal dryness with increased irritability can be treated in perennial rhinitis with ointments and inhalations or lavages.

In very severe cases of allergic rhinitis, sinusitis can occur. Recently "fungal allergic sinusitis," a disease corresponding to allergic bronchopulmonary mycosis, has seen renewed interest (see Sect. 5.4 on "Hypersensitivity Pneumonitis"). Interactions between allergic rhinitis and diseases of the ear (vestibular or tube ventilatory disturbances) have been reported without clear pathophysiological evidence. There is no good evidence for an allergic mechanism in morbus Menière, tinnitus, or chronic labyrinthitis, although anecdotal cases have been reported.

To summarize: Allergic rhinitis is not a neglectable bagatelle condition! It occurs with systemic symptoms and often represents the beginning of severe asthma ("united airway disease") [3, 4, 6, 7, 10, 12, 13, 16, 19].

Table 5.3. Irritative factors as elicitors of rhinitis

- Dust, smoke (particles)
- Chemical irritants (solvents, alcohol, washing powder)
- Kitchen vapors, odors, halogens, formaldehyde, ether, etc.
- Change of temperature (especially cold)
- Air draught
- Change of position
- Dryness
- Hormonal influence (e.g., rhinitis in the third pregnancy trimenon)

References

1. Bachert C, Hauser U, Prem B, Rudack C, Ganzer U (1995) Proinflammatory cytokines in allergic rhinitis. Eur Arch Otorhinolaryngol 1 [Suppl]: 44–49
2. Bachmann W, Bachert C (1984) Quantitative evaluation of rhinomanometric curves. A new simple method. Laryngol Rhinol Otol 63:58–61
3. Bousquet J, Vignola AM, Campbell AM, Michel FB (1996) Pathophysiology of allergic rhinitis. Int Arch Allergy Immunol 110:207–218
4. Busse WW, Holgate ST (eds) (1995) Asthma and rhinitis. Blackwell, Oxford
5. Canonica GW, Ciprandi G, Pesce GP, Buscaglia S, Paolieri F, Bagnasco M (1995) ICAM-1 on epithelial cells in allergic subjects: a hallmark of allergic inflammation. Int Arch Allergy Immunol 107: 99–102
6. Durham SR (1998) Mechanisms of mucosal inflammation in the nose and lungs. Clin Exp Allergy 28 [Suppl 2]:15–16
7. Ellegard E, Karlsson G (1999) Nasal congestion during pregnancy. Clin Otolaryngol 24:307–311
8. Heppt W (1998) Zytologie der Nasenschleimhaut. Springer, Berlin Heidelberg New York
9. Malm L, van-Wijk RG, Bachert C (1999) Guidelines for nasal provocations with aspects on nasal patency, airflow, and airflow resistance. Rhinology 37:133–135
10. Mygind N, Dahl R, Pedersen S, Thestrup-Pedersen K (1996) Essential Allergy. Blackwell Science, Oxford
11. Mygind N, Laussen LC, Dahl M (2000) Systemic corticosteroid treatment for seasonal allergic rhinitis: a common but poorly documented therapy. Allergy 55:11–15
12. Naclerio RM (1997) Pathophysiology of perennial allergic rhinitis. Allergy 52:41–44
13. Nolte D, Renovanz HD, Schumann K (1982) Nase und Respirationstrakt. Obere und untere Luftwege als funktionelle Einheit. Dustri, Munich
14. Passalacqua G, Bachert C, Davies RJ, Durham SR, et al. (2000) Inhaled and nasal corticosteroids: safety aspects. Position paper. Allergy 55:16–33
15. Simons FE (1996) Learning impairment and allergic rhinitis. Allergy Asthma Proc 17:185–189
16. Simons FE (1999) Allergic rhinobronchitis: The asthma-allergic rhinitis link. J Allergy Clin Immunol 104:534–540
17. van Cauwenberge P, Bachert C, Passalacqua G, Bousquet J, Canonica GW, Durham SR, Fokkens WJ, Howarth PH, Lund V, Malling HJ, Mygind N, Passali D, Scadding GK, Wang DY (2000) Consensus statement on the treatment of allergic rhinitis. European Academy of Allergology and Clinical Immunology. Allergy 55:116–134
18. Tas E, Bircher AJ (2001) Therapie der Rhinitis allergica. Ther Umsch 58:309–314
19. van Wijk RG, de Graaf-in 't Veld C, Garrelds IM (1999) Nasal hyperreactivity. Rhinology 37:50–55
20. World Health Organization (2004) Allergic rhinitis and its impact on asthma (ARIA). In: Bousquet J, et al. (eds) Executive summary. WHO (in press)
21. Wüthrich B, Schindler C, Leuenberger P, Ackermann-Liebrich U (1995) Prevalence of atopy and pollinosis in the adult population of Switzerland (SAPALDIA study). Swiss Study on Air Pollution and Lung Diseases in Adults. Int Arch Allergy Immunol 106:149–156

5.1.2 Bronchial Asthma

5.1.2.1 Definition

"Asthma is characterized by increased reactivity of the airway to various stimuli with decreased forced expiration changing in intensity either spontaneously or under therapy" (definition of the American College of Chest Physicians 1975). Newer definitions stress the bronchial hyperreactivity, defining asthma as airway disease with bronchial hyperreactivity [1, 17, 23, 35, 37]. "Reversible obstructive disturbance of ventilation" is the obligatory and central symptom of bronchial asthma, whereby two characteristic aspects are crucial:

- Attacks of dyspnea
- Hyperreactivity of airways against various stimuli

A new international definition of an expert group of the NIH [1] is:

"Asthma is a chronic inflammatory airway disease with participation of numerous inflammatory cells like mast cells, eosinophils, T lymphocytes, neutrophils, and epithelial cells. In sensitive individuals, inflammation leads to attacks of wheezing, dyspnea, tightness, and cough, especially during nights and early morning hours. These episodes go commonly with generalized but variable increased airway resistance which is reversible either spontaneously or following therapy. The airway inflammation causes increased airway sensitivity against a variety of different stimuli." Using this definition, bronchial asthma can be distinguished in the differential diagnosis from other conditions with dyspnea (Table 5.4).

Table 5.4. Differential diagnosis of bronchial asthma

- Mechanical ventilation disturbance (tumors, struma, mediastinal tumors, thymus hyperplasia, foreign body aspiration)
- Disturbance of ventilatory regulation (hyperventilation)
- Infection (bronchopneumonia, pertussis, acute epiglottitis ["pseudo-Krupp"], parasitoses)
- Gastroesophageal reflux
- Cardiac disease (left ventricular insufficiency with pulmonary edema, vitium cordis, coronary disease)
- Toxic or drug-induced bronchoconstriction
- Lung vessel disease (pulmonary embolism, pulmonary hypertension, vasculitis)
- Diseases of larynx and trachea (tracheal stenosis, tracheomalacia, acute laryngitis, functional laryngospasm)
- Other lung diseases (emphysema, fibrosis, sarcoidosis, interstitial lung disease, alveolitis)
- Sleep-apnea syndrome
- Chronic obstructive pulmonary disease (COPD)

The Deutsche Atemwegsliga (German Airway League) gives the following definition: "Asthma is an inflammatory airway disease with bronchial hyperreactivity and variable airway obstruction. Typical symptoms are cough and attacks of dyspnea, especially during the night and early morning, wheezing and clear viscous sputum" [46].

Bronchial asthma is the most common allergic lung disease, but can occur without detection of immune reactions ("intrinsic asthma"). In children, approximately 80% of asthma is allergic in origin, in adults approximately 60%.

5.1.2.2 Symptomatology

The major clinical symptom of an asthma attack is the sudden dyspnea (also tachypnea or orthopnea) with noisy breathing, characteristic dry noises (wheezing and humming), attacks of coughing and expectoration of a clear but viscous sputum. The attack often starts with tightness of the chest and a dry cough. Patients have difficulty speaking longer sentences.

Through the increasing difficulty in ventilation, respiratory auxiliary muscles are more intensely used. The suprathoracic veins are often filled, and cyanosis may occur. With an increased pulse rate, pulsus paradoxus often occurs. If an asthma attack persists in spite of therapy with beta-adrenergics and xanthine derivatives for more than 24 h, the term "status asthmaticus" ("acute severe asthma") is used. The breathing noises become less pronounced ("silent lung").

Sometimes an asthma attack occurs along with other symptoms of the upper respiratory airways (nasal blockage, sneezing, or itching eyes) as well as gastrointestinal complaints, increased diuresis, or fatigue [35, 36, 45, 46]. In the chest X-ray, few changes are seen, but in severe cases increased air with a pronounced inspiratory position of the thorax is seen. In contrast to lung emphysema, the lung vessels are not constricted in bronchial asthma. The characteristic finding in lung function is obstructive ventilatory disturbance with increased airway resistance and decreased forced expiratory volume (FEV_1).

The German Airway League has graded asthma according to severity (Table 5.5) [37, 46].

5.1.2.3 Different Forms of Bronchial Asthma

Bronchial asthma can be classified according to eliciting stimuli, sensitivity of the patient, test results or other underlying diseases [5, 11, 17, 18, 19, 23, 34, 35, 36, 37]. The best classification

Table 5.5. Classification of severity in bronchial asthma (German Airway League)

Grade	Term	Symptoms Day	Night	FEV1 or PEF (% normal)
I	Intermittent	≤2 times/week	≤2 times/month	>80%
II	Persistent, mild	<Once/day	>2 times/week	≥80%
III	Persistent, moderate	Daily	≥1 times/week	>60<80%
IV	Persistent, severe	Continuous	Frequent	<60%

Table 5.6. Forms of bronchial asthma

- Allergic (IgE-mediated, extrinsic)
- Physical-irritative, chemotoxic
- Intrinsic (cryptogenic, unknown etiology)
- Special forms[a]:
  Infection-associated
  Psychogenic
  Analgesic (additive) idiosyncrasy (Samter's triad)
  Pharmacologic (beta-blockers, histamine liberators)
  Exercise-induced
- Mixed forms

[a] These stimuli can trigger both allergic and intrinsic asthma

follows pathophysiologic criteria (Table 5.6). The frequent distinction between "extrinsic" (= allergic) and "intrinsic" (no antibodies detected) is not satisfactory since the term "intrinsic" is ill defined and would be better replaced by "cryptogenic." Mostly, the so-called infect-allergic or pathophysiologically unclear conditions are included. In intrinsic asthma, the typical signs and symptoms of atopy, such as increased serum IgE, detection of specific sensitizations in skin tests or RAST, are missing. However, eosinophilia in blood and sputum is often demonstrable.

Furthermore, asthma can be classified according to prognosis and therapeutic response. Intrinsic asthma responds to a lesser degree to beta-adrenergics, cromoglycate or theophylline. Sometimes, anticholinergics or ketotifen are effective; most patients, however, are glucocorticosteroid dependent [17, 20, 35].

The most important allergens in elicitation of extrinsic asthma are so-called inhalation or aeroallergens (pollen, animal epithelia, mold spores, housedust mites, etc.; see Sect. 3.4). The most important occupational triggers of allergic asthma are listed in Table 5.7 [6, 15, 16, 47]. In the differential diagnosis, allergic alveolitis (hypersensitivity pneumonitis), mostly caused by organic dusts, should be considered (see Sect. 5.4).

Exogenous toxic irritative factors able to trigger and maintain bronchial asthma comprise chemicals [ozone, chlorides, sulfur oxides, nitric oxides, isocyanates (partly also allergic)] and physical stimuli (cold, mechanical dust effects, cigarette smoke, etc.), which act

Table 5.7. Occupational IgE-mediated and irritative toxic asthma

Allergen	Occupation (examples)
Pollen	Agriculture, gardening, floristry
Storage mites	Agriculture
Animal epithelia	Zoology, laboratory research, bed clothing industry
Molds	Cheese-making
Enzymes	Washing powder, bakery
Castor oil	Agriculture
Cotton dust	Cotton harvesting
Silk	Textile industry
Coffee (raw)	Coffee harvesting
Flour and grain dust	Bakery, milling, pastry making, agriculture
Insect allergens	Zoology, food industry, cosmetics
Gum arabic	Printing
Lycopodium	Pharmacy
Rubber	Medical care, health workers
Metal salts (e.g., platinum)	Metal refinement, catalyzer production
Drugs	Health workers, pharmacy
Colophony	Paper production, printing
Wood dust	Forestry, woodcutting
Latex	Rubber industry, health personnel
Blooming plants	Gardening, kitchen
Small chemicals	Plastics, varnishes, furnishings, etc.
Irritative toxic substances	
Aliphatic amines	Chemical industry
Persulfates	Chemical industry, hairdressers, photo laboratory
Epichlorhydrine	Resins, softeners, hardeners
Acrylates	Plastic industry, dentistry

via cholinergic irritant receptors leading to bronchial constriction [4, 14, 17, 23, 27]. It is possible that the well-known exercise-induced asthma is caused by cold air or hyperosmolarity through water loss and can be improved by mouth protection. So-called psychogenic asthma (see Chap. 7) and infect-allergic asthma also belong here. Asthma in patients with analgesic or additive idiosyncrasy occurs together with polyposis nasi and sinusitis (Samter's triad) (see Sect. 5.7.2). All these stimuli can trigger both allergic and intrinsic asthma.

5.1.2.4 Pathophysiology

The reversible obstructive ventilation disturbance in bronchial asthma develops on the basis of bronchial hyperreactivity. This is due to inflammatory reactions caused either by allergen exposure or by other epithelial damage (infection, toxic agents, etc.) [4, 8, 14, 19, 21, 22, 23, 30, 35, 43, 45] (Figs. 5.3, 5.4).

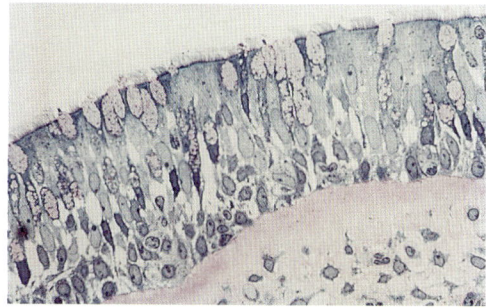

Fig. 5.3. Semi-thin-layer preparation of bronchial epithelia taken from a patient with bronchial asthma viewed under the light microscope (H. Behrendt)

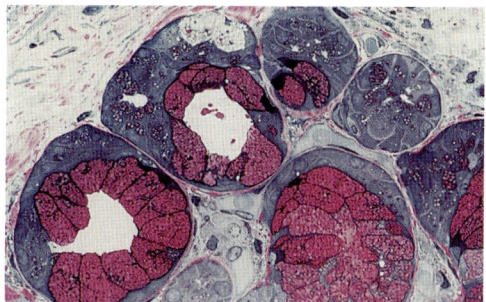

Fig. 5.4. Semi-thin-layer preparation of muciparous glands taken from a patient with bronchial asthma viewed under the light microscope (H. Behrendt)

In the development and maintenance of bronchial hyperreactivity, neurogenic factors play an increasing role (Table 5.8) [14, 19, 27, 31]. The nerve growth factor (NGF) induces neurotransmitters (Table 5.8) influencing neuronal plasticity of the airway nervous system. On the other hand, lymphocytes carry receptors for neurotransmitters or secrete neurotrophins as shown for TH2 cells secreting brain-derived neurotrophic factor (BDNF) [24]. These mechanisms might help to understand the well-known psychosomatic interactions in bronchial asthma (see Chap. 7).

The so-called Herxheimer's triad (mucous dyscrinia, mucosal edema, and bronchoconstriction) determines the intensity of clinical symptoms. In the sputum, Curschmann's spirales and Charcot-Leyden's crystals (crystalline forms of lysophospholipase from eosinophils) are found. The constriction affects both small and large bronchi.

Ventilation and perfusion rate are irregularly distributed with a decrease in CO_2 pressure (hypocapnia).

The airway resistance is increased, the flow rate decreased, and the ventilatory work increases, leading to premature closing of airways and lung emphysema. The intrathoracic gas volume and the functional residual capacity are increased.

Characteristic cardial symptoms in bronchial asthma comprise sinus tachycardia, signs of pulmonal hypertension (ECG changes) as well as pulsus paradoxus.

While previously in asthma the reversibility of acute bronchoconstriction was stressed, we know today that in chronic asthma, remodeling of the peribronchial tissue occurs with epithelial damage, and activation of myofibroblasts and fibroblasts (growth factors EGF, IGF, or TGF-β). This leads to a thickening of the basal membrane together with an increased fibrotic manteling and chronicity of the bronchial obstruction with persistent symptoms and deposits of collagens type I, III, and V [8, 23, 33, 39] (Fig. 5.5).

Table 5.8. Neurotransmitters (NT) and receptors in the airways

Substance	Receptor	Function
Sensory NT		
Tachykinins		
Substance P	NK 1	Vasodilation, plasma extravasation, mucus secretion, leukocyte infiltration
Neurokinin A	NK 2	Bronchoconstriction
Neurokinin B	NK 3	Autocrine inhibition (?)
CGRP	CGRP-1 and -2	Vasodilation
Bombesin	BB1-R, BB2-R	Mucus secretion, proliferation
VIP	VIP_1-R, VIP_2-R	Vasodilation, bronchoconstriction
Parasympathic postganglionic NT		
Acetylcholine (AC)	M_1	Reflex
M_2	Inhibition of AC release	
M_3	Bronchoconstriction, mucus secretion	
M_4	?	
Sympathic postganglionic NT		
Noradrenaline	α_1, α_2	Vasoconstriction
β_1	Cardial ino- and chronotropic effect	
β_2	Bronchodilation	
β_3	Lipid tissue regulation (?)	
NPγ	γ_{1-6}	Long-acting vasoconstriction
Opioids		
β-Endorphin	δ_1, δ_2, μ	Autocrine inhibition, mast cell degranulation (?)
Enkephalin	δ_1, δ_2, μ	
Proteolytic peptides		
Endothelin	ETA, -B	Vasoconstriction
Bradykinin	B_1, B_2	Vasodilation, sensory stimulation

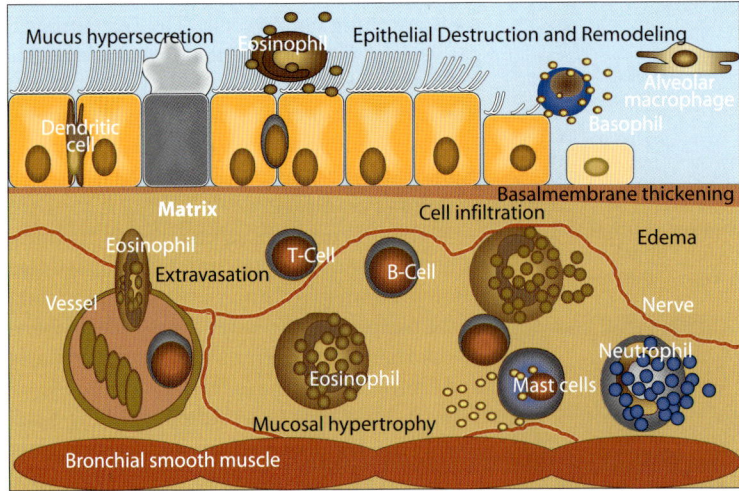

Fig. 5.5. Components of asthmatic inflammation (according to Schultze-Werninghaus)

5.1.2.5 Diagnosis

The diagnostic procedure in asthma is shown in Table 5.9. For allergy diagnosis in general, see Chap. 4. In bronchial provocation tests, unspecific stimuli like acetyl (or methyl) choline, histamine, dust, cold air, exercise or hyperventilation are used [1, 2, 13, 18, 34, 37, 41]. The following test concentrations are used: acetylcholine (1.0–100 mg/ml); methylcholine (0.05–50 mg/ml); carbamylcholine (0.05–50 mg/ml);

Table 5.9. Diagnostic procedure in allergic bronchial asthma

History
General history, allergy history, personal and family
General examination
Physical
Auscultation
Chest X-ray and sinuses
Lung function
Bronchial dilatation test
Unspecific provocation (acetylcholine, exercise, etc.) for bronchial hyperreactivity)
Blood count (eosinophils) and routine analysis, total IgE
Specific tests
Allergen avoidance (if possible)
Skin test
RAST
Bronchial allergen provocation (if necessary)
Additional procedures
Blood gas analysis
In vitro inflammatory parameters (ECP)
Sputum
Induced sputum
Bronchoalveolar lavage (BAL with cytology)
Exhalation analyses (e.g., NO)
Additional examinations
ECG
α_1-Antitrypsin
Parasites
Tb test

histamine (0.05–50 mg/ml) [17]. Cholinergic hyperreactivity is a cardinal symptom of asthma [40].

Bronchial provocation tests with allergens need to follow strict indications (see Sect. 4.4).

5.1.2.6 Differential Diagnosis

The most important differential diagnosis of bronchial asthma in adults is chronic obstructive bronchitis, which as persistent obstructive ventilation disturbance leads to chronic obstructive pulmonary disease (COPD) [4, 10, 15, 21, 26, 30, 33]. In some cases, the differential diagnosis from severe chronic asthma may be difficult (Table 5.10). The main risk factor for COPD is tobacco smoke, but also other indoor air pollutants or occupational toxic exposures play a role. In contrast to bronchial asthma, COPD responds only weakly to pharmacotherapy [30]. Steroids and thiotropin are used with moderate effect.

Differential diagnosis also comprises allergic bronchopulmonal aspergillosis as well as interstitial lung diseases such as hypersensitivity pneumonitis (see Sect. 5.3). Functional laryngospasm, also called "vocal cord dysfunction," may be triggered by physical and chemical stimuli and induce wheezing. Among the many forms of sleep apnea syndromes, there are obstructive variants similar to nightly asthma attacks.

5.1.2.7 Therapy

Avoidance Measures. The only causal therapy is avoidance of eliciting stimuli including all noxious influences. This implies careful allergy diagnosis. Apart from avoidance of occupational allergens, avoidance measures in daily life are of major importance (see Sect. 3.4 on "Aeroallergens"). Items to be avoided include:

Table 5.10. Differential diagnosis of bronchial asthma and "chronic obstructive pulmonary disease" (COPD)

Finding	Bronchial asthma	COPD
Age	Childhood, adults	Mostly over 50
Allergy	Frequent	Rarely
Smoking	Rare	Almost always
Nightly dyspnea	Yes	A little
Symptom-free intervals	Yes	No
Obstruction	Central and peripheral	Mostly peripheral
Eosinophilia (blood and sputum)	Frequent	Rare
Inflation	Sometimes reversible	Always irreversible
Blood gases	Normal	Abnormal
Variability of obstruction	Yes	No
Response to β-adrenergics	Good	Little
Response to steroids	Good	Little

Table 5.11. "Unspecific irritation syndrome" (according to H. Düngemann)

Physical
Temperature change, dust, fog
Chemical
E.g., exhaust, smog, odors, chemical irritants
Pharmacodynamic
E.g., histamine liberators, β-blockers, certain spices, drinks, and drugs
Infectious diseases
Infections of the upper airways
Psychological
Stress, emotional disturbance

feathers in bed clothing, animal or plant mattresses (horse hair, seaweed), pets (including furs!), carpets, old upholstery, humidity, moist walls, plants (mold), as well as all dust-collecting furniture, sprays, and certain humidifiers.

In all forms of asthma, the avoidance of nonspecific stimuli is important, which can lead to deterioration of any kind of asthma ("unspecific irritation syndrome" according to Düngemann [12]) (Table 5.11).

Finally, therapy of underlying infectious disease should be mentioned, for instance putrid sinusitis, polypectomy with impaired nose breathing, and short-term antibiotic treatment after microbiological examination (e.g., *Haemophilus influenzae*).

Allergen-Specific Immunotherapy (Hyposensitization). In uncomplicated allergic asthma, allergen-specific immunotherapy is effective when started early and with the right indications [38] (see Sect. 6.3).

Physical Therapy. Adequate breathing technique and correction of malposition of the thorax are important. Training of respiratory abdominal and back musculature; connective tissue massage and local heat application; and secretion drainage (deliverance of sputum in the downward position, etc.) are important [1, 3, 11, 20, 25, 38].

Psychosomatic Consultation. Psychosomatic consultation may help also with regard to avoidance of trigger situations and can imply behavioral therapy, group therapy, autogenic training, etc. (see also asthma schools below).

Climate Therapy. For rehabilitation of chronic asthma, climate therapy at sea level (North Sea) or at high altitude (e.g., Davos, Switzerland) has been shown to improve asthma by decreasing allergen exposure and unspecific climatic effects [7].

Mast Cell Blockers. Mast cell stabilizers (e.g., disodium cromoglycate) act prophylactically on the mucous membranes in preventing asthma attacks. Disodium cromoglycate is given either as a powder or as a 1% solution (4× daily every 6 h). Ketotifen acts both as a mast cell stabilizer and as an antihistamine, has no direct bronchodilating effect but is prophylactically effective. Nedocromil sodium has mast cell stabilizer and anti-inflammatory properties.

Antihistamines. Histamine H_1 antagonists do not play a major role in the treatment of asthma (see Sect. 6.2 on "Pharmacotherapy").

Leukotriene Antagonists and Inhibitors. Inhibitors of lipoxygenase as well as antagonists of sulfidoleukotrienes have a place in asthma therapy, especially in reducing glucocorticosteroids in severe asthma [44].

Xanthine Derivatives. Xanthine derivatives have been used for decades for bronchospasmolysis [23, 27]. New galenic formulas have decreased the problem of the small therapeutic range of theophylline. If side effects are suspected, the plasma level should be measured and kept between 10 and 20 µg/ml. Average daily dose for adults ranges between 10 and 15 mg/kg/day, with higher doses for smokers [46].

$β_2$ Adrenergics. While classical beta-adrenergics (e.g., isoproterenol) often lead to cardial side effects due to $β_1$-stimulation (tachycardia), selective $β_2$-adrenergics have predominant bronchodilatory effects. Furthermore, they have mast cell stabilizing properties and can be used orally or as an aerosol (one to two breaths every 4 h), and also in long-term therapy.

Long-acting β_2-adrenergics have greatly improved asthma therapy.

Anticholinergics. The atropine derivates ipratropium bromide and oxitropium bromide can be used as aerosols and act – more weakly than β-adrenergics – as bronchodilators, also prophylactically. They can be combined with β_2-agonists.

Secretolysis. Adequate volume replacement (2–3 l/day) and humidification of the inhaled air are important. Furthermore, detergents and mucolytics are used for secretolysis (acetylcysteine, bromhexine, or ambroxol as well as etheric oils).

Glucocorticosteroids. Glucocorticosteroids act at different levels in the asthmatic reaction: when given over longer periods they have a bronchodilatory and preventive effect on immediate reactions, decrease bronchial hyperreactivity, inhibit mucous secretion and increase the effect of β_2-adrenergics. Through the anti-inflammatory effect, mucosal edema and sputum viscosity will decrease. Systemic glucocorticosteroids are used in severe asthma, the dose depending upon the severity of the condition.

In *status asthmaticus* (acute asthma attack), doses of 250 mg up to 2 g prednisolone are indicated combined with β_2-adrenergics (with nebulizer) and theophylline (with perfusor). Persistent wheezing over more than 4 h, pulsus paradoxus, persistent tachycardia over 100/min, FEV_1 under 1 l/s, and abnormal blood gases are signs of an acute asthma attack. Immediate hospital admission is indicated. Therapy follows the above-mentioned rules; in addition, infusions, oxygen, sometimes anesthesia with mechanical ventilation and bronchoscopic removal of secretion are implied [26].

In cortisone-dependent chronic asthma, usually 40–80 mg prednisolone are given with a slow dose reduction (not more than 5 mg/week) until a minimal dose is "titrated."

Great progress for glucocorticosteroid therapy was achieved through the development of topical steroids (beclomethasone, budesonide, mometasone, triamcinolone). These are also prophylactically active and allow a reduction of systemic steroids in steroid-dependent asthma. Side effects comprise the possible occurrence of candida infection as well as changes in voice quality [28]; in children, a significant but small and reversible growth impairment has been observed. Topical Glucocorticosteroids can be combined with long-activity β-agonists.

Antibiotics. In intrinsic asthma and signs of infection, short-term antibiotic therapy may be helpful.

Surgical Treatment. Previously surgical measures such as vago- or sympathicotomy, cutting of the nervus laryngicus cranialis or resection of the glomus caroticum have been recommended, which today do not play a major role. The side effects of these operations are considerable; bronchial hyperreactivity can persist in spite of "denervation" of the lung [17].

New Immunotherapeutic Approaches. New approaches can be seen in the development of monoclonal humanized antibodies against IgE (omalizumab) [32]. Antagonists of interleukin-4 (soluble interleukin-4 receptor), adhesion molecules, tachykinins, as well as antibodies to other cytokines (anti-interleukin-5 = mepolizumab) are being tested in clinical trials (see Sect. 6.3).

Procedures Without Proven Efficacy. Often in asthma, so-called unconventional therapies are used such as acupuncture, use of certain bacterial "vaccines," homeopathy, standard gammaglobulins, and others (see Sect. 6.4).

Asthma Schools. The general concept of asthma management requires the cooperation of the informed patient. Schooling programs for children and adults have been proven helpful and are also paid for by insurance in some countries [40] (see also Sect. 6.5 on "Prevention"). Asthmatics may also do sports when treated properly [47].

References

1. National Institutes of Health (1997) Expert Panel Report 2: Guidelines for the diagnosis and management of asthma. Publication 97-4051, NIH, Bethesda
2. American Thoracic Society (2000) Guidelines for methacholine challenge and exercise challenge testing. Am J Respir Crit Care Med (2000) 161: 309–329
3. Bachert C (1997) Asthma and rhinitis: management implications. Eur Respir J 7:294–295
4. Barnes PJ, Chung F, Page CP (1998) Inflammatory mediators of asthma. An update. Pharmacol Rev 50:515–596
5. Baur X (1986) Asthma, alveolitis, aspergillose. Charakterisierung ursächlicher Allergene. Springer, Berlin Heidelberg New York
6. Bernstein DJ (1997) Allergic reactions to workplace allergens. JAMA 278:1907–1913
7. Borelli S, Düngemann H (eds) (1981) Fortschritte der Allergologie und Dermatologie. IMP-Verlag, Basel
8. Busse WW, Elias J, Sheppard D, et al. (1999) Airway remodeling and repair. Am J Respir Crit Care Med 160:1035–1042
9. Crapo RO (1994) Pulmonary function testing. N Engl J Med 331:25–30
10. Debelic M (ed) (1986) Bronchitis im Kindes- und Jugendlichenalter. Dustri, Munich
11. Doerschug KC, Peterson MW, Dayton CS, et al. (1999) Asthma guidelines. An assessment of physician understanding and practice. Am J Respir Crit Care Med 159:1735–1741
12. Düngemann H (1978) Karenz-Expositionsprophylaxe. Atemwegs Lungenkrankh 4
13. Dykewicz MS, Fineman S (eds) (1998) Diagnosis and management of rhinitis: Complete Guidelines of the Joint Task Force on Practice Parameters in Allergy, Asthma, and Immunology. Ann Allergy Asthma Immunol 81:478–518
14. Fischer A, McGregor GP, Saria A, Philipp B, Kummer W (1996) Induction of tachykinin gene and peptide expression in guinea pig nodose primary afferent neurons by allergic airway inflammation. J Clin Invest 98:2284–2291
15. Fruhmann G (1994) Sonstige Berufskrankheiten: Obstruktive Atemwegserkrankungen. In: Ferlinz R (ed) Pneumologie. Thieme, Stuttgart, p 622ff
16. Fuchs E (1982) Gewerbliche Allergene als Ursache obstruktiver Lungenerkrankungen. Früherkennung und Abklärung. Schweiz Med Wochenschr 112:185
17. Fuchs E, Schultze-Werninghaus G (1986) Asthma bronchiale. Themen der Medizin 7. Wander, Nürnberg
18. Gonsior E, Henzgen M, Jörres RF, Kroidl RF, Merget R, Riffelmann FW, Wallenstein GW (2001) Leitlinie für die Durchführung bronchialer Provokationstests mit Allergenen. Deutsche Ges für Allergologie und klinische Immunologie. Allergo J 10:193–199, 257–264
19. Hansen K (1957) Bronchialasthma (Bronchiolenasthma) und verwandte Störungen. In: Hansen K (ed) Allergie. Thieme, Stuttgart
20. Hansel TT, Bauer PJ (eds) (2001) New drugs for asthma, allergy and COPD. Progress in respiration research, vol 31. Karger, Basel
21. Henderson WR, Shelhamer JH, Reingold DB, Smith LJ, Evans R, Kaliner M (1979) Alpha-adrenergic hyper-responsiveness in asthma. N Engl J Med 300:642–647
22. Holgate ST, Davies DE, Lackie PM, Wilson SY, Puddicombe SL, Lordan JL (2000) Epitheliolmesenchymal interactions in the pathogenesis of asthma. J Allergy Clin Immunol 105:193–204
23. Kay AB, Austen KF, Lichtenstein LM (eds) (1984) Asthma. Physiology, immunopharmacology and treatment. Academic Press, London
24. Kerschensteiner M, Gallmeier E, Behrens L, Vargas Leal V, Misgeld T, Klinkert WEF, Kohlbeck R, Hoppe E, Oropeza-Wekerle RL, Bartke I, Stadelmann C, Lassmann H, Wekerle H, Hohlfeld R (1999) Activated human T cells, B cells, and monocytes produce brain-derived neutrophic factor in vitro and in inflammatory brain lesions: A neutroprotective role of inflammation? J Exp Med 189:865–870
25. Kjellmann N-IM (1976) Immunoglobulin E and atopic allergy in childhood. Linköping University Medicine Dissertation No. 36
26. König P (1985) Therapie des Status asthmaticus. Internist 26:208
27. Kunkel G (2001) Neurogene Aspekte der allergischen Entzündungsreaktion. In: Ring J, Darsow V (eds) Allergie 2000: Probleme, Strategien und praktische Konsequenzen. Dustri, Munich, pp 179–181
28. Kroegel C (ed) (1997) Moderne Therapie des Asthma bronchiale. Thieme, Stuttgart
29. Lebowitz MD, Barbee R, Burrows B (1984) Family concordance of IgE, atopy, and disease. J Allergy Clin Immunol 73:259–264
30. Magnussen H (1990) Überempfindlichkeit der Atemwege. Dtsch med Wochenschr 115:1604–1610
31. Middleton E Jr et al. (eds) (1998) Allergy: principles and practice, 5th edn. Mosby, St. Louis, pp 544–558
32. Milgrom H, Fick RB, Su JQ, et al. (1999) Treatment of allergic asthma with monoclonal anti-IgE antibody. N Engl J Med 341:1966–1973
33. Nadel JA (ed) (1980) Physiology and pharmacology of the airways. Marcel Dekker, New York
34. Niggemann B, Illi S, Madloch C (2001) Histamine challenges discriminate between symptomatic and asymptomatic children. MAS study group. Eur Resp J 17:246–253
35. Nolte D (1996) Asthma: Das Krankheitsbild, der Asthmapatient, die Therapie, 6th edn. Urban & Schwarzenberg, Munich

36. Reinhardt D (ed) (1996) Asthma bronchiale im Kindesalter. Springer, Berlin Heidelberg New York
37. Schultze-Werninghaus G (ed) (1999) Deutsche Atemwegsliga: Empfehlungen zur Allergiediagnostik bei Atemwegserkrankungen in der Praxis. Pneumologie 48:300–304
38. Schultze-Werninghaus G (1997) Die Immuntherapie (allergenspezifische Hyposensibilisierung) bei Asthma bronchiale. Atemw Lungenkrh 23: 701–707
39. Slavin RG, Reisman RE (eds) Expert guide to allergy and immunology. American College of Physicians, Philadelphia, pp 23–40
40. Szepanski R, Lecheler J (1995) Standard- und Qualitätssicherung der Asthmaschulung im Kindes- und Jugendalter. Präv Rehab 7:1–41
41. Tiffeneau R, Beauvallet M (1945) Production exclusive d'effets pulmonaires locaux par inhalation d'aerosol d'acetylcholine. Son utilisation comme test d'insuffacance respiratoire. Sem Hop (Paris) 21:154–166
42. Townsley RG (1976) IgE levels and methacholine inhalation responses in monozygous and dizygous twins. J Allergy Clin Immunol 57:227
43. Virchow JC, Kroegel C, Walker C, Matthyss H (1994) Cellular and immunological markers of allergic and intrinsic bronchial asthma. Lung 172:313–334
44. Virchow JC, Prasse A, Naya I, Summertin A, Harris A (2000) Zafirlukast improves asthma control in patients receiving high-dose inhaled corticosteroids. Am J Respir Crit Care Med 62:578–585
45. Wahn U, Seger S, Wahn V (eds) (1999) Pädiatrische Allergologie und Immunologie, 3rd edn. Urban und Fischer, Munich
46. Wettengel R, Berdel D, Cegla U, et al. (1994) Empfehlungen der Deutschen Atemwegsliga zum Asthmamanagement bei Erwachsenen und Kindern. Med Klin 89:57–67
47. Worth H, Meyer A, Folgering H, Kirsten D, Lecheler J, Magnussen H, Pleyer K, Schmidt S, Schmitz M, Taube K, Wettengel R (2000) Empfehlungen der Deutschen Atemwegsliga zum Sport und körperlichen Training bei Patienten mit obstruktiven Atemwegserkrankungen. Pneumologie 54: 61–67
48. Wüthrich B (1976) Zum Allergenkatalog beruflicher Inhalationsallergien. Berufsdermatosen 24: 123

5.1.3 Urticaria and Angioedema

5.1.3.1 Definition

Urticaria is a disease with occurrence of self-vanishing erythematous elevated skin lesions which disappear and blanch under pressure (wheals) (Figs. 5.6, 5.7). Identical skin lesions are observed after injection of histamine into the skin (Lewis' triad: mild redness = local vasodilation, edema = increase in capillary permeability, flare = axon reflex). When the reaction occurs in the subcutaneous tissue, the disease is called angioneurotic or angioedema (also "Quincke's edema") (Fig. 5.8). Urticaria comprises several clinical manifestations and may be caused by immunological and non-immune pathomechanisms.

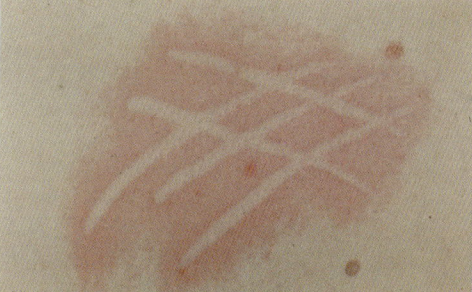

Fig. 5.6. Urticaria factitia caused by tangential application of force

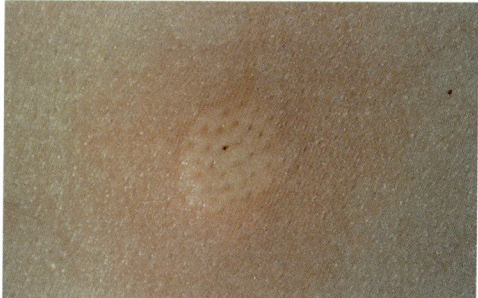

Fig. 5.7. Hive following a histamine injection

5.1.3.2 Classification

Clinically, urticaria can be classified according to:

1. The course: acute urticaria (<6 weeks) and chronic urticaria (>6 weeks). In between are acute intermittent urticaria (several acute episodes) and chronic relapsing urticaria (continuous relapses with short remissions of several days).

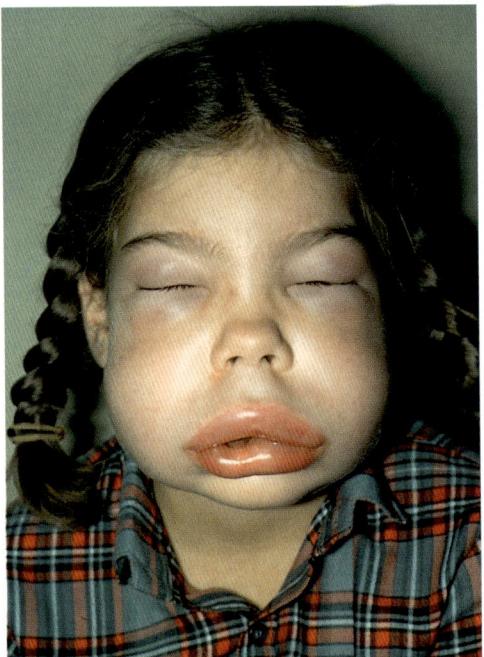

Fig. 5.8. Quincke's edema

Table 5.12. Classification of urticaria according to etiopathophysiology

Allergic
Foods
Drugs
Aeroallergens
Insect venoms
Plant allergens
Contact urticaria allergens
Others

Toxic-irritative
Insects, plants (*Urtica dioica*)
Drugs (e.g., opioids)
Enzymes (proteases)

Pseudo-allergic
Acetylsalicylic acid, analgesics
Additives
Colorings

Physical
Mechanical (urticaria factitia, pressure, vibration)
Thermal (cold, heat)
Cholinergic (exercise)
Water
Electromagnetic radiation (e.g., solar urticaria)

Focus reactions
Parasites
Mycoses
Bacterial and viral infections
Neoplasia

Enzyme defects
Angioneurotic edema
(C1 inactivator deficiency)
–Hereditary
–Acquired (neoplasia)
Serum carboxypeptidase B deficiency

Autoimmune diseases
Urticaria vasculitis
Systemic lupus erythematosus
Cryoglobulinemia

Psychosomatic conflicts
Stress
Depression
Other

Hormonal disturbances
Thyroid function disturbance
Urticaria during menstruation or pregnancy

Urticaria pigmentosa (mastocytosis)

"Idiopathic" urticaria

2. Pathophysiological aspects (Table 5.12): There are few epidemiological studies regarding the prevalence of urticaria. It seems that the incidence of urticaria has been constant during recent years [10]. Prevalence of chronic urticaria is estimated at 1–3% [4, 5, 9, 40]; in 1991, after German reunification, urticaria was more common in West German children compared to the East, following the pattern of hay fever and asthma prevalence (see Sect. 3.3.2).

Acute urticaria is the most common type of urticaria; it is estimated that 20–30% of the population suffer once in their life from an episode of acute urticaria. Mostly, acute urticaria heals spontaneously, and sometimes medical help is necessary. The etiopathogenesis often remains unclear: Apart from acute infections, allergic reactions need to be discussed. Histamine is one of the most important mediator substances [5, 11]. Often acute urticaria occurs after drug medication during acute infection. In these cases the suspected drugs are often tolerated at a later point in time. In up to 50% no cause for acute urticaria can be elucidated. There is an indication of more intense diagnosis in either very severe clinical manifestations (first degree of anaphylaxis), relapses, or when changing into chronic urticaria.

When *chronic urticaria* is subdivided according to pathophysiology (Table 5.12), approximately 5–10% is allergic in nature, 15–20% is pseudo-allergic, and 15–20% is triggered by physical stimuli. A large percentage (approximately 50%) remain etiopathophysiologically unclear (except for the rare cases of hereditary angioedema). Psychosomatic influences as well as so-called "focus reactions" are discussed when, e.g., gastrointestinal disturbance, chronic infectious disease, autoimmune disease, neoplasms, or parasitic infestation give rise to chronic urticaria. In recent years, a new concept of autoimmune pathogenesis has been postulated: Autoantibodies against the high-affinity IgE receptor may play a role which can be found in up to 50% of patients with severe chronic urticaria [9, 12, 28].

Chronic urticaria in adults is more frequent in females (f:m = 2:1).

5.1.3.3 Physical Urticaria

A common subgroup of urticaria is represented by the different forms of physical urticaria (Table 5.13) when specific physical stimuli induce wheals either:

- On the site of contact (e.g., contact cold urticaria) or
- Generalized in a reflex phenomenon (e.g., cholinergic urticaria, cold reflex urticaria)

The most common form of physical urticaria is *urticaria factitia* (also called "dermographic urticaria"), when tangentially acting forces in the upper dermis induce histamine release. This form is often associated with psychosomatic stress, but is also found in combination with IgE-mediated allergy. The occurrence of urticaria factitia is variable and sometimes directly stress dependent (a female colleague of mine only had urticaria factitia on Thursdays when Prof. Braun-Falco was doing his grand rounds). I sometimes try to console my patients: "Be glad that you are living today; some centuries ago, you would have been burnt as a witch!"

Cholinergic urticaria is characterized by the occurrence of small follicular wheals triggered by exercise, sweating, or strong psychologic stress.

The differential diagnosis of chronic urticaria comprises *localized heat urticaria,* where at the site of heat application (45–50°C) wheals can be triggered [31]. In vitro warming of a basophil suspension can induce histamine release [32].

Rather common is *exercise-induced urticaria,* which is often connected with food allergy and sometimes the first stage of anaphylaxis (see Sect. 5.1.4).

A frequent form (15% of physical urticaria) is *cold urticaria* (Fig. 5.9), which can rarely

Table 5.13. Classification of physical urticaria (*f*, frequent; *r*, rare; *vr*, very rare; *AH*, antihistamine; *TAD*, tricyclic antidepressant; *MS*, mast cell stabilizer; *GC*, glucocorticosteroid)

Elicitor		Pathophysiology	Therapy
Dermographism (urticaria factitia)	f	Psychosomatic influence, summation with IgE	AH_1 + AH_2, TAD, Counseling
Cholinergic (sweating)	f	Small follicular wheals, frequently psychosomatic	AH + anticholinergics
Localized heat	vr	?	AH
Exercise	f	Summation with food allergy, anaphylaxis	AH, MS
Cold	f	Rarely familiar, cryoglobulinemia, neutrophil infiltrate	AH, penicillin, dapsone
Pressure	f	4–6 h, neutrophils, ESR elevation	AH?, GC, dapsone
Vibration	vr	Angioedema	AH, GC
Electromagnetic radiation (solar urticaria)	r	Histamine not involved, specific eliciting wave lengths	AH?, photoprotection, chloroquine, hardening
Water	vr	Autoantigens in *S. corneum*?	Skin care, AH

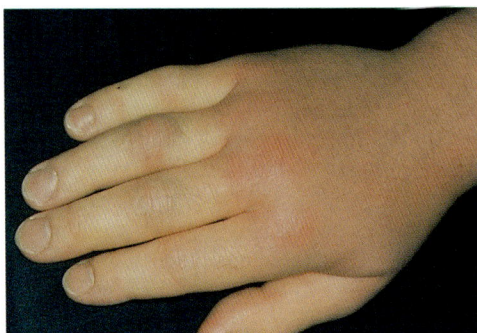

Fig. 5.9. Urticaria induced by cold

occur as a familial form, or be found along with cold-sensitive antibodies (e.g., cryoglobulinemia, cold hemagglutinins). In dermatohistopathology, neutrophil infiltrates are found; sometimes ESR is increased. Cold urticaria can be a sequel of chronic infection (e.g., borreliosis). Antihistamines have little effect. High-dose intravenous penicillin has led to improvement without the mechanisms being known [13].

Pressure urticaria occurs mostly in young men (22–50 years) doing heavy physical work. There is an immediate type where wheals develop acutely within minutes up to 1 h and a delayed type which only 4–6 h after pressure application (5–10 kg over 10–20 min) elicits massive whealing. Antihistamines have little effect; dapsone has been tried successfully.

Light urticaria summarizes all forms of urticaria where the effect of electromagnetic radiation (from X-rays to visible light) induces whealing. The most common form is solar urticaria, where radiation mostly in the UV-A range elicits whealing. Histamine and mast cell reactions do not seem to play a major role; possibly direct nerval stimulation takes place (E. Hölzle, H. Behrendt, personal communication).

For therapy, UVA rush-hardening can be used in solar urticaria [2].

Aquagenic urticaria is rare (not to be confused with the much more common aquagenic pruritus); it has been speculated that a water-soluble autoantigen is released from the stratum corneum and induces histamine release [11]. Prophylactic skin care prior to water contact may help.

In the treatment of all forms of physical urticaria, one should warn patients not to do "heroic self-experiments" (for hardening), since anaphylactic reactions may occur (my first patient with solar urticaria suffered anaphylactic shock in a solarium).

5.1.3.4 Special Forms of Urticaria and Angioedema

Contact Urticaria. In these patients, epidermal contact of the unlesional skin with eliciting agents (either irritative like nettle, *Urtica dioica*, or allergenic like latex proteins) leads to wheal formation, sometimes deteriorating into anaphylaxis ("contact anaphylaxis") [19].

Urticaria Pigmentosa (Mastocytosis). This type differs from the other urticarias since there are irreversible long-lasting skin lesions corresponding to local accumulations of mast cells in the skin. In childhood, isolated mastocytomas are common, which after physical stress (hot baths or thumb sucking) can trigger generalized urticaria, sometimes local bulla formation. The prognosis is good.

In adulthood, urticaria pigmentosa with characteristic brownish red disseminated skin lesions is common, which show after rubbing urticarial dermographism (Darier's sign). The brownish color is not postinflammatory hyperpigmentation but corresponds to activation of epidermal melanocytes through stem cell factor (SCF).

Mastocytosis may be limited to the skin or be found along with systemic involvement (bone marrow, gastrointestinal tract). Very rare are mast cell leukemias or precursors such as "aggressive mastocytosis" with lymphadenopathy.

Recently cases of "occult mastocytosis" have been reported where without visible skin lesions patients were suffering from relapsing urticaria or anaphylactoid reactions; diagnosis can be made from the strongly elevated mast cell tryptase level in the serum (see also Sect. 3.1.4).

A rare form of mastocytosis is teleangiectasia eruptiva macularis perstans.

Urticaria Vasculitis. Here the single wheals do not vanish within hours but persist over 12–48 h, being found along with painful large erythematous swellings. Histologically, leukocytoclastic vasculitis as well as immune complex deposits with direct immunofluorescence is found [16, 21]. Urticaria vasculitis sometimes is a precursor of autoimmune disease such as lupus erythematosus and can be concomitant with petechial bleeding (see Sect. 5.3).

Hereditary Angioneurotic Edema (HANE). This genetically determined disease is characterized by acute attacks of circumscribed giant edema formation especially in the face (eyelids, lips), but also in the genitals without concomitant urticaria. Sometimes attacks are triggered by local trauma (e.g., at the dentist). There is a chemical or functional defect of C1-inactivator (C1-esterase inhibitor) in the complement system leading to a decrease of C4 and C2 with activation of the complement and the kallikrein kinin system. HANE is a severe and life-threatening disease (note: laryngeal edema), sometimes manifesting only as acute colic-like abdominal pain (angioedema of the GI tract). In rare cases the disease is acquired in the context of neoplasia [3]. There is a third form of HANE without detectable C1 inactivator deficiency and a still unknown pathophysiology [3].

Severe attacks of angioedema have also been observed in patients under angiotensin-converting enzyme inhibitors (ACE inhibitors) where a pathophysiological role of kallikrein kinin activation has been speculated [15, 16].

Idiopathic Urticaria. The diagnosis "idiopathic urticaria" only should be made when all other (Table 5.12) possible causes have been excluded. Diagnosis of chronic urticaria is often tedious for the physician and patient [4, 5, 9, 10, 11, 23, 27, 34, 36].

5.1.3.5 Diagnosis

In the diagnosis of chronic urticaria, a three-step program has proven helpful and practical, increasing the intensity of diagnostic work-up according to the intensity of the disease [27] (Fig. 5.10). Between the single diagnostic steps,

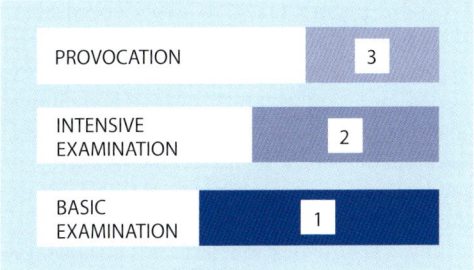

Fig. 5.10. Three-step plan for urticaria diagnostics (according to Ring and Przybilla)

apart from possible causal therapy of the pathological findings detected, symptomatic treatment with H_1 antihistamines over 1 month is employed. If – after stopping pharmacotherapy – new lesions occur, the next step is started. Each step of the three-step program comprises history, clinical examination, laboratory examination and special test procedures.

Urticaria Diagnosis: Step 1 (Basic Examination). Step 1 comprises basic examinations performed in all patients with chronic urticaria (Table 5.14).

Table 5.14. Urticaria diagnosis: step 1 (basic examination)

History
Time course
Family history (atopy, HANE)
Contact urticaria
Drugs, foods
Psychological factors
Clinical examination
Skin lesions
Localization
Duration of single lesions
Physical tests
Dermographism
Cold/warm, ice cube contact
Exercise (ergometer)
Pressure test
Phototesting (minimal erythema dose, MED)
Laboratory
Blood count, ESR
Stool
Serum IgE
(C1 inactivator if suspected)
Allergy diagnosis
Atopy screen
Skin prick test with standard food allergens

A careful history taken by experienced allergists/dermatologists is crucial. Psychosocial factors should be considered. HANE can be excluded by a careful family history and clinical observation (almost never wheals!). In the differential diagnosis of lid edema, sinusitis or emphysema of the orbita should also be excluded.

Physical provocation tests are an essential part of urticaria diagnosis and comprise provocation with cold, warmth, pressure, exercise, as well as dermographism. Phototests with UV light are only done when there is a history of light urticaria. History should also cover contact urticaria [9]. HANE is characterized by a deficiency in C1 inactivator, which can be detected immunochemically, although in 15% only functionally [3, 15, 24].

Urticaria Diagnosis: Step 2 (Intensive Examination). In step 2 the history is repeated. In addition, the patient is advised to keep a diary of diet and symptom course. A clinical examination search for "foci" (Table 5.15) is performed in cooperation with the relevant other disciplines. Especially gastrointestinal disturbances (e.g., *Helicobacter pylori*) may play a role. Urticaria vasculitis as the precursor of autoimmune disease should be excluded. In the serum, autoantibodies against the high-affinity IgE receptor (FcεRI) of classes IgG 1 and IgG 3 can be detected by immunoblot or functionally with the autologous serum test ("Greaves test") [8, 9, 12, 23]. These patients may represent a subgroup where only systemic steroids or immunosuppression is effective. For the autologous serum test, we recommend a serum dilution of 1:100 in the intradermal test in order to avoid false-positive results [23]).

Examination of thyroid function is also recommended (4–6% show disturbed thyroid function or autoantibodies) [11, 17]. Amplification of in vitro histamine release through thyroid hormones has been described [22].

Urticaria Diagnosis: Step 3 (Provocation Tests). Step 3 comprises provocation testing using different dietary approaches sometimes employed under inpatient conditions in order to standardize other environmental conditions and guarantee possible emergency therapy for anaphylaxis (Table 5.16). Provocation tests include suspected foods as well as food additives ("oral provocation test for idiosyncrasy," OPTI) (see Sect. 5.1.5 on "Food allergy"). The marker substance in the provocation of chronic urticaria is acetylsalicylic acid; a high percentage (20–30%) of patients have significant and partly dramatic exacerbation of skin lesions, sometimes together with anaphylactoid reactions [5, 6].

Table 5.15. Urticaria diagnosis: step 2 (intensive examination)

History
Diary for diet and symptoms
Clinical examination
Search for "foci" (ENT, teeth, gastrointestinal tract, thyroid, urology, gynecology, others)

Laboratory
Serum and urine analysis (routine)
Antinuclear antibodies
Antistreptolysin, rheuma factor
Others (e.g., cryoglobulins)

Allergy tests
Food allergens (intradermal)
Drugs (e.g., penicillin)
In vitro tests (RAST)

Possibly open patch test (contact urticaria)

Table 5.16. Urticaria diagnosis: Step 3 (provocation tests)

History
Elimination and provocation diets

Clinical examination
Skin biopsy with direct immunofluorescence

Laboratory
Complement levels
Thyroid hormones and antibodies
Others

Allergy tests
Avoidance diet
Provocation tests (food challenge)
Oral provocation test for idiosyncrasy (OPTI) with additives and ASA
Autoimmune diagnostics ("Greaves test," antibodies against FcεRI)

5.1.3.6 Therapy

Treatment of acute urticaria is done using H_1 antihistamines [25], in severe cases preferably intravenously (dimetinden maleate or clemastine fumarate); if the patient does not respond glucocorticosteroids (e.g., 100 mg prednisolone) are given. For severe cases see treatment of anaphylaxis (Sect. 5.1.4).

In therapy of chronic urticaria, H_1 antagonists are the first choice [30]. Often they are not dosed adequately [13, 30]. Obviously, the dose to suppress urticaria has to be higher than doses applied for hay fever. During the day, non-sedating antihistamines should be used (fexofenadine, loratadine, desloratadine, mizolastin, cetirizine, levocetirizine); if people suffer from nightly attacks the use of classical sedating antihistamines in the evening is an option (see also Sect. 6.2 on "Pharmacotherapy"). Antihistamines with a mast cell stabilizing effect (ketotifen) are sometimes helpful.

Some patients respond better to a combined use of H_1 plus H_2 antagonists. Doxepin as a tricyclic antidepressant has both H_1 and H_2 antagonizing effects. Antihistamines also showing antiserotonin effects may be helpful in some cases of physical urticaria (cold urticaria) (e.g., cyproheptadiene, hydroxyzine), and some cases of cold urticaria can be improved by parenteral penicillin therapy.

β_2-Adrenergics (e.g., terbutaline) have been found helpful in some cases of chronic urticaria, as has dapsone [14].

Leukotriene antagonists (Montelukast) have been used with controversial effects [15]; a subgroup of patients has been reported to experience possible improvement [7]. Some studies have also recommended using calcium antagonists especially when flush attacks are predominant [15].

Due to the strong psychosomatic interaction in chronic urticaria, tricyclic antidepressants with antihistamine effects (e.g., opipramol) as well as psychosomatic counseling can be helpful.

Systemic glucocorticosteroids should only be used in severe cases together with antihistamines.

In very severe cases (sometimes with a positive autologous serum test and autoantibodies), immunosuppressive treatment (cyclosporin) or high-dose intravenous immunoglobulin G infusions have been effective [9, 23].

In some patients, alterations of the gastrointestinal flora may induce improvement. Braun-Falco recommended the "Munich scheme" with a combination of antibiotic (tetracycline), antimycotic (amphotericin B, nystatin), anthelmintic, and antihistamine followed by restoration of the GI flora with lactobacilli and other agents [1, 4]. When there is evidence of *Helicobacter pylori* involvement, eradication may be helpful.

There is no specific urticaria diet; however, if food allergy has been proven, a specific avoidance diet is indicated (see Sect. 5.1.5 on "Food Allergy).

In rare cases of HANE, androgens like danazol [3, 24] or stanazolol induce an increase in the decreased C1 inhibitor concentration in serum. In acute attacks, purified C1 inactivator can be given as a life-saving infusion. Patients

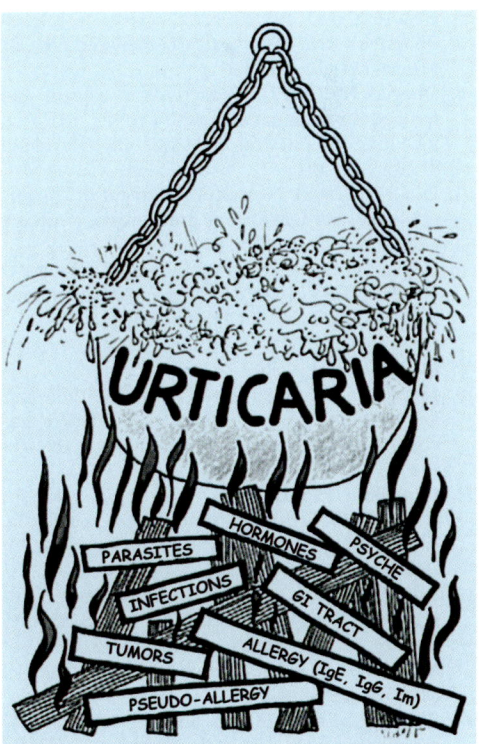

Fig. 5.11. The "witches'" cauldron of urticaria

and physicians need to know where they can get this preparation!

In solar urticaria and mastocytosis, UV hardening (UV-A or PUVA) can be used.

The general principle of any kind of urticaria management is the elimination of triggering or maintaining factors, which keep the process "boiling" (Fig. 5.11)!

References

1. Abeck D, Thomsen S, Plötz S, Ring J (1999) Die Biologische Urtikaria-Therapie. Acta Biol 38:3–23
2. Beissert S, Stauder H, Schwarz T (2000) UVA rush hardening for the treatment of solar urticaria. J Am Acad Dermatol 42:1030–1032
3. Bork K, Witzke G (1989) Long-term prophylaxis with C_1-inhibitor (C_1INH) concentrate in patients with recurrent angioedema caused by hereditary and acquired C_1-inhibitor deficiency. J Allergy Clin Immunol 83:677
4. Braun-Falco O (1976) Entwicklungen in der Dermatologie. In: Braun-Falco O, Marghescu S (eds) Fortschritte der praktischen Dermatologie und Venerologie, vol 8. Springer, Berlin Heidelberg New York, p 417
5. Champion RH (1988) Urticaria then and now. Br J Dermatol 119:427–436
6. Doeglas HMG (1975) Reactions to aspirin and food additives in patients with chronic urticaria, including the physical urticarias. Br J Dermatol 93:135
7. Ellis MH (1998) Successful treatment of chronic urticaria with leukotriene antagonists. J Allergy Clin Immunol 102:876–877
8. Fiebiger E, Hammerschmid F, Stingl G, Maurer D (1998) Anti-FcεRIα autoantibodies in autoimmune-mediated disorders. J Clin Invest 101:243–251
9. Greaves M (2000) Chronic urticaria. J Allergy Clin Immunol 105:664–671
10. Haas N, et al. (1995) Vergleichende Studie zur Häufigkeit, Diagnostik und Therapie der Urtikaria in einer Hautpoliklinik. Allergologie 18:110–113
11. Henz BM (1996) Das Spektrum der Urtikaria. In: Henz BM, Zuberbier T, Grabbe J (eds) Urtikaria. Klinik, Diagnostik, Therapie. Springer, Berlin Heidelberg New York, pp 1–17
12. Hide M, Francis DM, Grattan CE, Hakimi J, Kochan JP, Greaves MW (1993) Autoantibodies against the high-affinity IgE receptor as a cause of histamine release in chronic urticaria. N Engl J Med 328:1599–1604
13. Illig L, Paul E (1978) Die Stellung der Antihistaminika in der Urtikaria-Therapie. Hautarzt 29:407
14. Juhlin L (1981) Modem approaches to treatment of chronic urticaria. In: Ring J, Burg G (eds) New trends in allergy. Springer, Berlin Heidelberg New York, p 279
15. Kaplan AP (1981) The pathogenic basic of urticaria and angioedema: Recent advances. Am J Med 70:755–757
16. Kumar SA, Martin BL (1999) Urticaria and angioedema: diagnostic and treatment considerations. J Am Osteopath Assoc 99 [Suppl]:1–4
17. Leznoff A, Sussmann GL (1989) Syndrome of idiopathic chronic urticaria and angioedema with thyroid autoimmunity: A study of 90 patients. J Allergy Clin Immunol 84:66
18. Leznoff A (1998) Chronic urticaria. Can Fam Physician 44:2170–2176
19. Maibach HI, Johnson HL (1975) Contact urticaria syndrome. Contact urticaria to diethyltoluamide. Arch Dermatol 111:720–730
20. Merk H (1992) Urticaria und Rhinitis allergica: In: Hornbostel H, Kaufmann W, Siegenthaler W (eds) Innere Medizin in Praxis und Klinik, 4th edn. Thieme, Stuttgart, pp 3281–3293
21. Meurer M (1981) Urticaria vasculitis. In: Ring J, Burg G (eds) New trends in allergy. Springer, Berlin Heidelberg New York, pp 148–151
22. Müller J, Vieluf D, Ring J (1993) Schilddrüsenhormone als Amplifikatoren der Histamin-Freisetzung unter Insektengift-Hyposensibilisierung. Allergo J 2 [Suppl 2]:77–80
23. Ollert M, Ring J (2000) Urtikaria und Angioödem. In: Przybilla B, Bergmann K, Ring J (eds) Praktische allergologische Diagnostik. Steinkopff, Darmstadt, pp 328–334
24. Opferkuch W, Kövary PM, Jaeger U, Echternacht-Happle K, Gronemeyer W, Hammar C, Niemczyk H, Rieger C (1981) Clinical aspects and therapy of hereditary angioneurotic edema. In: Ring J, Burg G (eds) New trends in Allergy. Springer, Berlin Heidelberg New York, p 272
25. Paul E, Bödeker R-H (1987) Behandlung der chronischen Urticaria mit Terfenadin und Ranitidin. Allergologie 10:113
26. Ring J, Brockow K, Ollert M, Engst R (1999) Antihistamines in urticaria. Clin Exp Allergy 29 [Suppl 1]:31–37
27. Ring J, Przybilla B (1987) Diagnostik der chronischen Urtikaria. Med Welt 38:256–259
28. Sabroe RA, Grattan CE, Francis DM, Barr RM, Kobza Black A, Greaves MW (1999) The autologous serum skin test: A screening test for autoantibodies in chronic idiopathic urticaria. Br J Dermatol 140:446–452
29. Schäfer T, Ring J (1996) Epidemiology adverse food reactions due to allergy and other forms of hypersensitivity. In: Eisenbrand G et al. (eds) Food allergies and intolerances. DFG, VCH Weinheim, pp 40–54
30. Schmutzler W (1997) Histamin als Mediator allergischer Reaktionen. Allergologie 20:536–542

31. Skrebova N, Takiwaki H, Miyaoka Y, Arase S (2001) Localized heat urticaria: a clinical study using laser Doppler flowmetry. J Dermatol Sci 26:112–118
32. Schrallhammer-Baenkler S, Ring J, Landthaler M (1985) Localized heat urticaria. Arch Dermatol Res 277:406
33. Toubi E, Blant A, Kessel A, Golan TD (1997) Low dose cyclosporin A in the treatment of severe chronic idiopathic urticaria. Allergy 52:312–316
34. Warin RP, Champion RH (1974) Urticaria. Saunders, London
35. Wüthrich B (1989) Therapie der akuten und chronischen Urtikaria und des Quincke-Ödems. Schweiz Rundschau Med 78:576–581
36. Zuberbier T, Henz BM (1996) Diagnostik der Urtikaria. In: Henz BM, Zuberbier T, Grabbe J (eds) Urtikaria. Klinik, Diagnostik, Therapie. Springer, Berlin Heidelberg New York, pp 137–156
37. Zuberbier T, Aberer W, Grabbe J, Hartmann K, Merk H, Ollert M, Rueff F, Wedi B, Wenning J (2004) Diagnostik und Therapie der Urtikaria. Leitlinie der DDG und DGAI. Allergo J (in press)

5.1.4 Anaphylaxis

5.1.4.1 Definition

Anaphylaxis is the maximal variant of allergic immediate-type reaction involving the whole organism. Usually the allergen is transmitted through the blood (by injection or oral ingestion). However, anaphylaxis can also be induced after intense contact with the skin or mucous membrane surfaces (contact urticaria, contact anaphylaxis, also by aeroallergens).

When Richet and Portier (1902) first observed the condition while doing animal experiments on the yacht of the Prince of Monaco and later on in Paris, they wanted to name it "condition without protection" [28]; this was, however, both linguistically and pathophysiologically wrong ("without protection" should have been "aphylaxis"). Today anaphylaxis is best translated as "excessively deviated defense reaction" ("ανα" = up, over; "φυλαξ" = guardian, protection).

Some authors restrict the term anaphylaxis to IgE-mediated reactions. However, there are other mechanisms such as immune complex anaphylaxis by circulating IgG or IgM antibodies (e.g., against IgA or dextran); furthermore, there are non-immunological reactions leading to identical clinical symptoms (see Sect. 5.7.2 on "Pseudo-allergy"). Therefore the term "anaphylactoid reaction" is also used as a clinical entity before pathophysiological investigations can be done [31].

Recently, the term anaphylaxis has been defined as also comprising non-immune reactions as a "maximal variant of an acute generalized hypersensitivity reaction" [15]. With this definition, the term "anaphylactoid" becomes superfluous.

5.1.4.2 Clinical Symptomatology and Elicitors

Clinically, anaphylaxis represents a syndrome of different symptoms involving different organs which may develop either alone or simultaneously or subsequently. The acute occurrence is characteristic, and the rapid progression within a few minutes is according to route of contact and resorption characteristics.

Case Report. Patient M.H., female, 53 years old, received an infusion of 5% human serum albumin on the 3rd day after colectomy. After a few minutes, the patient complained of nausea, and on the face and the trunk patchy wheals developed. At the same time, tachycardia and hypotension were present. The doctor starting the infusion was still present and stopped the infusion after 30 ml and replaced it with physiological saline. The patient became unconscious, blood pressure was no longer measurable, peripheral pulses were not palpable, and there was no carotid pulse. Cardiac noises were no longer audible. Immediate resuscitation including cardiac massage, artificial respiration, oxygen and volume replacement together with 500 mg prednisolone i.v. led to a restoration of the cardiac and respiratory function. The patient survived this severe anaphylactic reaction (grade IV) without sequelae [31].

For this example, human serum albumin as elicitor was selected on purpose to show that practically there is no "a priori" innocent drug in allergy! Of course some drugs have a higher and some a lower risk of anaphylaxis. In the United States 100–500 fatalities annually are attributed to penicillin (see Sect. 6.7 on "Drug Allergy"). Apart from drugs, foods (e.g., nuts, celery, poppy seeds, rarely also ethanol [25], fish, etc.) can elicit anaphylaxis. Insect venom anaphylaxis will be considered in a separate section (Sect. 5.1.6).

Aeroallergens or vapors (e.g., fish odor) may elicit anaphylaxis in highly sensitized individuals as well as contact urticariogens (contact anaphylaxis against rubber gloves, ointments, or in the open patch test) [33]. Similarly, all the elicitors of physical urticaria (see Sect. 5.1.3) may in severe cases lead to anaphylaxis (anaphylactic shock in the solarium in solar urticaria). Finally, so-called "idiopathic anaphylaxis" exists where people suffer repeatedly from anaphylactic episodes without clear-cut reasons, sometimes following exercise [32, 36].

Not infrequently, the combination of different simultaneously acting stimuli (e.g., exercise or psychological stress together with certain otherwise tolerated foods) elicit a reaction which we call "summation anaphylaxis" [21, 32]. Beta-blockers may enhance anaphylaxis [13].

Symptoms of anaphylaxis comprise mainly:

- The skin (itch, flush, urticaria, angioedema) and the neighboring mucous membranes; itchy palms, paresthesia in the pharynx, or genital mucosa are often the first symptoms
- The respiratory tract (sneezing, rhinorrhea, hoarseness, dysphonia, laryngeal edema, cough, bronchospasm, respiratory arrest)
- Abdominal symptoms (nausea, cramps, vomitus, defecation, also miction and uterus cramps occur)
- The cardiovascular system (tachycardia, blood pressure changes – not necessarily hypotension, but also transient hypertension has been observed as first symptoms – arrhythmia, shock, cardiac arrest). Primary cardiac manifestation in anaphylaxis has been observed in ECG changes (T-flattening, supraventricular arrhythmia, AV block) [20, 24, 43, 44]. Marked changes of central-venous pressure are common [39]. During anaphylaxis, myocardial infarction may occur [1, 6, 24, 31, 34, 43].

Prodromi of anaphylaxis comprise paresthesia on palms and soles, metallic "fishy" taste, anxiety, sweating, headache, or disorientation.

According to the intensity of anaphylactic symptoms, a severity grading from I to IV has proven helpful (Table 5.17) [30].

Table 5.17. Severity grading of anaphylactic reactions (according to [30])

Grade	Skin	Abdomen	Airways	Cardiovascular system
I	Itch Flush Urticaria Angioedema	–	–	–
II	Itch Flush Urticaria Angioedema (not obligatory)	Nausea Cramps	Rhinorrhea Hoarseness Dyspnea	Tachycardia (>20/min) Hypotension (>20 mm Hg syst.) Arrhythmia
III	Itch Flush Urticaria Angioedema (not obligatory)	Vomitus Defecation	Laryngeal edema Bronchospasm Cyanosis	Shock
IV	Itch Flush Urticaria Angioedema (not obligatory)	Vomitus Defecation	Respiratory arrest	Cardiac arrest

Autopsy of fatal cases has shown few specific findings; sometimes there is inflation of the lung, and pulmonary edema with peribronchial eosinophilic infiltrates. Sometimes hemorrhages in the gastric mucosa as well as hepatosplenomegaly are reported [1]. In immune complex anaphylaxis, fibrinoid deposits in the lung have been observed [38].

Some authors define anaphylaxis exclusively by the occurrence of cardiovascular symptoms. For these cases, of course, grade I and II will be missed, which, however, often turn into more severe anaphylaxis at the next contact. Rohrer and Pichler examined 118 patients with cardiovascular involvement and found skin symptoms in 88 %, respiratory reactions in 72 %, and gastrointestinal symptoms in 44 % [35].

5.1.4.3 Pathophysiology

Classical anaphylaxis is mediated by IgE antibodies on the surface of mast cells and basophil leukocytes, which after bridging with an at least bivalent allergen trigger the secretion reaction of preformed and newly synthesized mediators (see Chap. 2). In spite of our knowledge of mast cell activation and IgE antibodies, the exact mechanisms of amplification are not yet understood, which make it possible that a healthy individual may be killed by a few micrograms of an allergen within minutes.

The extent of mediator release reaction differs between individuals but also in one and the same individual at different times. The term "releasability" describes this phenomenon. Factors influencing releasability comprise cyclic nucleotides, cytokines, psychoneurogenic (autonomic nervous transmitters, neuropeptides) and hormonal influences (e.g., thyroid). Among the cytokines, interleukin-3 has special importance in priming mast cells and basophils and enhancing releasability. These phenomena are not only of scientific interest, but gain practical relevance in helping to explain the often confusing variability of symptomatology underlying the term "summation" or "augmentation anaphylaxis" (see below).

Apart from IgE, other antibody classes may elicit anaphylactic reactions: There is immune complex anaphylaxis with high concentrations of circulating IgG or IgM antibodies with complement activation and formation of anaphylatoxins. Clinical examples are anaphylactic reactions after blood products, e.g., in IgA-deficient persons after plasma replacement, anaphylaxis in serum sickness, or after xenogenic proteins (antilymphocyte serum) as well as dextran anaphylaxis [17, 29, 31, 38].

Besides immunological there are non-immune mechanisms, which will be considered in Sect. 5.7.2 on "Pseudo-allergic Reactions."

Neuropsychogenic reflex mechanisms should be considered especially when we know that psychic stress alone can lead to increased plasma histamine (see Chap. 7 on "Psyche and Allergy").

In the end phase of an anaphylactic reaction, similar mechanisms lead to clinical symptoms: postcapillary plasma exudation and microcirculatory disturbance leads to decreased capillary pressure and perfusion [9, 22].

Mast cell dependent anaphylactic reactions occur with an increase of mast cell tryptase in the serum (see Chap. 4), which can be detected even hours (sometimes also postmortem) after a reaction [3].

The mediator release reaction from mast cells and basophils is not a cytolytic process but energy, calcium, and temperature dependent and can be inhibited by specific antagonists (e.g., via cAMP-elevating agents) (see Chap. 2). The concomitant use of beta-blockers and possibly also angiotensin-converting enzyme inhibitors (ACE inhibitors) may lead to an enhancement of anaphylactic symptoms [13]. In patients with insect venom anaphylaxis, we found a significant inverse correlation between the plasma angiotensin II level and the severity of anaphylactic symptoms in history [14]. Under allergen-specific immunotherapy, the previously lowered angiotensin II levels normalized [14].

5.1.4.4 Allergens and Elicitors

The most common elicitors of anaphylaxis are drugs, proteins, foods, aeroallergens, additives, body fluids, latex, microbial antigens, but also physical factors (Table 5.18).

Table 5.18. Elicitors of anaphylactic reactions

Drugs (all forms!)
Additives
Foods
Occupational agents (e.g., latex)
Insect venoms
Aeroallergens
Contact urticariogens
Seminal fluid
Echinococcal cysts
Cold, heat, UV radiation
Exercise
Summation (infection, stress, exercise, other allergen concomitant exposure, medication as β-blockers, NSAIDs, ACE inhibitors, etc.)
Idiopathic (?)
Underlying diseases:
C1 inactivator deficiency
Systemic mastocytosis

Table 5.19. Differential diagnosis of anaphylaxis

Pharmacologic-toxic effects
Cramps
Syncope (cardial, cerebral)
Pulmonary embolism
Bolus aspiration
Hypoglycemia
Hyperventilation
Vasovagal reflexes
Vocal cord dysfunction
Hysterical fit
"Anaphylaxis factitia" (Münchhausen's syndrome)

Rare cases of passive transfer of IgE antibodies via blood transfusion as well as suicide attempts (penicillin-allergic nurse) have been reported. Murder has been attempted by eliciting anaphylaxis in the detective literature. Also anaphylaxis factitia ("Münchhausen's syndrome") exists [I remember the case of a 17-year-old girl with repeated severe anaphylactic (grade III and IV) episodes on the basis of serious somatoform disturbance]. Epidemiology of anaphylaxis mostly focuses on the elicitors. The rate of drug-induced anaphylaxis ranges from 0.001% up to 10% per dose applied [2, 31]. Rarer reactions have been observed after poppy seeds, beer (hops and barley), but also due to ethanol [25].

The elicitor of anaphylaxis may be transmitted to the organism via the air (fish allergens in vapors around fish stores, latex allergens in rooms decorated with air balloons). The application of an ointment on unlesional skin may elicit contact anaphylaxis in sensitized individuals [33]. In recent years, increasing reports describe patients who only suffer anaphylaxis after combined action of different stimuli, for instance, physical exercise, mental or emotional stress, acute infection, or concomitant exposure against other relevant allergens. We call this phenomenon "summation" or "augmentation anaphylaxis" and think that it may be much more common than generally suspected. Possibly, this type of reaction is the rule and that explains why fortunately many sensitized individuals tolerate allergen contact without clinical incompatibility symptoms! We believe that many cases of so-called idiopathic anaphylaxis may thus be explaianed [32, 45].

5.1.4.5 Diagnosis and Differential Diagnosis

The clinical symptomatology of anaphylaxis is so characteristic that diagnosis usually is not difficult. Nevertheless several differential diagnoses need to be considered (Table 5.19).

Patients having survived an anaphylaxis have to undergo allergy diagnosis! This diagnostic procedure has three aims:

1. Determination of the eliciting agent
2. Description of the relevant pathomechanism (e.g., IgE)
3. Offering of a compatible alternative (see Sect. 5.7 on "Drug Allergy").

5.1.4.6 Prophylaxis and Therapy

For prophylaxis (Table 5.20), abstaining from polypragmatic pharmacotherapy is as important as the endeavors of the pharmaceutical industry to produce better and less allergenic drugs.

Knowledge of possible complications is the best basis for successful therapy. Being prepared for such complications enables one to react more quickly. This also implies knowledge of additives (stabilizers, preservatives, colorings, etc.) in drugs against which people can react.

The question regarding adverse drug reactions in the history allows the risk groups to be pinpointed. The importance of atopic diathesis

Table 5.20. Prophylaxis of anaphylactic reactions

Exact diagnosis
Avoidance strategies
Information from the patient ("allergy passport")
Strict indication for pharmacotherapy
Avoidance of β-blockers
If possible oral administration
Observance of the patient after injection
"Prophetic" testing in selected cases
Hyposensitization (or "adaptive deactivation")
Tolerance induction
Hapten inhibition
Premedication (e.g., with histamine H_1 and H_2 antagonists or antihistamines plus steroids)
Emergency set (for self-medication)

as a risk factor is controversial and is probably limited to IgE-mediated reactions.

Only in a few cases is specific prophylaxis possible such as induction of tolerance against xenogenic immunoglobulin in heterologous protein therapy [31] or by hapten inhibition in dextran anaphylaxis [17, 29, 31].

The combined administration of H_1 and H_2 antagonists or antihistamines together with glucocorticosteroids is recommended for the prophylaxis of anaphylactoid reactions after volume substitutes or radiographic contrast media [19] (see Sect. 5.7.2 on "Pseudo-allergic Reactions").

Observation of the patient in the first minutes after parenteral drug administration is the basis of prophylaxis. *General rule: The more severe the anaphylactic symptoms to be expected, the sooner they will become manifest!* Of course, there are exceptions from the rule in the form of "tricky" late anaphylactic reactions after several hours [31, 41]; often, however, mild symptoms occur within the first 20 min which tend to be overlooked.

5.1.4.7 Therapy

The treatment of anaphylaxis follows the severity of symptoms (Fig. 5.12). If the reaction only involves the skin (urticaria) with a stable cardiovascular system, antihistamines may be sufficient. In any case, an intravenous catheter should be placed and an infusion prepared.

If the reaction proceeds (and the differential diagnosis is easy!) glucocorticoids and epinephrine (0.3 mg i.m., in children 0.1 mg/kg body wt.) should be given, in dyspnea together with theophylline (0.24–0.48 mg) plus $β_2$-adrenergics.

In fully developed anaphylactic shock, the general principles of shock therapy are applied [8, 10, 11, 22, 26, 27, 37, 42]. Epinephrine can be given intravenously (dilute the commercial ampule 1 ml in 10 ml saline for slow infusion of 1–3 ml under pulse control; if needed, up to 10 ml and more) or more practically subcutaneously. In patients on β-blockers, i.v. glucagon

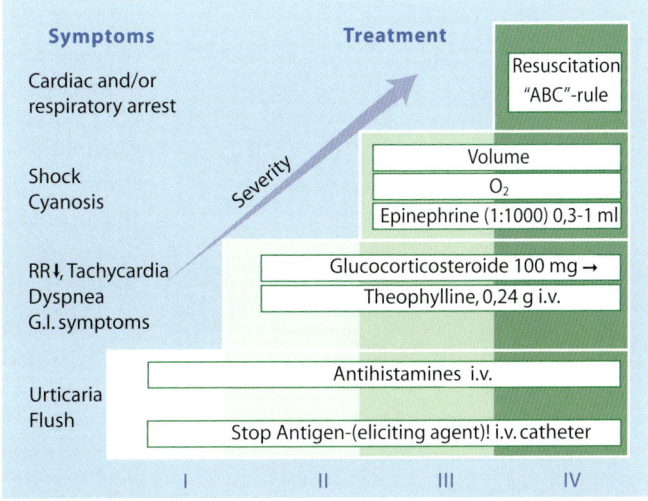

Fig. 5.12. Immediate action to be taken in the event of anaphylactic reactions of varying severity

(1–2 mg) is beneficial [46] in restoring β-receptor responsiveness. For self-medication, epinephrine as autoinjector ("Epi-pen" or "Fastject") is recommended. The undoubted effect of epinephrine, however, does not guarantee a successful outcome: in spite of early epinephrine, fatal anaphylactic reactions have been observed [18]. Furthermore, epinephrine may induce severe cardiac arrhythmia until ventricular fibrillation occurs especially in elderly patients [4, 23, 39, 40, 44].

In severe hypotension, intensive volume replacement (e.g., crystalloids or hydroxyethyl starch up to 1,000 ml as rapid infusion) is vital. Levarterenol [12], metaraminol, or dopamine may also be applied. In grade IV reactions (cardiac or respiratory arrest), only immediate and adequate resuscitation measures are life-saving [8] (Table 5.21).

In addition to the classical rule of resuscitation (ABC rule), the treatment of severe anaphylaxis requires the AAC rule (Fig. 5.13) [31].

The use of glucocorticosteroids in anaphylaxis is controversial (see references cited in [31, 34]). Steroids need some time until they act (approximately 15 min). They are not as useful for monotherapy as antihistamines in the treatment of grade I and II reactions. Possibly, H_2 antagonists have an additional beneficial effect in anaphylaxis [7]. We recommend in severe anaphylaxis the additional administration of high-dose glucocorticosteroids (e.g., 1 g prednisolone i.v.), if only to avoid late complications [31].

The necessary emergency equipment for treatment of anaphylaxis is listed in Table 5.22.

Patients who have suffered an anaphylactic reaction of grade III and IV should be kept un-

Table 5.21. Basic rules of resuscitation

Diagnosis (evaluation of severity, carotid pulses)
Airways (clearing and respiration)
Oxygen
Call help (get someone to call)
Cardiac massage/respiration
Venous catheter plus volume therapy (pressure infusion)
Intubation
ECG (?)
Defibrillation (?)
Pharmacotherapy (epinephrine, sodium bicarbonate, dopamine, lidocaine, possibly atropine, etc.)

Table 5.22. Emergency equipment for the allergist's office

Tourniquet, disinfectant
Syringes, cannulas, infusion sets, connecting pieces
Blood pressure, stethoscope
Laryngoscope
Guedel and intratracheal tubes (size 0–5 Guedel, 28–32 Wendel, 3–8 mm intratracheal)
Oxygen
Breathing masks (for children and adults)
Ventilation device (Ambu)
Suction pump
ECG (possibly with defibrillator)
Infusion solutions (NaCl, human serum albumin, hydroxyethyl starch, sodium bicarbonate)
Antihistamines (e.g., clemastine, dimetinden, ranitidine ampules)
Glucocorticosteroids (e.g., prednisolone hemisuccinate 250 mg, triamcinolone 1 g)
Atropine (0.5-mg ampules)
Theophylline (0.24-g ampules)
Epinephrine (e.g., Suprarenin ampules = epinephrine 1:1,000)
Beta-adrenergics (e.g., fenoterol, salbutamol)
Glucagon (ampules)
Spasmolytics (e.g., diazepam)
Antiemetics (e.g., metoclopramide)
Analgesics (tramadol)
Antihypertensives (α-blockers)
Antiarrhythmics (lidocaine 2% ampules, digoxin ampules)
Calcium ampules, glucose ampules, saline, aqua dest. ampules

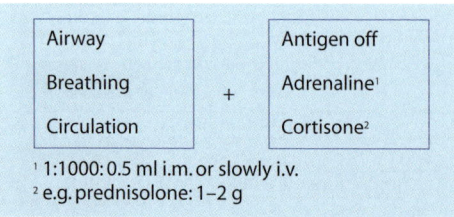

[1] 1:1000: 0.5 ml i.m. or slowly i.v.
[2] e.g. prednisolone: 1–2 g

Fig. 5.13. The "AAC Rule"

der supervision in hospital at least overnight; occasional cases of "late shock," e.g., second anaphylactic episode after 6–12 h, are dangerous complications [31, 40]. These patients also represent a risk group for skin testing, which should only be done under emergency conditions.

References

1. Barnard JH (1973) Studies of 400 Hymenoptera sting deaths in the United States. J Allergy Clin Immunol 52:259–264
2. Bochner BS, Lichtenstein LM (1991) Anaphylaxis. N Engl J Med 324:81–88
3. Brockow K, Kiehn M, Riehtmüller C, Vieluf D, Berger J, Ring J (1997) Efficacy of antihistamine pretreatment in the prevention of adverse reactions to Hymenoptera venom immunotherapy: a prospective randomized placebo-controlled trial. J Allergy Clin Immunol 100:458–463
4. Brown MJ, Brown DC, Murphy MB (1983) Hypokalemia from beta-2-receptor stimulation by circulating epinephrine. N Engl J Med 309:1414–1419
5. Capurro N, Levi R (1975) The heart as target organ in systemic allergic reactions. Circ Res 36:520–528
6. Delage C, Irey HC (1972) Anaphylactic deaths: a clinicopathologic study of 43 cases. J Forens Sci 17:525
7. De Soto H, Turk P (1989) Cimetidine in anaphylactic shock refractory to standard therapy. Anesth Analg 69:264–265
8. Eisenberg MS, Mengest TJ (2001) Cardiac resuscitation. N Engl J Med 344:1304–1313
9. Endrich B, Ring J, Intaglietta M (1979) Effects of radiopaque contrast media on the microcirculation of the rabbit omentum. Radiology 132:331–339
10. Fisher MMD (1986) Clinical observations on the pathophysiology and treatment of anaphylactic cardiovascular collapse. Anesth Intensive Care 17:17–21
11. Fuchs E, Ferlinz R (1986) Allergische Krankheiten. In: Wolff HR v, Weihrauch TR (eds) Internistische Therapie, 6th edn. Urban und Schwarzenberg, Munich, pp 275–288
12. Gronemeyer W (1980) Noradrenalin statt Adrenalin beim anaphylaktischen Schock. Dtsch Med Wochenschr 102:101
13. Hannaway PJ, Hoppler GDK (1983) Severe anaphylaxis and drug induced beta-blockage. N Engl J Med 308:1536
14. Hermann K, Ring J (1997) The renin-angiotensin system in patients with repeated anaphylactic reactions during Hymenoptera venom hyposensitization and sting challenge. Int Arch Allergy Immunol 11:251–156
15. Johansson SGO, Hourihane JOB, Bousquet J, Bruijnzeel-Koomen, Dreborg S, Haahtela T, Kowalski ML, Mygind N, Ring J, van Cauwenberge P, van Hage-Hamsten M, Wüthrich B (2001) A revised nomenclature for allergy. An EAACI position statement from the EAACI nomenclature task force. Allergy 56:813–824
16. Kleinhans D (1987) Anstrengungs-induzierte Urtikaria und Anaphylaxie. Med Klein 82:103–104
17. Laubenthal H (1986) Dextrananaphylaxie, Pathomechanismus und Prophylaxe. Ergebnisse einer multizentrischen Studie. Springer, Berlin Heidelberg New York
18. Lockey RF, Benedict LM, Turkeltaub TB, Bukantz SC (1987) Fatalities from immunotherapy (IT) and skin testing (ST). J Allergy Clin Immunol 79:666–677
19. Lorenz W, Doenicke A, Dittmann I, Hug P, Schwarz B (1977) Anaphylaktoide Reaktionen nach Applikation von Blutersatzmitteln beim Menschen. Verhinderung dieser Nebenwirkung von Haemaccel durch Praemedikation mit H_1- und H_2-Antagonisten. Anaesthesist 26:644
20. Marone G, Patelle V, Crescanzo A de, Genovese M (1995) Human heart mast cells in anaphylaxis and cardiovascular disease. Int Arch Allergy Immunol 107:72–75
21. Maulitz RM, Pratt DS, Schocket AL (1979) Exercise-induced anaphylactic reaction to shellfish. J Allergy Clin Immunol 63:433
22. Meßmer K (1983) Plasma substitutes and indications for their use. In: Tinker J, Rapin M (eds) Care of the critically ill patient. Springer, Berlin Heidelberg New York, pp 569–575
23. Müller U (2001) Spätkomplikationen bei Anaphylaxie. In: Ring J, Darsow U (eds) "Allergie 2000: Probleme, Strategien und praktische Konsequenzen". Dustri, Munich, pp 249–252
24. Pavek K, Wegmann A, Nordström L, Schwander D (1982) Cardiovascular and respiratory mechanisms in anaphylactic and anaphylactoid shock reactions. Klin Wochenschr 60:941–947
25. Przybilla B, Ring J (1983) Anaphylaxis to ethanol and sensitization to acetic acid. Lancet 1:483
26. Pumphrey RS (2000) Lessons for management of anaphylaxis from a study of fatal reactions. Clin Exp Allergy 30:1144–1150
27. Reimers A, Müller U (2000) Behandlung des anaphylaktischen Schocks. Ther Umschau 58:325–328
28. Richet C (1904) De l'anaphylaxie ou sensibilite croissante des organismes a des doses successives de poison. Arch Fisiol 1:129
29. Richter W, Hedin H, Ring J, Kraft D, Messmer K (1980) Anaphylaktoide Reaktionen nach Dextran I. Immunologische Grundlagen und klinische Befunde. Allergologie 3:9
30. Ring J, Messmer K (1977) Incidence and severity

of anaphylactoid reactions to colloid volume substitutes. Lancet 1:466–468
31. Ring J (1978) Anaphylaktoide Reaktionen nach Infusion natürlicher und künstlicher Kolloide. Springer, Berlin Heidelberg New York
32. Ring J, Darsow U (2002) Idiopathic anaphylaxis. Curr Allergy Asthma Rep 2:40–45
33. Ring J, Galosi A, Przybilla B (1986) Contact anaphylaxis from emulgade F. Contact Dermatitis 15:49–40
34. Ring J, Behrendt H (1999) Anaphylaxis and anaphylactoid reactions. Classification and pathophysiology. Clin Rev Allergy Immunol 17:387–399
35. Rohrer CL, Pichler WJ, Helbling A, et al. (1998) Anaphylaxie: Klinik, Ätiologie und Verlauf bei 118 Patienten. Schweiz Med Wochenschr 128:53–63
36. Sheffer AL, Austen KF (1980) Exercise-induced anaphylaxis. J Allergy Clin Immunol 66:106
37. Simons FE, Gu X, Johnston LM, Simons KJ (2000) Can epinephrine inhalations be substituted for epinephrine injection in children at risk for systemic anaphylaxis? Pediatrics 106:1040–1044
38. Smedegard G, Revenäs B, Arfors KE (1979) Anaphylaxis in the monkey: hemodynamics and blood flow distribution. Acta Physiol Scand 106:191
39. Smith PL, Kagey-Sobotka A, Blecker ER, Traystman R, Kaplan AP, Gralink H, Valentine MD, Permut S, Lichtenstein LM (1980) Physiologic manifestations of human anaphylaxis. J Clin Invest 60:1072
40. Sullivan TJ (1982) Cardiac disorders in penicillin-induced anaphylaxis: association with intravenous epinephrine therapy. J Am Med Assoc 248:2161
41. Stark BJ, Sullivan TJ (1986) Biphasic and protracted anaphylaxis. J Allergy Clin Immunol 78:76–83
42. Tryba M, Ahnefeld FW, Barth J, Dick W, Doenicke A, Fuchs T, Gervais H, Laubenthal H, Löllgen H, Lorenz W, Mehrkens HH, Meuret GH, Möllmann H, Piepenbrock S, Przybilla B, Ring J, Schmutzler W, Schultze-Werninghaus G, Schüttler J, Schuster JP, Sefrin P, Zander J, Zenz M (1994) Akuttherapie anaphylaktoider Reaktionen. Ergebnisse einer interdisziplinären Konsensuskonferenz. Allergo J 3:211–222
43. Waldhausen E, Keser G, Marquardt B (1987) Der anaphylaktische Schock. Anästhesist 36:150–158
44. Wegmann A, Reuker H, Pavek K, Schwander D (1983) Katecholamintherapie und Herzrhythmusstörungen im anaphylaktischen und anaphylaktoiden Schock. Anaesthesist 32 [Suppl]:320
45. Wiggins CA, Dykowicz MS, Patterson R (1988) Idiopathic anaphylaxis. Classification, evaluation and treatment of 123 patients. J Allergy Clin Immunol 82:849–855
46. Zaloga GP, Delacey W, Holmboe E, Chernow B (1986) Glucagon reversal of hypotension in a case of anaphylactoid shock. Ann Intern Med 105: 65–66

5.1.5 Food Allergy and Other Adverse Food Reactions

5.1.5.1 Classification and Symptomatology

Adverse food reactions represent an increasing problem in allergy practice. The clinical symptoms range from nausea, vomiting, abdominal pain, gastroenteritis, diarrhea, urticaria, asthmoid complaints, allergic rhinitis to full anaphylaxis or serum sickness type reactions with arthralgia and vasculitis [9, 26, 42, 67–70] (Table 5.23).

As in all fields of allergology, clinically similar but pathophysiologically different non-immunologically elicited conditions (pseudo-allergic reactions) need to be distinguished Table 5.24); in this chapter, particularly enzyme deficiency (e.g., lactase) as well as toxic effects of contaminants (bacterial toxins) should be considered. Diseases due to malnutrition will not be covered here [11, 12, 48, 51].

Table 5.23. Clinical manifestation of adverse food reactions

Skin	Panniculitis?
Itching	Melkersson-Rosenthal
Flushing	Syndrome?
Urticaria	
Angioedema	**Eye and airways**
Atopic eczema	Rhinoconjunctivitis
Lip swelling and swelling	Laryngeal edema
of oral mucosa	Bronchial asthma
Stomatitis, glossitis	
(papillitis linguae)	**Gastrointestinal tract**
Relapsing aphthae	Nausea
Immune complex vascu-	Vomiting
litis	Meteorism
Purpura pigmentosa	Acute gastroenteritis
progressiva	Diarrhea
Hematogenous (system-	Colitis?
ic) contact dermatitis	**Cardiovascular system**
Protein contact dermatitis	Anaphylaxis
Phototoxic and photo-	
allergic reactions	
Exanthematous eruptions	
Dermatitis herpetifor-	
mis Duhring (gluten)	

Table 5.24. Classification of adverse food reactions

Mechanism	Allergy IgE	IgG/M	IgA (?)	Lympho-cytes	Mediator release	Enzyme defects	Pseudo-allergy/intolerance
Examples	Immediate reaction	Serum sickness	Gluten-sensitive enteropathy	Cellular allergy	Colorings, preservatives, salicylates	Lactase • Inherited • Secondary Galactokinase Gal-1-PO_4 Uridyltransferase	Poisons, histamine Serotonin, catecholamines, psychoactive substances
Clinical symptoms: (selection)	Urticaria, anaphylaxis, diarrhea Colics Anaphylaxis (atopic eczema)	Vasculitis, arthralgia	Diarrhea, malabsorption	Systemic contact Contact dermatitis Exanthematous eruption Colitis (?) Diarrhea	Urticaria, angioedema Anaphylaxis	Diarrhea, malabsorption Blood pressure changes	Anaphylaxis/anaphylactoid reaction Mental confusion (?)

Food allergies manifest frequently on the skin (60%), the GI tract (20%), the airways (20%) and the cardiovascular system (10–15%) [29]. Food-induced contact urticaria or contact dermatitis represent special forms.

Adverse food reactions are a frequent problem (Sect. 3.1.2).

Few fields of allergology have comparable difficulties with parascientific practices such as food allergy, especially when patients only suffer from subjective complaints elicited through foods (tension, fatigue, behavioral changes, etc.). The movement of "clinical ecology" has focused interest on so-called allergic reactions against pollutant chemicals especially in foods manifesting as psychiatric diseases [14, 19] (see Sect. 5.10 on "Eco-syndrome").

5.1.5.2 Food Allergens

The most common food allergens in Central Europe are cow's milk, hen's eggs, nuts, spices, vegetables, cereals, fish, meat, and fruits. Regional, ethnic-cultural aspects play an important role as well as age and underlying diseases.

Of practical importance are cross-reactions between different fruits (e.g., apple, peach, cherry) and tree pollen (e.g., hazel, birch, alder) as well as between mugwort pollen and spices (anis, curry, etc.) and celery (see Sect. 3.3.4 on "Allergens") [1, 57, 67].

Food allergens may be altered by preparatory procedures (e.g., boiling) [20]. Many allergens, however, are relatively resistant to pH changes, heat, and proteases.

IgE-inducing food allergens are glycoproteins. Small chemicals may elicit systemic contact dermatitis (e.g., nickel, fragrances) [32]. Elicitors of pseudo-allergic reactions comprise additives and biogenic amines [29, 31, 39].

Gene Technology and Food Allergy. Gene technology can lead to food changes of allergological relevance. This can be either as increased risk as in the introduction of the major allergen of Brazil nuts into soy [38] or as chance (production of hypoallergenic rice). The recommendations of the German Society for Allergology and Clinical Immunology (DGAI) regarding gene technology and foods are listed in Table 5.31.

In the following, the most important food allergens are briefly discussed:

Cow's Milk. Milk is the secretion product of the mammary glands of mammals. The species

Table 5.25. Dietary recommendations employed in food allergy and other adverse food reactions

1. Diagnostic diets
Allergy diet no. 1 ("allergen-free"): short-term, up to 10 days, prior to provocation or after acute reaction
Allergy diet no. 2 ("allergen-poor"): up to 3 weeks, basis for provocation tests
Allergy diet no. 3 ("additive-free"): can be given over months, basis for provocation with additives
2. Stepwise diets (diagnostic and therapeutic)
Stepwise elimination (interval days or weeks)
Stepwise provocation (interval days or weeks)
3. Therapeutic diets
Specific allergen avoidance
Additive-free diet (hypersensitivity to additives)
Nickel- or fragrance-free diet (in patients with positive oral provocation test and systemic contact dermatitis)
Gluten-free diet (in sprue, dermatitis herpetiformis)
4. Prophylactic diets (general antiallergic diet)
Breastfeeding in infants
Hydrolyzed cow's milk formula
Hypoallergenic (oligoantigenic) diet of the mother during lactation

is important. Plant extracts should not be falsely called "milk" (e.g., "soy milk"). Cow's milk contains up to 30–35 g protein/ml, 80% of which is casein and 20% whey protein (beta-lactoglobulin, alpha-lactalbumin, bovine serum albumin, as well as immunoglobulins). The most common allergens are whey proteins (beta-lactoglobulins) but also casein, which is not species-specific and shows cross reactions between cattle, goat, sheep, etc. During milk preparation, whey proteins remain in solution while casein coagulates; in spite of this, whey proteins may be present in cheese or butter as well as casein in whey. Casein is heat-stable, whereas whey proteins are partly denatured.

Allergenic proteins may be denatured to different degrees by hydrolysis, leading to so-called hypoallergenic infant formulas. The term "hypoallergenic" is not well defined. One distinguishes between prophylactically hypoallergenic preparations (a low degree of hydrolysis) and strongly hydrolyzed products, which can be used for therapy of cow's milk allergic individuals. This needs to be evaluated using a prick test [3].

Cross reactions between cow's milk and beef or veal are possible but rare (most likely due to BSA). Allergies against horse mare's milk (also after topical application) can occur.

The common dietary recommendation of pork avoidance in allergic individuals or atopics is rarely based on manifest allergy, but is rather of historic, cultural origin.

Hen's Eggs. Specific IgE antibodies against hen's eggs are the best marker of atopy risk in the newborn (even if the child has been exclusively breast-fed); obviously, small amounts of allergens reach the infant through the maternal nutrition and breast milk. The major allergen is ovomucoid (Gal d 1) from the clear part besides ovalbumin (Gal d 2) and ovotransferrin (Gal d 3) and lysozyme (Gal d 4). In the yellow part of the egg, livetin, apovitillin, and vosviten can be found, which may play a role in adult hen's egg allergics. Cross-sensitizations between hen's eggs and poultry meat (chicken, turkey, duck, goose) have been described.

Cereals. Here we have to distinguish between the food and the respiratory allergy (in bakers). It is interesting that most asthmatic flour-allergic bakers may be able to eat cereals without problems. Cross-reactions between different flours are less frequent than between pollen allergens of the same species. The most frequent cereal allergy is wheat allergy; patients are not required to avoid other cereals. In one-fourth of patients cross-reactions exist to grass pollen and other cereal flours without symptoms of food allergy. Cereals may elicit exacerbation of atopic eczema which may be diagnosed using the atopy patch test (see Sect. 5.5.3).

Vegetables/Fruit. Many patients with pollen allergy are also allergic against fruit and vegetables on the basis of the known cross-reactions (see Sect. 3.4). The relevant plant proteins exert different functions (hydrolases, carrier proteins, enzyme inhibitors, stress proteins).

One of the most common pathogenesis-related proteins is the major allergen from birch pollen (Bet v 1), which is not only present in pollen of different trees (hazel, alder, oak, beech, etc.) but also in foods (apple, prunes, carrots, nuts, celery). It is heat-sensitive. Many apple-allergic individuals tolerate apple mousse. Bet v 2 = profillin as a structural protein is heat-stable [13].

Celery represents a major problem for many food-allergic individuals; minute amounts may elicit severe reactions (anaphylaxis) (e.g., celery salt in salad).

Patients with latex allergy often show cross-sensitization to certain foods such as kiwifruit, avocado, buckwheat, chestnut, and lychee.

Among the legumes, the most common allergens are soy and peanut (peanuts are not nuts!). Severe reactions to minute amounts of peanut allergen in other foods prepared in the same machines where peanut butter has been prepared have been reported.

Soy not only is a relevant allergen for children (supplement for cow's milk) but also for adults. Often, allergic individuals do not recognize soy in the food ("hidden allergens") (allergic reactions to peas and lentils are rather rare).

Fish and Seafood. Fish allergy is especially common in populations on the coast. The first chemically defined food allergen was the major allergen of codfish (Gad c 1) [1]. There are multiple cross-reactivities to other fish but rarely to crustaceans and mollusks. The fish allergen is very heat-stable and also volatile (patients with severe asthmatic reaction and anaphylaxis over 50 m distance from a fish food store).

While seafood represents a delicacy in some countries, it is a basic food for large populations of the world. The major allergen of shrimps (Met e 1) corresponds chemically to a tropomyosin and shows cross-reactivity to some arthropods (housedust mites).

5.1.5.3 Pathomechanisms

Little is known about the mechanism of sensitization in food allergy [2, 24, 25, 56]. Apart from the genetic predisposition, acute inflammatory diseases of the gut may play a role in the development of food allergy perhaps through enhanced resorption as well as absorption-enhancing substances (alcohol, spices) or hectic and excessive monoalimentation (e.g., case of hen's egg allergy after the intake of 24 raw eggs during a bet) [66].

Immune reactions play a role in normal gastrointestinal physiology; this has been shown in experiments when sensitized dogs digested orally applied proteins much better, probably due to gastrin release, stimulated via antigen-presenting cells and T cells in the gastric mucosa and release of cytokines [41]. Gastrin itself acts on mast cells as a histamine liberator. It is not yet clear whether allergens need to be absorbed totally in order to elicit food-allergic reactions. Normally proteins and high molecular weight food constituents are enzymatically digested in the gut. Only the gut of the infant and small child shows a higher permeability. Experimental investigations, however, show that also in adult organisms, a small percentage of high molecular weight proteins passes the gut undigested and with immunologic activity [53].

Food allergies may develop via different mechanisms (Table 5.24). The most important clinical conditions are due to IgE-mediated allergic or corresponding pseudo-allergic immediate-type reactions [29, 31, 47, 62].

Rare forms of IgG- or IgM-mediated reactions manifesting a serum sickness, arthralgia, or vasculitis and fever can occur [17]. Cellular hypersensitivity against microbial or mucosal antigens has been discussed in the pathogenesis of ulcerative colitis or m. Crohn [9, 30].

The obvious relationship between the gastrointestinal tract and skin in food allergy has not been explained pathophysiologically. Pichler [40] distinguishes three types of food allergy:

Type A: The sensitization occurs orally and in early life; major allergens are cow's milk, hen's eggs, fish, peanut, etc. Each foreign protein in foods is specifically recognized, but induces tolerance in normal individuals. In early life, there is a risk of IgE formation in the special conditions of "immune deviation." While cow's milk and hen's egg allergy are mostly reversible during childhood, fish and peanut allergies are often lifelong conditions.

Type B: Here the sensitization occurs in adulthood against aeroallergens with cross-reacting food allergens (see Sect. 3.4) (celery-mugwort-carrot-spice syndrome). A high percentage of pollinosis patients are also sensitized against foods.

Type C: The sensitization is acquired orally in adulthood (isolated cow's milk allergy of the adult with anaphylaxis).

5.1.5.4 Diagnosis

The diagnostic recommendations for food allergy are:

1. Reproducible elicitation of symptoms by the suspected food
2. Exclusion of other possibilities of incompatibility
3. Demonstration of immunological sensitization

Taking the history for food allergy may be difficult (e.g., to obtain the recipe for certain dishes). We were able to solve a case of severe anaphylaxis after the patient had partaken of "*Prinzregententorte*" (a Bavarian delicacy without nuts) as being due to nut allergy only after obtaining the recipe from the pastry maker, who had used a coconut-derived lipid for the glazing [60].

The diagnostic workup in a patient with severe anaphylaxis after a breakfast including the Munich delicacy "white sausage" (obtainable from only one special butcher) was successful only by demonstrating chicken meat in the sausage (I) in RAST inhibition [54] (Fig. 5.14a,b).

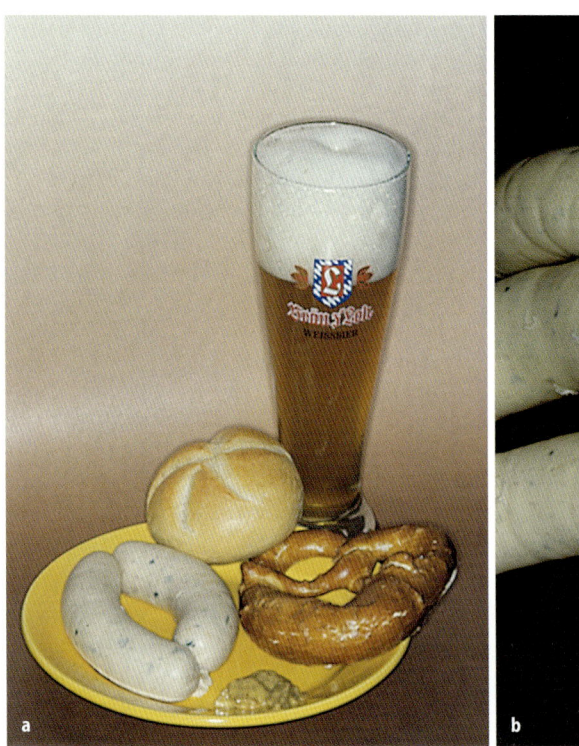 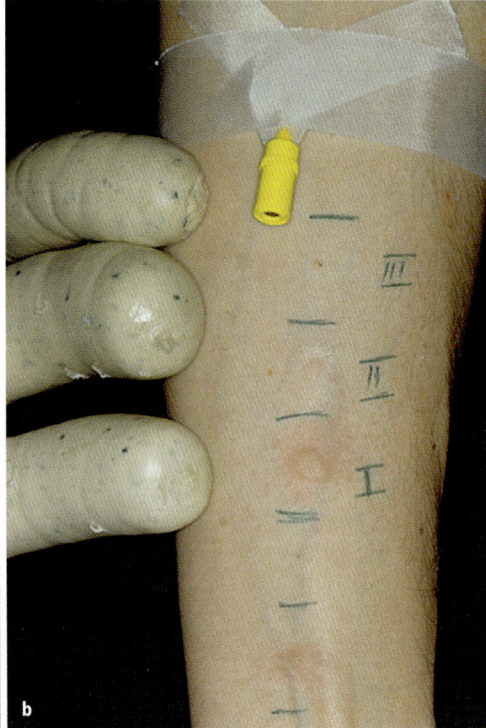

Fig. 5.14a,b. The cause of a severe anaphylactic reaction occurring after a breakfast of Munich white sausage in a patient who regularly ate white sausage from the same butcher's shop was elucidated with the RAST inhibition test [54]: Chicken allergens (due to the non-declared addition of turkey meat to the sausage meat) proved to be the culprit!

Table 5.26. Stepwise diet for adults (according to Ring and Braun-Falco [47])

Step 1	Cow's milk and cow's milk products
Step 2	Carbohydrates and vegetables
Step 3	Meat
Step 4	Poultry and hen's eggs
Step 5	Fish and seafood
Step 6	Mixed food containing additives

Table 5.27. Stepwise diet in small children

Step	Foods to be added
1	Tea (fennel) with glucose plus mineral water
2	Carrots
3	Oats
4	Potatoes
5	Bread (wheat)
6	Noodles
7	Pears
8	Rice
9	Soy
10	Cow's milk
11	Veal
12	Beef
13	Pork
14	Chicken
15	Hen's eggs
16	Leguminosae
17	Citrus fruits
18	Chocolate, lemonade, sweets

Table 5.28. Oral provocation test for idiosyncrasy (OPT1) (according to Ring and Przybilla)

Day 1	Tartrazine 10–50 mg, PHB ester 500 mg
Day 2	Color mixture I–II Color mixture I (5 mg each): quinoline yellow E104, yellow-orange S110, azorubine E122, amaranth E123, cochineal red E124 Color mixture II (5 mg each): erythrosin E127, patent blue E131, iron oxide E172
Day 3	Sodium benzoate 50–250–500 mg
Day 4	Potassium metabisulfite 10–50–100 (–300) mg
Day 5	Acetylsalicylic acid 50–250–500 (–1,000) mg
Day 6	Possibly repetition, nitrites, tyramine, propionate, other benzoates or colorings, glutamate, etc., placebo

In cases with an unclear history, patients should keep a diet diary and try to certain avoidance diets [47] (Table 5.25). In parallel, allergy diagnosis in vivo and in vitro should be done. After avoidance diets (most suspected substances), provocation diets with a slow reintroduction of different foods (Tables 5.26, 5.27) are tried out, which need to be individually tailored [6, 21, 47].

If necessary, oral provocation tests with foods and food additives should be performed such as the oral provocation test for idiosyncrasy (OPTI) (Table 5.28). Preservatives such as benzoates and sulfites sometimes are not declared properly and can elicit pseudo-allergic reactions (see Sect. 5.1.3 on "Urticaria"). Sulfites are contained especially in dried fruit, fruit juice, wine, but also deep-frozen vegetables (e.g., potatoes) and at the salad bar [54].

Provocation tests should be done blinded, at least single-blind, in order to reduce the psychosomatic influence [6, 10, 15, 37]. Placebo capsules contain coal, mannose or silicate. Foods can be blinded with carob and colored juices (blackcurrant). In severe reactions or multiple allergies, food challenges should be performed under inpatient conditions in order to guarantee optimal standardization and avoidance of additional allergens.

Provocation parameters include subjective and objective complaints (pulse, blood pressure, inspection of the skin, platelet and leukocyte count, sometimes measurement of vasoactive mediators for, e.g., histamine, ECP, tryptase).

After oral provocation, alterations of the mucosal surface have been observed on X-ray [66]. Using intragastral provocation under endoscopic control (IPEC), local mucosal reactions can be visualized [43]. Similarly, intramucosal allergen injection into the colon (colonic allergen application = COLAP) has been performed [7]. These investigations cannot be recommended for routine diagnosis and should be used for rare cases with unclear test results. From our experience with IPEC, however, we know that double-blind placebo-controlled food challenge can have false-negative results: In spite of massive erythema and petechial bleeding of the gastric mucosa, there were no subjective complaints felt by the patient!

5.1.5.5 Therapy

Avoidance is the most important principle in the management of food allergy. This may be difficult when basic foods are involved. In patients with additive hypersensitivity, knowledge of the E-numbers is important (Table 5.29). In occasional cases, oral (or even subcutaneous) immunotherapy with allergen extracts after careful allergy diagnosis has been attempted [22, 30, 34, 35] with success, but side-effects can occur and may lead to changes in doses. Of course, during hyposensitization strict avoidance should be kept. After reaching a maintenance dose, natural foods can be tried. In cow's milk allergy, for instance, a daily dose of 200 ml cow's milk needs to be drunk. After longer intervals (5–7 days), the effect may be lost.

Therapy and prophylaxis of cow's milk allergy plays a major role in infants (Table 5.30). A

Table 5.29. Food additives and European (E) numbers

Colorings	E No.	Preservatives	E No.
Lactoflavin (riboflavin)	E101	Sorbic acid	E200
Beta-carotene	E160a	Sodium sorbate	E201
Caramel	E150	Potassium sorbate	E202
Silver	E174	Calcium sorbate	E203
Gold	E175	Benzoic acid	E210
Curcumin	E100	Sodium benzoate	E211
Tartrazine	E102	Potassium benzoate	E212
Quinoline yellow	E104	Calcium benzoate	E213
Riboflavin-5-phosphate	E106	Ethyl *p*-hydroxybenzoate	E214
Orange yellow S	E110	Sodium ethyl *p*-hydroxybenzoate	E215
Carmine (carminic acid, cochineal)	E120	Propyl *p*-hydroxybenzoate	E216
Azorubine	E122	Sodium propyl *p*-hydroxybenzoate	E217
Amaranth	E123	Methyl *p*-hydroxybenzoate	E218
Cochineal red A (Ponceau 4R)	E124	Sodium methyl *p*-hydroxybenzoate	E219
Erythrosine	E127	Sulfur dioxide	E220
Patent blue V	E131	Sodium sulfite	E221
Indigotin I (indigo carmine)	E132	Sodium hydrogen sulfite	E222
Chlorophyll	E140	Sodium metabisulfite	E223
Copper-containing chlorophyll complexes	E141	Potassium metabisulfite	E224
Brilliant acid green BS (lisamine green)	E142	Calcium sulfite	E226
Brilliant black BN	E151	Calcium hydrogen sulfite	E227
Vegetable carbon	E153	Formic acid	E236
Alpha-carotene	E160a	Sodium formiate	E237
Gamma-carotene		Calcium formiate	E238
Bixin, norbixin (Annatto, Orlean)	E160b	Propionic acid	E280
Capsanthian, Capsorubin	E160c	Sodium propionate	E281
Lycopene	E160d	Calcium propionate	E282
Beta-apo-8'-carotenal	E160e	Potassium propionate	E283
Beta-apo-8'-carotenoic acid ester	E160f	Biphenyl	E230
Xanthophyll	E161	Orthophenyl phenol	E231
Flavoxanthin	E161a	Sodium orthophenyl phenol	E232
Lutein	E161b	Thiabendazol	E233
Cryptoaxanthin	E161c	Potassium ascorbate	E303
Rubixanthin	E161d	Tocopherols	E306
Violaxanthin	E161e	Alpha-tocopherol	E307
Rhodoxanthin	E161f	Delta-tocopherol	E309
Canthaxanthin	E161g		
Betanin	E162		
Anthocyanin	E163		
Aluminum	E173		
Calcium carbonate	E170		
Titanium dioxide	E171		
Iron oxides and hydroxides	E172		

Table 5.29. (Cont.)

Antioxidants	E No.	Carriers	E No.
Propyl gallate	E310	Ammonium alginate	E403
Octyl gallate	E311	Potassium alginate	E402
Dodecyl gallate	E312	Sodium alginate	E401
Butylated hydroxyanisole (BHA)	E320	Glycerol	E422
Butylated hydroxytoluol (BHT)	E321	Pectin	E440
Ascorbic acid	E300	Sorbitol	E420
Sodium L-ascorbate	E301	Carrageenan	E407
Calcium ascorbate	E302	Gum arabic	E414
Citric acid	E330		
Sodium citrate	E331		
Potassium citrate	E332		
Calcium citrate	E333		
Lactic acid	E270		
Sodium lactate	E125		
Potassium lactate	E326		
Calcium lactate	E327		
Lecithin	E322		
Glycerides of fatty acids esterified with citric acid	E472c		
Sodium orthophosphate	E339		
Potassium orthophosphate	E340		
Orthophosphate	E341		
6-Palmitoyl-L-ascorbic acid	E304		
Tartric acid	E334		
Sodium tartrate	E335		
Potassium tartrate	E336		
Sodium potassium tartrate	E337		

distinction should be made between prophylactic and therapeutic hypoallergenic formulas (Table 31). Strongly hydrolyzed products have been proven in a large epidemiological study (GINI) as being equivalent to breast feeding [3, 61].

It is open for discussion whether the addition of probiotic lactobacillae with immunomodulating effects in the gastrointestinal tract plays a role in atopy prevention [27].

For pharmacotherapeutic prevention, mast cell stabilizers have been used successfully (oral cromoglycate) [28, 54], possibly also antihistamines.

Food-allergic individuals do not have to spend the rest of their life with appalling restrictions and impairment of quality of life. If correctly diagnosed, there are recipes for each kind of food allergy in order to allow for an agreeable diet [5, 52].

Table 5.30. Hydrolyzed cow's milk formulas for infant food

Protein basis	Hydrolysis	Name	Producer
Whey	Partial	Beba HA	Nestlé
		Aletemil HA	Nestlé
	Strong	Alfaré	Nestlé
	Partial	Humana HA	Humana
	Partial	Nutrition Pepti	Milupa
		Hipp HA	Hipp
	Strong	Nutramigen	Mead-Johnson
Casein	Partial	Aptamil HA	Milupa
Soy	Strong	Pregomin	Milupa
Carob, amino acids	–	Sinlac, Neocate	Nestlé

Table 5.31. Statement published by the German Society for Allergology and Clinical Immunology (DGAI) regarding gene technology and food allergy

Many people are worried by the introduction of gene technologically altered foods. In this context, the question regarding the risk of food allergy through gene technological procedures is real. The German Society for Allergology and Clinical Immunology (DGAI), therefore, publishes the following statement:

1. Food allergies are a real and widely prevalent clinical problem, independent of gene technology. The prevalence of food allergy in the total population is not precisely known. Estimates range from 2% to 4% in adults and from 5% to 10% in childhood. The symptoms of allergic food reactions are multiple and cover mild reactions (itching, nausea, etc.) up to life-threatening shock conditions (anaphylaxis).

2. In the cultural development of mankind "artificial" procedures have been used for millennia by which the nature of possible allergens is changed through technological procedures (e.g., boiling of food). On the other hand, classical breeding techniques in botany have led to the creation of new species characterized by a multitude of altered proteins (500–1,000 genes involved); this phenomenon has never led to anxiety in the general population.

   Through the progress in gene technology, for the first time it is exactly known which genes are involved and how they are altered and expressed in foods. The major novel aspect of this technology is the tremendously improved state of knowledge.

3. Gene technological procedures may lead to changes in foods with possible relevance for allergy; this regards both the risk (e.g., Brazil nut allergen in soy beans) and chance (e.g., hypoallergenic rice).

4. Therefore, it is important prior to the introduction of a novel product to fulfill specific safety criteria regarding allergy:
   - Sequence homology of the altered proteins has to be compared with well-known allergens
   - Immune reactivity against positive sera or skin test reactions in sensitized individuals has to be tested
   - Stability against enzymatic digestion has to be studied.
   - Unless these safety data exist, gene technologically altered products should not be used for the prevention of allergic disease in infants.
   - One actual problem has to be seen in the fact that the evaluation of immunoreactivity in humans can only be tested with known allergens in defined sensitized populations. New proteins cannot be tested in this manner. Here, animal experiments or in vitro models for predictive testing need to be developed.

5. The German Society for Allergology and Clinical Immunology has recommended for many years an improvement in the declaration not only of additives, but also of food contents, independently of technological procedures. It remains open whether the "gene technologically produced" procedure should be especially declared in identical proteins.

6. The German Society for Allergology and Clinical Immunology recommends the presence of persons with allergological expertise on the relevant committees involved with food production and control.

References

1. Aas K (1978) The diagnosis of hypersensitivity to ingested foods. Reliability of skin prick testing and the radioallergosorbent test with different materials. Clin Allergy 8:39–50
2. André C (1984) L'allergie digestive, concept ou realité? Presse Med 27:1667–1669
3. Bauer CP Grübl A (2002) Hypoallergene Babynahrung. In: Behr-Völtzer C, Hamm M, Vieluf D, Ring J (eds) Diät bei Nahrungsmittelallergien und -intoleranzen, 2nd edn. Urban & Vogel, Munich, pp 105–111
4. Ballmer-Weber BK, Wüthrich B (2001) Die Nahrungsmittelallergie und ihre diätetische Behandlung. Aktuell Ernähr Med 26:196–201
5. Behr-Völtzer C, Hamm M, Vieluf D, Ring J (eds) (2002) Diät bei Nahrungsmittelallergien und -intoleranzen, 2nd edn. Urban & Vogel, Munich
6. Balmer-Weber B, Bengtsson U, et al. (2004) Standardization of food challenges in patients with immediate reactions to foods. Position paper EAACI. Allergy (in press)
7. Bischoff SC, Mayer J, Wedemeyer J, et al. (1997) Colonoscopic allergen provocation (CO-LAP): a new diagnostic approach for gastrointestinal food allergy. Gut 40:745–753
8. Bock SA, Sampson HA, Atkins FM, Zeiger RS, et al. (1988) Double-blind, placebo-controlled food challenge (DBPCFC) as an office procedure: a manual. J Allergy Clin Immunol 82:986–997
9. Brostoff J, Challacombe SJ (eds) (1987) Food allergy and intolerance. Bailliere Tindall, London
10. Bruijnzeel-Koomen C, Ortolani C, Aas K, et al. (1995) Adverse reactions to food. European Academy of Allergology and Clinical Immunology Subcommittee. Allergy 50:623–635

11. Deutsche Gesellschaft für Ernährung (ed) (1995) Richtig essen. F+G Rollendruck, Berlin
12. Diätverband – Bundesverband der Hersteller von Lebensmitteln für besondere Ernährungszwecke (ed) (1998) Product & Diät. Presto, Hemmingen
13. Ebner C, Hirschwehr R, Bauer L, et al. (1995) Identification of allergens in fruits and vegetables: IgE cross-reactivities with the important birch pollen allergens Bet v 1 and Bet v 2 (birch profilin). J Allergy Clin Immunol 95:962–969
14. Egger J, Carter CM, Wilson J, Turner MW, Soothill JF (1983) Is migraine food allergy? A double blind controlled trial of oligoantigenic diet treatment. Lancet 2:865–869
15. Ehlers I, Henz B, Zuberbier T (1996) Diagnose und Therapie pseudo-allergischer Reaktionen der Haut durch Nahrungsmittel. Allergologie 19:270–276
16. Eisenbrand G, Aulepp H, Dayan AD, et al. (1996) Food allergies and intolerances. VCH Verlagsgesellschaft, Weinheim
17. Eisenmann A, Ring J, Helm D von der, Meurer M, Braun-Falco O (1988) Vasculitis allergica durch Nahrungsmittelallergie. Hautarzt 39:318–321
18. Ewan PW, Clark AT (2001) Long-term prospective observational study of patients with peanut and nut allergy after participation in a management plan. Lancet 357:111–115
19. Feingold B (1975) Why your child is hyperactive. Random, New York
20. Franck P, Moneret Vautrin DA, Dousset B, et al. (2002) The allergenicity of soybean-based products is modified by food technologies. Int Arch Allergy Immunol 128:212–219
21. Häberle M (1987) Klinische und lebensmittelchemische Aspekte bei Unverträglichkeits-Reaktionen auf Salicylat- und Additiva-haltige Lebensmittel. Zbl Haut 153:75–95
22. Henzgen M, Schlenvoigt G, Diener C, Jäger L (1991) Nahrungsmittelallergie bei Frühblüherpollinose und deren Beeinflussung mittels Hyposensibilisierung. Allergologie 14:90–94
23. Hjorth N, Roed-Petersen J (1976) Occupational protein contact dermatitis in food handlers. Contact Dermatitis 2:28–42
24. Holt PG (1998) Mucosal immunity in relation to the development of tolerance/sensitization. Allergy 53:6–19
25. Host A (1991) Importance of the first meal on the development of cow's milk allergy and intolerance. Allergy Proc 12:27–32
26. Hourihane JO, Kilburn A, Dean P, Warner JO (1997) Clinical characteristics of peanut allergy. Clin Exp Allergy 27:634–639
27. Isolauri E (2001) Probiotics in the prevention and treatment of allergic disease. Pediatr Allergy Immunol 12 [Suppl 14]:56–59
28. Jäger L, Wüthrich B (1998) Nahrungsmittelallergien und -intoleranzen. Gustaf Fischer, Ulm
29. Jarisch R, Pirker C, Möslinger T, Götz M (1997) The role of histamine in wine intolerance. J Allergy Clin Immunol 89:197
30. Jorde W (1980) Orale Desensibilisierung. In: Fillipp G (ed) Allergologie, vol 2. Banaschewski, Munich, pp 53
31. Kanny G, Hatahet R, Moneret-Vautrin A, Kohler C, Bellut A (1994) Allergy and intolerance to flavouring agents in atopic dermatitis in young children. Allerg Immunol 6:204–210
32. Klaschka F (1987) Hämatogenes Kontaktekzem durch Nahrungsmittel. Allergologie 10:93–96
33. Kurek M, Janowska E (2001) Allergische und pseudoallergische Reaktionen auf Aromastoffe in der Nahrung. Z Hautkrankheiten H+G 76:699–703
34. Mempel M, Rakoski J, Ring J, Ollert M (2003) Severe anaphylaxis to kiwi fruit: Immunologic changes related to successful sublingual allergen immunotherapy. J Allergy Clin Immunol 111:1406–1409
35. Möller C (1989) Effect of pollen immunotherapy on food hypersensitivity in children with birch pollinosis. Ann Allergy 62:343–345
36. Montes RG, Perman JA (1991) Lactose intolerance: pinpointing the source of nonspecific gastrointestinal symptoms. Postgrad Med 89:175–178
37. Niggemann B, Reibel S, Roehr CC, et al. (2001) Predictors of positive food challenge outcome in non-IgE-mediated reactions to food in children with atopic dermatitis. J Allergy Clin Immunol 106:1053–1058
38. Nordlee JA, Taylor SL, Townsend JA, Thomas LA, Bush RK (1996) Identification of a Brazilnut allergen in transgenic soybeans. N Engl J Med 334:688–692
39. Ortolani C, Ballmer-Weber BK, Hansen KS, et al. (2000) Hazelnut allergy: a double-blind, placebo-controlled food challenge multicenter study. J Allergy Clin Immunol 105:577–581
40. Pichler WJ, Stich O (1993) Nahrungsmittelallergien bei Pollensensibilisierungen, part II: Kreuzreaktionen bei Beifußpollen-Sensibilisierungen. Allergologie 16:494–501
41. Pratschke E (1986) Mediatoren der immunologischen Stimulation gastraler Funktionen: Experimentelle Untersuchungen am Beispiel der Gastrinfreisetzung. Habilitationsschrift, München
42. Przybilla B, Ring J (1990) Food allergy and atopic eczema. Semin Dermatol 9:220–225
43. Reimann HJ, Ring J, Ultsch B, Wendt P (1985) Intragastral provocation under endoscopic control (IPEC) in food allergy. Clin Allergy 15:195–202
44. Ring J (1984) Nahrungsmittelallergie und andere Unverträglichkeitsreaktionen durch Nahrungsmittel. Klin Wochenschr 62:795–802
45. Ring J (1999) Nahrungsmittel-Allergie und Gentechnik. In: Steinhart H, Tanner W (eds) Bayerische Akademie der Wissenschaften. Rundgespräche der Kommission für Ökologie, vol 16. Lebens-

mittel und Gentechnik. Dr. Friedrich Pfeil, Munich, pp 61–72
46. Ring J (1997) Gentechnologie und Lebensmittelallergie (DGAI-Stellungnahme). Allergo J 6:214
47. Ring J, Braun-Falco O (1987) Allergie-Diät Verfahren zur Diagnostik und Therapie von Nahrungsmittel-Allergien und -Pseudo-Allergien. Hautarzt 38:198–205
48. Roe DA (1986) Nutrition and the skin. Liss, New York
49. Sampson HA (2001) Utility of food-specific IgE concentrations in predicting symptomatic food allergy. J Allergy Clin Immunol 107:891–896
50. Schäfer T, Bohler E, Ruhdorfer S, et al. (2001) Epidemiology of food allergy/food intolerance in adults: associations with other manifestations of atopy. Allergy 56:1172–1179
51. Schauder P, Ollenschläger G (2002) Ernährungsmedizin. Prävention und Therapie, 2nd edn. Urban & Fischer, Munich
52. Schindler H, Bräckle J, Karch B (1981) Kochbuch für Allergiker. Ehrenwirth, Munich
53. Seifert J, Ring J, Brendel W (1975) Prolongation of skin allografts after oral application of antilymphocyte serum in rats. Nature 249:776
54. Stefanini GF, Saggioro A, Alvisi V, et al. (1995) Oral cromolyn sodium in comparison with elimination diet in the irritable bowel syndrome, diarrheic type. Multicenter study of 428 patients. Scand J Gastroenterol 30:535–541
55. Stevenson DD, Simon RA (1981) Sensitivity to ingested metabisulphites in asthmatic subjects. J Allergy Clin Immunol 68:26–32
56. Strobel S, Hourihane JO (2001) Gastrointestinal allergy: clinical symptoms and immunological mechanisms. Pediatr Allergy Immunol 12 [Suppl 14]:43–46
57. Thiel CL, Fuchs E (1981) Über korrelative Beziehungen bei Kräuterpollen- und Gewürzallergenen, RAST 3. Berichtsband. Grosse, Berlin, pp 178–185
58. Turjanmaa K (2001) Atopy patch test, an additional new tool in the diagnosis of food allergy. Acta Dermatovenerol Croat 9:69–71
59. Vieths S, Meyer AH, Ehlers I, et al. (2001) Zur Deklaration "versteckter Allergene" in Lebensmitteln. Allergo J 10:130–136
60. Wagner G, Ring J (1981) Anaphylaktische Reaktionen bei Nuß- und Mohnallergie. Notfallmedizin 7:361
61. Wahn U, Seger R, Wahn V (1999) Pädiatrische Allergologie und Immunologie, 3rd edn. Urban & Fischer, Munich
62. Warin RP, Smith RJ (1975) Challenge test battery in chronic urticaria. Br J Dermatol 94:401–406
63. De Weck AL, Griot-Wenk M, Schneider H, et al. (2002) Human allergogeneticists should listen to their dog's barking. In: Ring J, Behrendt H (eds) New trends in allergy V. Springer, Berlin Heidelberg New York, pp 27–36
64. Werfel T (2000) Allergenspezifische T-Zell-Antwort bei Ekzemkrankheiten. Dustri, München-Deisenhofen
65. Werfel T, Wedi B, Kleine-Tebbe J, et al. (1999) Vorgehen bei Verdacht auf eine pseudoallergische Reaktion auf Nahrungsmittelinhaltsstoffe. Allergo J 8:135–341
66. Werner M (1967) Krankheiten infolge peroraler Allergeninvasion. In: Hansen K, Werner M (eds) Lehrbuch der klinischen Allergie. Thieme, Stuttgart, p 179
67. Wüthrich B (1986) Nahrungsmittelallergien. Internist 27:362–371
68. Wüthrich B, Ballmer-Weber BK (2001) Food-induced anaphylaxis. Allergy 56 [Suppl 67]:102–104
69. Wüthrich B (2000) Lethal or life-threatening allergic reactions to food. J Invest Allergol Clin Immunol 10:59–65
70. Wüthrich B (2002) Nahrungsmittel und Allergie. Dustri, München-Deisenhofen

5.1.6 Insect Venom Allergy

Allergic reactions against insect venoms are not infrequent: 0.8–5% of the population react to the venoms of wasps, bees, and hornets with systemic allergic symptoms (19% with hypererergic local reactions) [31, 33, 47, 49]. In Germany, 10–40 fatalities per year are estimated with a high "hidden number" of cases of unexplained cardiac death [2, 11, 37, 52]. Most reactions arise on the basis of IgE-mediated sensitization against insect venoms. Rare cases of immune complex anaphylaxis as well as pseudoallergic reactions should be distinguished.

5.1.6.1 Insect Venoms

The most important insects honeybee (*Apis mellifera*) and certain wasps (*Vespula germanica, V. vulgaris, Dolichovespula*) belong to the order of Hymenoptera [12, 29, 34] (Figs. 5.15, 5.16). Rarer elicitors are bumblebees (*Bombus*), hornets (*Vespa crabro*), field wasps (*Polistes*), ants (Formicidae), and mosquitos (Diptera). Insect venoms contain toxic and allergenic substances.

A painful, itching, or burning sensation with a surrounding wheal and flare at the sting site is normal. Moreover, in certain localizations (upper airways) or after an excessive

5.1 Diseases with Possible IgE Involvement

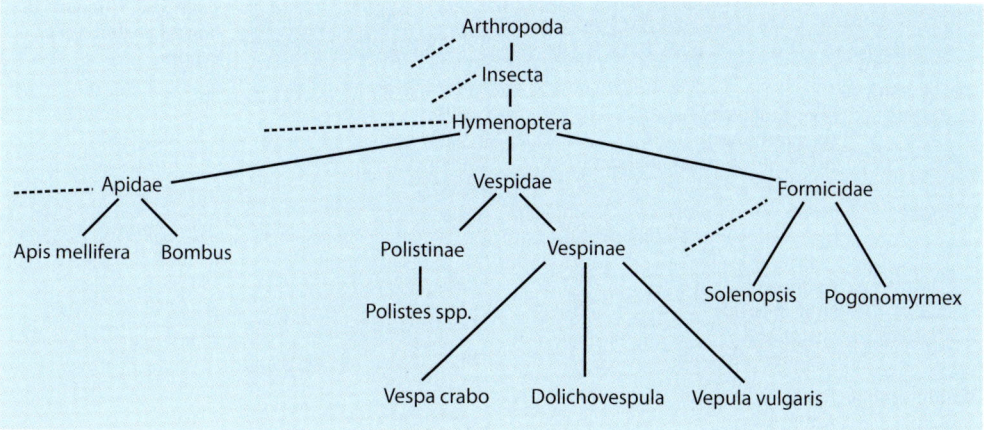

Fig. 5.15. Taxonomic classification of the most important *Hymenoptera* species responsible for insect venom allergies

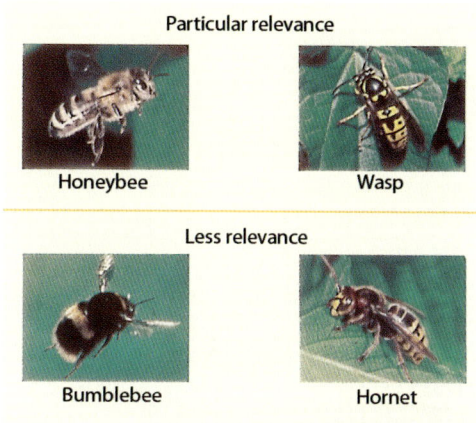

Fig. 5.16. The most important *Hymenoptera* species responsible for insect venom allergies (R. Jarisch)

amount of stings, individuals who are not sensitized may be in danger [44]. Table 5.32 shows the contents of bee and wasp venom [5, 12]. In bee venom, the peptide melittin represents the major product, characterized by a strongly basic group on one end and a hydrophobic sidechain on the other end, of the molecule. This detergent effect leads to lysis of cells. Melittin is a weak allergen. Only 3% of bee-venom-allergic individuals are sensitized to melittin. The major allergen of bee venom is the enzyme phospholipase A_2. Apamin has neurotoxic effects. The phospholipase A_2 from wasp venom shows no cross-reaction to the corresponding enzyme in bee venom. Wasp venom also contains antigen 5 as well as hyaluronidase. There is a marked cross-reactivity between the venoms of different species of the order Vespidae [19, 34, 35, 50, 51]. Hornet venom also contains kinins and acetylcholine.

5.1.6.2 Symptomatology

Allergic reactions against insect stings have been known for a long time [26] and range from hyperergic local reactions to anaphylactic shock. Strong local reactions also are often IgE mediated [1], but do not represent an indication for allergen-specific immunotherapy. They are more frequent in hematologic disease (e.g., lymphatic leukemia) [54, 58]. Anaphylactic symptoms can be classified according to severity (see Sect. 5.1.4 on "Anaphylaxis"; Table 5.17). The severity scale proposed by H.L. Mueller et al. is more complicated in practice [30].

5.1.6.3 Diagnosis

History. Often the eliciting insect species cannot be remembered [28, 29]. The severity of the reaction also needs to be determined through cooperation with the physician treating the reaction and the therapy given. The question regarding atopy is important for interpretation of skin test and RAST results [39]. There are standardized questionnaires [47].

Table 5.32. Contents of honeybee and wasp venom

Contents		Molecular weight	Percentage
Bee venom			
Proteins	Phospholipase A_2	15,800	12%
	Hyaluronidase	45,000	2%
	Acid phosphatase (allergen B)	49,000	?
	Allergen C	105,000	?
Peptides	Melittin	2,840	50%
	Mast cell degranulating peptide (MCDP)	2,593	2%
	Apamine	2,038	2%
	Other peptides	?	15%
Mediators	Histamine	111	1%
	Leukotriene B_4 and C_4	336	<0.001%
Vespid venom			
Proteins	Antigen 5	25,000	15%
	Phospholipases	~35,000	10%
	Hyaluronidase	45,000	2%
	Proteases	?	?
Peptides	Kinins	~2,000	?
Mediators	Histamine	111	4%
	Serotonin		~1%
	Leukotriene B_4 and C_4	336	~0.001%
	Dopamine		~5%
	Acetylcholine[a]		5%

[a] Only for *Vespa cabro*

Skin Tests. Skin tests (4 weeks after the sting) are performed under emergency conditions using endpoint titration with venom extracts (skin prick test beginning with 1 µg/ml and increasing the concentration to 300 µg/ml; if negative, intradermal tests are performed with 0.01–1 µg/ml). A second reading after 24 h for documentation of non-IgE-mediated reactions is sensible.

In Vitro Allergy Tests. Apart from total serum IgE, specific IgE – possibly also IgG subclasses – against bee and wasp venom is determined [9]. Using cellular tests as in vitro histamine release or basophil activation (CD 63) or CAST ELISA, additional information can be obtained [47] (see Chap. 4 on "Allergy Diagnosis").

Indication for Allergen-Specific Immunotherapy. On the basis of history, skin test, and in vitro tests, the indication for immunotherapy is evaluated by considering possible ris factors (Table 5.33). Allergen-specific immunotherapy is indicated in patients with an objective generalized systemic reaction and demonstration of IgE-mediated sensitization. For general contraindications, see Sect. 6.3 ("Immunotherapy"). Age alone does not represent a contraindication [18].

Table 5.33. Risk factors for insect venom allergy (according to [46])

Risk factors regarding exposure
Occupations with increased exposure to Hymenoptera (e.g., fruit and pastry workers, firefighters, forestry workers, agriculture workers, gardeners, refuse disposal workers)
Intense outdoor leisure activities (e.g., gardening, swimming, tennis, biking, jogging, golf)
Beekeeping by the patient himself, neighbors or family members
Motor cycling

Risk factors due to underlying disease
Diseases such as cardiovascular disease, asthma, mastocytosis
Elderly age
High physical or psychological stress
Medication with β-blockers or ACE inhibitors (possibly also NSAIDs)
Severe systemic reaction after insect stings (>severity grade III) in the history

Sting Provocation. Sting challenge with honeybees or wasps should not be used as a diagnostic instrument in patients prior to allergen-specific immunotherapy! It is an instrument of control of therapeutic efficacy. Severe complications have been observed [3].

5.1.6.4 Allergen-Specific Immunotherapy (Hyposensitization)

In 1930, Benson and Semenov reported the case of a beekeeper suffering from asthma and anaphylaxis while working with bees [4]. After immunotherapy with a whole-body extract of homogenized honeybee, the asthma improved. Based on this report, a worldwide practice of immunotherapy of insect venom allergy with whole-body extracts started with reports of therapeutic effects in up to 75% of cases [30]. Early evidence of possible hyposensitization with purified bee venom [17, 26] was probably not followed because of anaphylactic complications [10, 27]. Only after it was shown that bee venom and whole-body extracts contain very different allergens [23] and that the relevant allergens are in the venom [22] was hyposensitization with venom extracts proposed [9, 14, 22, 40, 43, 56]. Lichtenstein et al. pioneered the work with a double-blind study: From three groups of 20 patients each, 58% of the placebo-treated, 64% of the whole-body extract treated, but only 5% of the bee venom extract treated patients reacted to sting challenge. This study was only possible through the production of purified venom extracts in larger amounts. Bee venom is produced by electrical stimulation of bees [5]; wasps have to be killed, operated on, and the venom sac removed. For 500 g wasp venom, 250 collectors have to work for 1 year and need 74 million insects (= 6,000 kg).

The future will show the place of recombinant allergens (recombinant phospholipase A_2 from bee venom) in practical allergy [32].

There are various methods of allergen-specific immunotherapy (Table 5.34) by which the standard maintenance dose of 100 μg every 4 weeks is reached. According to a schedule of rush hyposensitization with up to four injections a day the maintenance dose can be reached in approximately 1 week.

We start with 0.1 ml of a concentration corresponding to 1/100 of the lowest prick test positive allergen solution and increase the dose by 0.2, 0.4, and 0.8 ml to the next higher concentration. "Ultrarush" schedules have been published [6, 42, 57], increasing the dosis over 1 or 2 days. Conventional immunotherapy protocols with weekly injections should only be performed preseasonally [15]. After reaching the maintenance dose, intervals are slowly increased from 1, 2, 3 to finally 4 weeks.

Table 5.34. Dose schedule (in micrograms) for rush hyposensitization. The schedule holds true for patients with optimal dose increases

Day	Conventional	Hamburg schedule	"Ultrarush"
1	0.02	0.001	0.01
	0.04	0.01	0.1
	0.08		1.0
	0.2		10.0
			20.0
			40.0
			80.0
2	0.4	0.1	100.0
	0.8	0.4	100.0
	1.0	0.7	
	4.0		
3	8.0	1.0	
	10.0	4.0	
	20.0	7.0	
	30.0		
4	10.0	10.0	
	20.0	40.0	
	60.0	70.0	
	70.0		
5	40.0	100.0	
	50.0		
	60.0		
	70.0		
6	80.0		
	90.0		
	100.0		
8			100.0
15	100.0	100.0	
22	100.0	100.0	
36	100.0	100.0	100.0
50	100.0	100.0	
71	100.0	100.0	(Day 43) 100.0
92	100.0	100.0	(Day 71) 100.0
120	100.0	100.0	(Day 99) 100.0
(to be continued every 4 weeks)			

Therapeutic Efficacy. As demonstrated by sting challenge under emergency conditions, allergen-specific immunotherapy with Hymenoptera venoms is effective in 80–100% of pa-

Systemic anaphylactic reactions after sting provocation (severity grade)	Systemic reactions in history (severity grade)				
	I n (%)	II n (%)	III n (%)	IV n (%)	Total
None	19 (90.5)	61 (78.2)	40 (75.5)	4 (80.0)	125 (79.6)
I	2 (9.5)	13 (16.7)	6 (11.3)	0 (0)	20 (12.7)
II	0 (0)	4 (5.1)	4 (7.5)	1 (20.0)	9 (5.8)
III	0 (0)	0 (0)	3 (5.7)	0 (0)	3 (1.9)
Total	21 (100)	78 (100)	53 (100)	5 (100)	157 (100)

Table 5.35. Results of sting provocation and severity grades (highest individually stated severity grades) of anaphylaxis in history (from [30])

tients. In our own experience, only 5% showed reactions equally as strong as before immunotherapy. When increasing the dose from 100 to 200 µg, most of these patients tolerated the subsequent sting challenge [40] (Table 5.35).

Side Effects: Local Reactions. Local reactions occur as swelling with wheal and redness and are observed in most patients, sometimes lasting 6–12 h. The reactions occur mostly during the course of the dose increase at higher concentrations (10–100 µg) and sometimes slow the further increase of dose. Local treatment with moist wraps and topical corticosteroids leads to improvement. Subsequent injections are usually well tolerated.

Side Effects: Systemic Reactions. In 3–35% of patients, systemic reactions are observed [39, 46], which occur more frequently in bee than wasp venom allergic individuals [48]. After treatment, immunotherapy is continued with reduced dose (see Sect. 6.2). In patients with repeated systemic reactions, prophylaxis with H_1 antihistamines can be considered [7, 15]. Rarely, serum sickness or immune complex reactions occur [8]; then therapy has to be discontinued.

5.1.6.5 Therapy Control

Under allergen-specific immunotherapy, most patients show an increase of specific IgE together with specific IgG antibodies (Fig. 5.17). However, in the individual case IgG concentrations do not give reliable prognostic information [3]. Possibly, the ratio sIgG4/sIgE in the immunoblot may be relevant regarding the protective effect of immunotherapy [36].

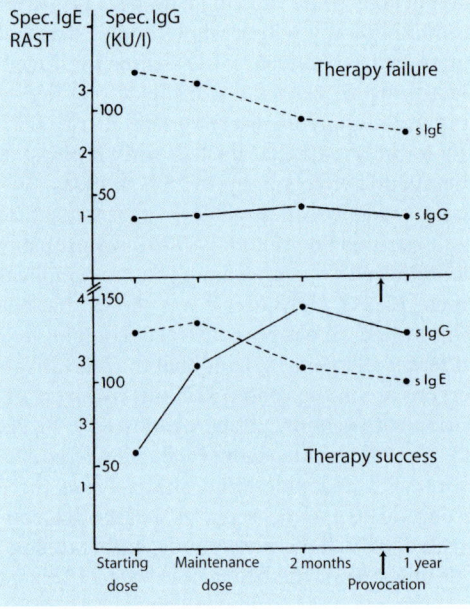

Fig. 5.17. Bee-venom-specific antibodies of the IgE and IgG class demonstrated in two patients undergoing hyposensitization treatment with bee venom extract

Sting Challenge. After reaching the maintenance dose and maintaining it over at least 3 months, sting challenge can be performed with a living insect in emergency conditions (Fig. 5.18). Sting challenge represents the only objective method for evaluation of therapeutic efficacy [40]. In patients still reacting to sting challenge, we increase the dose up to 200 µg every 4 weeks or shorten the interval (3 weeks).

Duration of Treatment. Since there is no reliable prognostic marker which gives solid information on the duration of protection, some authors recommend lifelong immunotherapy. International recommendations vary between 3 and 5 years at least. In patients with risk factors (systemic reaction after sting challenge, mastocytosis, repeated anaphylactic reactions to immunotherapy injection), an increase in dose and a longer treatment duration is necessary [32, 47].

Double Sensitizations to Bee/Wasp Venom
Some patients are positive in skin test and/or RAST against both bee and wasp venom and the history remains doubtful. If cellular tests do not give additional information and only one anaphylactic episode was seen in the history, we usually use the species with stronger skin or RAST reactivity for immunotherapy. In unclear cases, immunotherapy against both Hymenoptera species has to be performed. Watching the kinetics of IgE response immediately after the sting event (anaphylaxis) and 4 weeks later, additional information about the relevant insect species may be obtained.

Passive Immunotherapy. Intramuscular administration of hyperimmunoglobulin from beekeepers has been proven to be protective and may also enhance efficacy of active immunotherapy [21, 38].

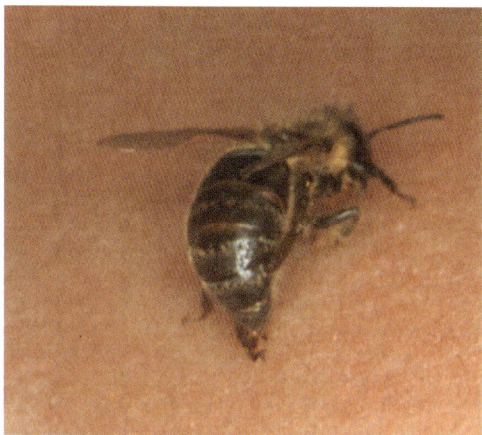

Fig. 5.18. Sting provocation with a living insect

Table 5.36. Patient information in honeybee and wasp venom allergy (according to [28, 47])

Avoidance measures
- Repellents (chemical agents) do not give protection.
- Avoid eating of sweets, ice cream, lemonade, fruits in the open, flower picking, presence near dustbins, animals, fallen fruits, as well as fragrance or perfumed cosmetics. After eating, wash hands and wipe mouth.
- Do not drink from bottles or open cans, cover glasses, use straws.
- Do not chase away insects from their food sources, avoid hectic movements.
- Cover your skin by adequate clothing (especially when gardening), avoid going barefoot, open shoes. When motorbiking wear helmet, gloves, and adequate clothing. Open biking helmets should be covered with a net.
- On humid warm days, exert extreme caution since insects may be especially aggressive.
- Avoid too loose clothing and dark colors, rather wear light colors.
- Keep apartment windows closed during the day or use insect protection (shutters). Do not open the window when you have a light on inside in the evening (attractive to hornets).
- Watch out for hidden insects (bed, shoes, etc.).
- Avoid bee and wasp nests and their environs. Nests near your permanent living place should be removed (by beekeepers or firefighters).
- When you find yourself in the vicinity of insects, avoid hectic movements, withdraw slowly! Do not tremble, never breathe into a nest opening.
- When attacked by bees or wasps, cover your head with arms or clothing. Withdraw slowly. If stung, remove the sting with a fingernail without emptying the sac. Cover the sting site.

Behavior after being stung
- Keep calm! Inform people around you about your situation.
- Remove sting carefully using the fingernail. Never squeeze the sac.
- Take the drugs from your emergency kit

Immediately after the sting (if not successfully hyposensitized) take:
- Oral antihistamine
- Oral cortisone
- If dyspnea, tachycardia, lip or tongue swelling occur: Inhale epinephrine or use an epinephrine injector.

After allergen-specific immunotherapy, drugs only need to be used when systemic symptoms are observed

Problems. Rare allergic reactions against other insects such as mosquitos, ants, etc., represent an increasing problem due to the non-availability of adequate amounts of purified extracts.

There are controversial opinions regarding indications for immunotherapy in patients with HIV infection and other immunodeficiencies or with malignancy. While this earlier was regarded as a contraindication – the problem was very rare in allergy praxis; however, due to the increasing allergy prevalence, more patients with this combination come and ask for a decision. We perform allergen-specific immunotherapy if criteria for indication are given and if known neoplasms have been surgically removed or HIV infection is under control with triple therapy. However, future studies are required to answer these questions.

5.1.6.6 Patient Information

Independently of immunotherapy, patients should be informed about sensible behavior after insect stings and also about prevention of stings (Table 5.36) [25, 28, 29, 43, 47], especially about the relevant risk factors [35]. All patients should carry with them an "emergency kit" (see Sect. 5.1.4 on "Anaphylaxis") with epinephrine for inhalation or self-injection (in severe cases).

References

1. Albrecht I, Eichler G, Müller U, Hoigné R (1980) On the significance of severe local reactions to hymenoptera stings. Clin Allergy 10:675
2. Barnard JH (1973) Studies of 400 hymenoptera sting deaths in the United States. J Allergy Clin Immunol 52:259
3. Bauer CP (1986) Stichprovokationen zur Diagnostik von Insektengift-Allergien? Allergologie 9:14
4. Benson R, Semenov H (1930) Allergy in its relation to bee sting. J Allergy 1:105
5. Benton AW, Morse RA, Stewart JD (1963) Venom collection from honey bees. Science 142:228
6. Brehler R (1999) Ultra-Rush-Hyposensibilisierung. Allergologie 22 [Suppl 2]:570–571
7. Brockow K, Kiehn M, Riethmüller C, et al. (1997) Efficacy of antihistamine treatment in the prevention of adverse reactions to Hymenoptera immunotherapy: A prospective, randomized, placebo-controlled trial. J Allergy Clin Immunol 100:458–463
8. De Bandt M, Atassi-Dumont M, Kahn MF, et al. (1997) Serum sickness after wasp venom immunotherapy: clinical and biological study. J Rheumatol 24:1195–1197
9. Forck G, Kästner H, Kalveram C (1981) Insect venom tolerance: IgG-"blocking" antibodies and sting provocation. In: Ring J, Burg G (eds) New trends in allergy. Springer, Berlin Heidelberg New York, p 269
10. Fuchs E (1959) Allergie. Münch Med Wochenschr 100:1711
11. Golden DBK, Valentine MD, Kagey-Sobotka A, Lichtenstein ML (1982) Prevalence of hymenoptera venom allergy. J Allergy Clin Immunol 69:124
12. Habermann E (1972) Bee and wasp venoms. Science 177:314
13. Hemmer W, Focke M, Jarisch R (1999) In-vitro-Doppelpositivität gegen Bienen- und Wespengift. Allergologie 22 [Suppl 2]:63–64
14. Hunt KJ, Valentine MD, Sobotka AK, Benton AW, Amodio FJ, Lichtenstein LM (1978) A controlled trial of immunotherapy in insect hypersensitivity. N Engl J Med 299:157
15. Jarisch R (1980) Die Bienengiftallergie (Modell einer IgE-mediierten Soforttypallergie). Wien Klin Wochenschr 92 [Suppl 122]:3
16. Jeßberger B, Habig J, Karl S, et al. (1994) Hymenopterengiftallergie: Hyposensibilisierungstherapie trotz vorhandener Kontraindikationen. Allergologie 17:255–260
17. Kämmerer H (1941) Fragekasten. Münch Med Wochenschr 88:939
18. Kiehn M, Ring J (1993) Hyposensibilisierung mit Insektengiftextrakten bei Patienten mit Hymenopterengift-Allergie im höheren Lebensalter. Allergo J 2 [Suppl 2]:90–94
19. King TP, Lu G, Gonzalez M, Qian N, Soldatova L (1996) Yellow jacket venom allergens, hyaluronidase and phospholipase: Sequence similarity and antigenic cross-reactivity with their hornet and wasp homologues and possible implications for clinical allergy. J Allergy Clin Immunol 98:588–600
20. Lerch E, Müller UR (1998) Long-term protection after stopping venom immunotherapy: results of restings in 200 patients. J Allergy Clin Immunol 101:606–612
21. Lessof M, Sobotka AK, Lichtenstein LM (1976) Protection against anaphylaxis in hymenoptera-sensitive patients by passive immunization. J Allergy Clin Immunol 57:246
22. Lichtenstein LM, Valentine MD, Sobotka AK (1974) A case for venom treatment in anaphylactic sensitivity to hymenoptera sting. N Engl J Med 290:1223
23. Light WV, Reismann RE, Rosario NA, Arbesman CE (1976) Comparison of the allergenic properties of bee venom and whole bee body extract. Clin Allergy 6:293
24. Lockey RF (1975) Systemic reactions to stinging ants. J Allergy Clin Immunol 54:132

25. Lonsdorf G, Ring J, Burg G (1981) Anaphylaktische Reaktionen nach Insektenstichen. Notfall Medizin 7:409
26. Lotter G (1939) Sensibilisierung für Bienengift durch Typhus-Antitoxin und Desensibilisierung mit Forapin. Münch Med Wochenschr 86:330–331
27. Loveless MH, Fackler WR (1956) Wasp venom allergy and immunity. Ann Allergy 14:347
28. Mauss V (1999) Einfluß von Lebensweise, Populationsdynamik und Abwehrverhalten aculeater Hymenopteren auf das Stichrisiko für den Menschen. Allergologie 22 [Suppl]:542–545
29. Mauss V, Treiber R (1994) Betreuungsschlüssel für die Faltenwespen (Hymenoptera: Masarinae, Polistinae, Vespinae) der Bundesrepublik Deutschland. Deutscher Jugendbund für Naturbeobachtung, Hamburg
30. Mueller HL, Schmid WH, Rubinstein R (1975) Stinging-insect hypersensitivity. A 20-year old study of immunologic treatment. Pediatrics 55:530
31. Müller UR (1988) Insektenstichallergie. Klinik, Diagnostik und Therapie. G. Fischer, Stuttgart
32. Müller U (2001) New development in the diagnosis and treatment of hymenoptera venom allergy. Int Arch Allergy Immunol 124:447–499
33. Müller U, Mosbech H (1993) Position paper: Immunotherapy with hymenoptera venoms. Allergy 48 [Suppl 2]:37–46
34. Mumcuoglu Y, Rufli T (1980) Dermatologische Entomologie. 12. Apidael Bienen. 13. Vespidae Wespen. Schweiz Rundsch Med 69:1317, 1574
35. O'Connor R, Peck ML (1978) Venoms of Apidae. In: Handbook of experimental pharmacology, vol 48. Springer, Berlin Heidelberg New York, p 613
36. Ollert M, Ring J (1999) Prognostische Bedeutung von Immunoblot-Untersuchungen bei Hymenopterengift-Allergie. Allergologie 22 [Suppl 2]: 578–579
37. Parrish HM (1963) Analysis of 460 fatalities from venomous animals in the United States. Am J Med Sci 245:129
38. Przybilla B, Ring J, Galosi A, Geursen RG, Stickl HA (1986) Bee-venom immunoglobulin for prophylaxis of anaphylactic reactions during bee venom immunotherapy (rush hyposensitization). Immunol Allergy Practice 8:107–111
39. Przybilla B (1986) Pathophysiologische und klinische Aspekte der allergischen Reaktion vom Soforttyp und der Immunglobulin-E-Immunantwort: Untersuchungen unter besonderer Berücksichtigung der Bienen- und Wespengiftallergie. Habilitationsschrift, Munich
40. Przybilla B, Ring J, Grießhammer B, Braun-Falco O (1987) Schnellhyposensibilisierung mit Hymenopterengiften – Verträglichkeit und Therapieerfolg. Dtsch Med Wochenschr 112:416
41. Przybilla B, Ring J, Rieger B (1992) Die Indikation zur Hymenopterengift-Hyposensibilisierung kann nicht anhand eines diagnostischen Parameters bewertenden Punkteschemas gestellt werden. Allergologie 13:114–119
42. Rakoski J, Mayenburg J von (1986) Das Ultra-Rush-Verfahren – eine neue Methode zur Überprüfung der Aktualität von Insektengiftallergien. Allergologie 9:73–74
43. Ring J, Lonsdorf G, Schury W, Burg G (1982) Bienen- und Wespengift-Allergie. Klinik Prophylaxe und Therapie. Münch Med Wochenschr 124:587
44. Ring J, Gottsmann M, Przybilla B, Eisenmenger W (1986) Tod nach 1000 Bienenstichen. Münch Med Wochenschr 128:339
45. Ring J, Przybilla B, Müller U (1997) Insektengiftallergie: Aktuelles für die Praxis. Allergo J 6 [Suppl 1]:571–572
46. Rueff F, Reißig J, Przybilla B (1997) Nebenwirkungen der Schnellhyposensibilisierung mit Hymenopterengift. Allergo J 6 [Suppl 1]:659–664
47. Rueff F, Przybilla B, Fuchs T, Gall H, Rakoski J, Stolz W, Vieluf D (2000) Diagnose und Therapie der Bienen- und Wespengiftallergie. Positionspapier der Deutschen Gesellschaft für Allergologie und klinische Immunologie (DGAI). Allergo J 9:458–472
48. Rzany B, Przybilla B, Jarisch R, et al (1991) Clinical characteristics of immunotherapy with Hymenoptera venoms. A retrospective study. Allergy 46:251–254
49. Schäfer T, Przybilla B (1996) IgE antibodies to hymenoptera venoms in the serum are common in the general population and are related to indications of atopy. Allergy 51:372–377
50. Schumacher MJ, Tveten MS, Egen NB (1994) Rate and quantity of delivery of venom from honeybee stings. J Allergy Clin Immunol 93:831–835
51. Schuberth KC, Golden DBK, Kagey-Sobotka A, Valentine M, Lichtenstein LM (1981) Evaluation and treatment of insect sting allergy. In: Ring J, Burg G (eds) New trends in allergy. Springer, Berlin Heidelberg New York, p 260
52. Settipane GA, Newstead GJ, Boyd GK (1972) Frequency of hymenoptera allergy in an atopic and normal population. J Allergy Clin Immunol 50:176
53. Stibich AS, Carbonaro PA, Schwartz RA (2001) Insect bite reactions: an update. Dermatology 202:193–197
54. Tokura Y (1994) Lymphocyte populations associated with exaggerated insect bite reactions. J Am Acad Dermatol 31:298
55. Tunget CL, Clark RF (1993) Invasion of the "killer" bees. Separating fact from fiction. Postgrad Med 94:92–102
56. Urbanek R (1979) Neue Konzepte der Behandlung von Insektengiftallergien. Derm Beruf Umwelt 27:44
57. Van der Zwan JC, Flintermann J, Jankowski IG, et al. (1983) Hyposensitisation to wasp venom in six hours. Br Med J 287:1329–1331
58. Weed RI (1965) Exaggerated delayed hypersensitivity to mosquito bite in chronic lymphocyte leukemia. Blood 26:257–268

5.1.7 Allergy and the Eye

5.1.7.1 Introduction

Allergic eye diseases are sometimes only marginally covered in allergy textbooks, e.g., "rhinoconjunctivitis." Often, the most common elicitors of allergic conjunctivitis are called "inhalation allergens." Attempts to classify allergic eye diseases are difficult, partly due to different understandings of diseases as well as lack of knowledge of histopathophysiology of common conditions. The term "conjunctivitis" – used by many allergists as a synonym for type I allergy – only has a descriptive character and is used for clinical conditions of quite different pathophysiology; it can be best compared with the term "dermatitis" in dermatology.

Transparency of the central part of the eye is the major basic condition for visual function. In cornea, anterior chamber, lens, and vitreous body, there are no lymph or blood vessels and no immunocompetent cells. The barrier between blood and chamber fluid as well as blood and retina is physiological. The anterior chamber of the eye is an immunologically privileged site [2, 5, 6, 11, 14, 21]. Inflammatory reactions occur mostly in the neighboring tissue, especially conjunctiva, where 90 % of the mast cells of the eye are situated [2, 20].

5.1.7.2 Atopic Eye Diseases

5.1.7.2.1 Type I Allergic Conjunctivitis

This acute form of allergic conjunctivitis is classically combined with hay fever, but also in perennial allergy against airborne allergens without nasal symptoms. Pathophysiology corresponds to IgE-mediated allergic rhinitis and allergic bronchial asthma (type I). The clinical symptoms comprise itching, burning, photophobia, immediate hyperemia, and chemosis of the conjunctiva (often aggravated by rubbing) and increased lacrimation. There is no papillary reaction and no corneal involvement. All the symptoms can be elicited by local histamine application. In animal experiments, this type of allergy is also called ocular anaphylaxis [2, 6, 22]. Prophylaxis and therapy comprise allergen avoidance, mast cell stabilizers, antihis-

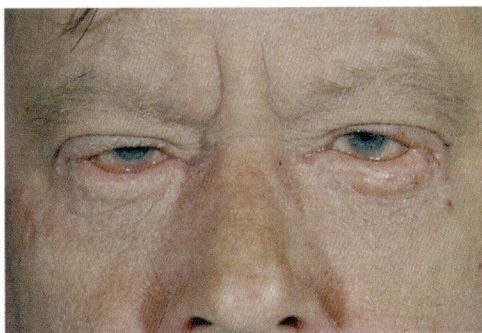

Fig. 5.19. Atopic keratoconjunctivitis

tamines, as well as vasoconstrictors [20]. Rarely, steroids are necessary. Occasionally, cyclooxygenase inhibitors such as ketorolac can help against itch [20].

5.1.7.2.2 Atopic Keratoconjunctivitis

Chronic atopic conjunctivitis (Fig. 5.19) often occurs with other manifestations of atopy and is predominantly observed in medium-aged males; the pathophysiology may be similar to that of atopic eczema with increased cellular infiltrates and high IgE in serum and tear fluid [6, 9]. The conjunctiva is thickened, rather pale and chemotic. Not infrequently, the cornea can be affected, sometimes vascularized. Almost all patients also suffer from intense lid eczema with common superinfections. Mast cell stabilizers and glucocorticosteroids are recommended, generally topically (sometimes also systemically).

The so-called atopic cataract (prevalence of up to 25 %; in our opinion this has been overestimated in the past) is associated with atopic eczema [2, 21]. This cataract involves the lens epithelium of the anterior lens capsule and can be clearly differentiated from steroid-induced posterior subcapsular cataract.

5.1.7.2.3 Vernal Keratoconjunctivitis

This chronically relapsing general conjunctivitis occurs predominantly in southern countries often seasonally in spring and summer and is characterized by papillary hyperplasia of the tarsal upper lid conjunctiva [8]. The disease begins often before the 10th year and subsides spontaneously after puberty. In 70–80% of cases, it occurs with other atopic diseases; boys are more often affected than girls (3:1). Two anatomic forms are differentiated: a palpebral form with typical "cobblestone conjunctivitis" of the upper lid and a limbal form (more common in colored people and American Indians).

Symptoms are characterized by intense itching. Patients feel like "scratching out their eyes." Furthermore, burning, redness, swelling, photophobia and in 50% also corneal involvement as superficial keratitis occur. Rarely, ulcus vernalis occurs by loosening of the cornea epithelium through eosinophil products [22].

A thick white mucous secretion can be seen containing numerous eosinophils. Histologically, mast cells are increased, and eosinophils and basophil leukocytes can be found in conjunctival epithelium [2]. In the tear fluid, histamine and complement products are elevated [1].

There is no clear-cut relation to aeroallergens in spite of sometimes positive prick test results. Therefore, specific immunotherapy mostly remains unsuccessful. As basic therapy, mast cell stabilizers are used, in acute exacerbation steroids, in severe cases even cyclosporin topically. Occasionally with massive mucous secretion, topical administration of mucolytics (acetylcysteine 10–20%) has been tried. In corneal involvement, surgical removal of papillae with subsequent coagulation of the conjunctiva is helpful.

5.1.7.2.4 Giant Papillary Conjunctivitis in Contact Lens Wearers

This conjunctivitis is observed in people wearing predominantly soft – sometimes after some latency also hard – contact lenses as well as plastic eye prostheses and corresponds clinically and histologically to conjunctivitis vernalis in the early stage. There is no evidence for atopy. Allergic reactions against unknown allergens from contact lenses or cleaning fluid in the mucus are suspected [6, 17].

Avoidance of contact lenses is the first step, and renewal of contact lenses and changing to preservative-free lens fluids (especially enzymes!) are recommended.

5.1.7.3 Contact-Allergic Conjunctivitis (Type IV)

This common form of ocular allergy occurs with itching, redness and infiltration (sometimes "follicular") conjunctivitis; often simultaneous allergic contact dermatitis of the lid (blepharo-conjunctivitis) is seen. Pathophysiologically, type IV hypersensitivity corresponding to allergic contact dermatitis is present (see Sect. 5.5.2). The most common elicitors are therapeutics (antibiotics, local anesthetics, preservatives in eyedrops), but also chemicals, cosmetics, and phytoallergens [10, 11, 21].

5.1.7.4 Blepharitis and Lid Eczema

The differential diagnosis of blepharitis and lid eczema comprises apart from allergic conditions (mostly type IV) and atopic eczema also irritative reactions such as cumulative toxic eczema (especially when eyedrops or wet wraps are applied too frequently), psoriasis, rosacea, seborrheic eczema, as well as infectious diseases with inflammatory reactions.

A common disease is microbial-allergic conjunctivitis: On the basis of an initiating staphylococcal infection, blepharoconjunctivitis occurs with hypersensitivity against bacterial exotoxins and the formation of conjunctival phlyctena or keratitis marginalis.

5.1.7.5 Cicatricial Conjunctivitis in Erythema Exsudativum Multiforme or Lyell's Syndrome

In rare cases, erythema exsudativum multiforme can occur with massive conjunctival swelling and cicatricial conjunctivitis ("syndroma muco-cutaneo-oculare Fuchs" or "Stevens-Johnson syndrome").

In the acute phase, bullous, partly pustular changes can be seen, leading to erosions with cicatricial healing. Conjunctiva is affected with hyperemia, chemosis, bulla formation, and ulceration. Sometimes scarring of the conjunctiva with entropium, trichiasis, and synechia occurs. Secondary disturbance of lacrimation and bacterial superinfection lead to severe corneal ulcers. The pathophysiology of this reaction is unclear. Apart from a postherpetic form ("infect allergy"), drug-induced Stevens-Johnson syndrome has been described with subepithelial vesiculation, epithelial necrosis, and superficial inflammatory reaction [11].

A similar condition is observed in toxic epidermal necrolysis (TEN), also called drug-induced Lyell's syndrome. The pathophysiology is unclear; type III and IV reactions as well as apoptotic processes are discussed (see Sect. 5.7.3 on "Drug Eruptions").

Early ophthalmologic counseling is the primary recommendation. Hourly nursing with steroids, topical artificial tears and regular prophylaxis of symblepharon is important; however, sometimes serious changes cannot be prevented. Early systemic corticosteroids are controversial. In cases with corneal involvement and opacification, prognosis quoad visum is poor. The cornea transplantation in these cases is often unsuccessful, synechiolysis shows a high relapse rate, mucous membrane transplantation is difficult, and sometimes amnion transplants succeed.

Ocular (Scarring) Mucous Membrane Pemphigoid. The processes in scarring pemphigoid are pathogenetically similar where autoantibodies against basement membrane have been formed. The disease manifests as chronic progredient scarring conjunctivitis with mostly severe corneal complications responding poorly to therapy (local therapy together with systemic immunosuppression with steroids, cyclophosphamide, dapsone, etc.).

5.1.7.6 Eye Diseases of Questionable Allergic Origin

Sympathetic Ophthalmia. Sympathetic ophthalmia is a diffuse granulomatous inflammation of the uvea of both eyes – also of the unlesional eye – as a consequence of a perforating trauma or intraocular surgery and represents a classic autoimmune disease [12]. The organism is sensitized against proteins with which the immune system because of the privileged anatomical site was previously not in contact. The time interval between primary trauma and occurrence of sympathetic ophthalmia is variable; 90% of cases occur within 1 year. The resulting uveitis may destroy the eye. Therapeutically, high-dose glucocorticosteroids with or without immunosuppressives, which are sometimes lifelong, are indicated [11, 18, 19]. Enucleation of the traumatized eye after the occurrence of sympathetic ophthalmia is rarely helpful.

Endogenous Autoimmune Uveitis. It has been discussed as to what degree certain forms of endogenous uveitis correspond pathophysiologically to an immune complex vasculitis [18].

Paraneoplastic Retinopathy. In patients with neoplasia or melanoma-associated retinopathy, autoimmune processes in the sense of a cross-reaction between tumor antigens and retinal proteins have been found with the formation of antibodies against retinal constituents, leading to disturbance of retinal function. There is little therapy of these conditions, and in occasional cases plasmapheresis has been used.

Graft Versus Host Reactions. A rare complication of bone marrow transplantation in leukemia is severe keratoconjunctivitis with opacification and vascularization of the cornea.

5.1.7.7 Therapy

If possible, treatment should be topical – except for the severe autoimmune diseases. Table 5.37 lists some antiallergic eyedrops with different drugs. Long-term steroid treatment should be avoided. For lid eczema the new topical calcineurin inhibitors (tacrolimus and pimecrolimus) (see Sect. 5.5.3) are promising.

Table 5.37. Antiallergic eyedrops

Active substances	
DSCG (disodium cromoglycate)	Flurbiprofen
	Diclofenac
Lodoxamide	**Glucocorticosteroids**
Nedocromil	Betamethasone
Azelastine	Dexamethasone
Emedastine	Fluorometholone
Levocabastine	Prednisolone
	Rinaxolone
Non-steroidal anti-inflammatory drugs (NSAIDs)	
Ketorolac	
Indometacin	

References

1. Abelson MB, Schaefer K (1993) Conjunctivitis of allergic origin: immunologic mechanisms and current approaches to therapy. Surv Ophthalmol 38:115–132
2. Allansmith MR (1982) The eye and immunology. Mosby, St. Louis
3. Allansmith MR, Ross RN (1986) Ocular allergy and mast cell stabilizers. Surv Ophthalmol 30:229–244
4. Anderson DF (1996) The conjunctival late-phase reaction and allergen provocation in the eye. Clin Exp Allergy 26:1105–1107
5. Bialasiewicz AA (1998) Augenheilkunde. In: Heppt W, Renz H, Röcken M (eds) Allergologie. Springer, Berlin Heidelberg New York, pp 262–271
6. Bielory L (2000) Allergic and immunologic disorders of the eye, part II: ocular allergy. J Allergy Clin Immunol 106:1019–1032
7. Bonini S, Bucci MG, et al. (1990) Allergen dose response and late symptoms in a human model of ocular allergy. J Allergy Clin Immunol 86/6:869–876
8. Bonini S, Bonini S, Lambiase A, et al. (2000) Vernal keratoconjunctivitis revisited: a case series of 195 patients with long-term followup. Ophthalmology 107:1157–1163
9. Foster CS, Rice BA, Dutt JE (1991) Immunopathology of atopic keratoconjuncitvitis. Ophthalmology 98:1190–1196
10. Friedlaender MH (1988) Contact allergy and toxicity in the eye. Int Ophthalmol Clin 28/4: 317–320
11. Friedlaender MH (1993) Allergy and immunology of the eye. Raven, New York
12. Fuchs E (1905) Über sympathisierende Entzündung. Albrecht v. Graefes Arch Ophthal 61:365
13. Hatinen A, Terasvirta M, Fakj JE (1985) Contact allergy to components in topical ophthalmologic preparations. Acta Ophthalmol 63:424–426
14. Jay JL (1981) Clinical factors and diagnosis of atopic keratoconjunctivitis and the effect of treatment with sodium cromoglycate. Br J Ophthal 60:335–340
15. McGill J (2000) Conjunctival cytokines in ocular allergy. Clin Exp Allergy 30:1355–1357
16. Montan PG, Biberfeld PJ, Scheynius A (1995) IgE, IgE receptors and other immunocytochemical markers in atopic and nonatopic patients with vernal keratoconjunctivitis. Ophthalmology 102:725–732
17. Neuhann T (1983) Papillomatös-hyperplastische Konjunktivitis durch Kontaktlinsen. Mbl Augenheilkunde 8:46–50
18. Ring I, Dechant W, Seifert J, Lund O-E, Grette J-H, Stefani FH, Brendel W (1978) Immunosuppression with antilymphocyte globulin (ALG) in the treatment of ophthalmic disorders. Ophthal Res 10:82–97
19. Silverstein AM, O'Connor GR (eds) (1979) Immunology and immunopathology of the eye. Masson, New York
20. Solomon A, Pe'er J, Levi-Schaffer F (2001) Advances in ocular allergy: basic mechanisms, clinical patterns and new therapies. Curr Opin Allergy Clin Immunol 1:477–482
21. Theodore FH, Schlossmann A (1958) Ocular allergy. Williams & Wilkins, Baltimore
22. Trocme SD, Aldave AJ (1994) The eye and the eosinophil. Surv Ophthalmol 39:241–252

5.2 Allergic Diseases by Cytotoxic Antibodies (Type II)

5.2.1 Mechanisms of Antibody-Mediated Cytotoxicity

The cytotoxic reaction (type II) is mediated by antibodies with or without complement activation directed against markers on hematologic cells. The classical type II reaction is the transfusion reaction (hemolytic reaction caused by natural mostly IgM and complement-binding antibodies) against foreign blood group antigens [10]. The antigens of the AB0 system differ by the terminal sugar residue on a common glycolipid (paragloboside) with a terminal fucose (= H-antigen in group 0), to which either N-acetyl-D-galactosamine (group A) or D-galactose (group B) are bound [29].

Another form of type II reaction is the *hyperacute rejection* after organ transplantation, mediated by specific antibodies [5].

Theoretically, some autoimmune diseases also have to be classified under this type of reaction when organ-specific antibodies play a role (certain forms of glomerulonephritis = Masugi nephritis, pemphigus vulgaris, bullous pemphigoid, Goodpasture's syndrome, autoimmune hemolytic anemia).

Cytotoxic antibodies may destroy cells via different mechanisms (Fig. 5.20).

- **Complement-mediated cytotoxicity**
  Binding of the antibody molecule to the cell surface leads to activation of complement via the classical pathway with subsequent cell lysis (activation of C6 to C9).

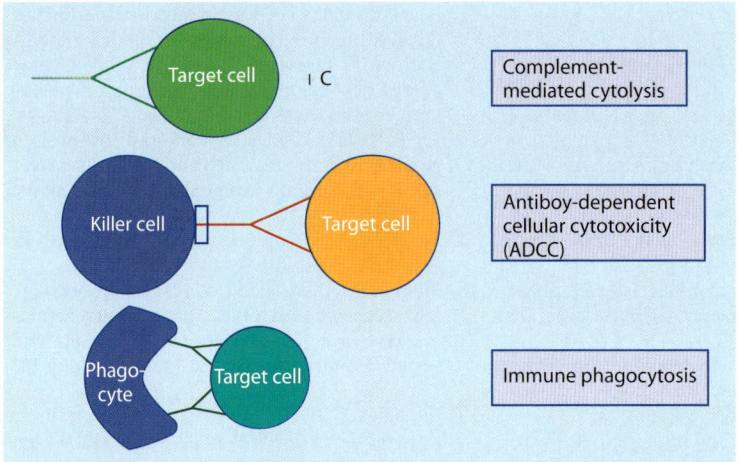

Fig. 5.20. Mechanisms of allergic cytotoxicity

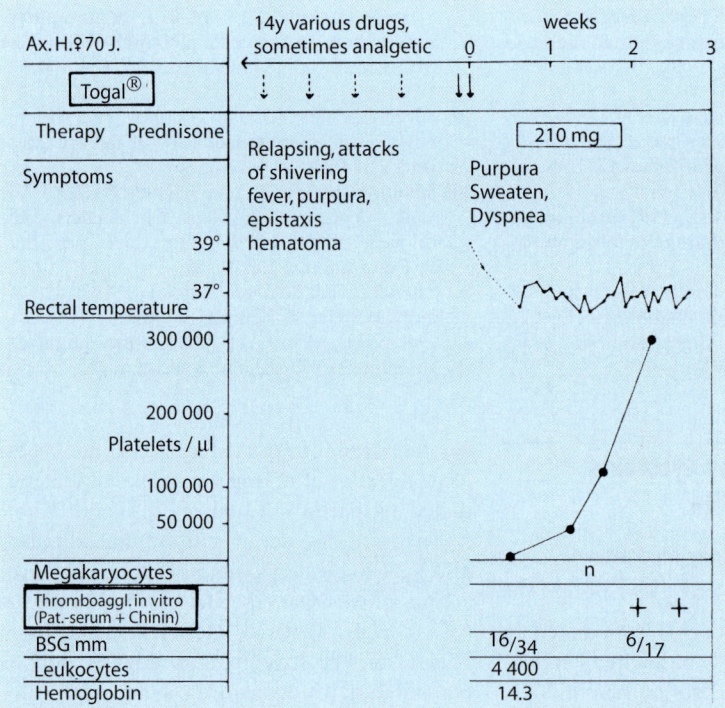

Fig. 5.21. Course of a thrombocytopenia induced by quinine (in Togal). Remission followed termination of the drug (reprinted with the permission of Raif and Schubothe [20])

- Antibody-dependent cellular cytotoxicity (ADCC)
  Here the antibody acts together with the so-called killer cell, to which it is bound. These cells represent a subgroup of lymphocytes with large granules showing neither typical T- nor B-cell characteristics. The cell destruction follows similar mechanisms such as T-cell-mediated cytotoxicity (perforin, etc.).
- Antibody-dependent phagocytosis (immune phagocytosis)
  Here cytotoxic antibodies are bound via Fc-receptors to the surface of macrophages. After binding of antigens on the target cell, the latter will be phagocytosed.

5.2 Allergic Diseases by Cytotoxic Antibodies (Type II)

These mechanisms are best investigated in peripheral blood cells; however, it is speculated that tissue destruction in parenchymatous organs occurs in a similar manner (e.g., hepatitis).

The most important allergic diseases of the blood (Figs. 5.20–5.22a) are triggered by drugs; similar conditions may also be elicited by infections (especially virus), lymphoproliferative diseases, other neoplasias or "idiopathically." The complex interaction between drug and target cell occurs in different ways (types of cytotoxic reaction) [1, 14, 20]:

1. *"Hapten" type.* Here the drug is bound to the cell surface leading to a new antigen; with or without complement activation, specific antibodies lead to cell destruction (e.g., penicillin, cephalosporins). Hemolysis occurs extravascularly after high-dose administration; IgG can be detected on the surface of erythrocytes without complement products (e.g., C3d).

2. *"Immune complex" type* (not to be confused with immune complex reaction of type III!). Here a complex of antibody and antigen formed intravascularly with activation of complement leads to cell destruction [15] most likely via Fc receptors. Since the target cells only are lysed through secondary absorption of immune complexes, this reaction was also called "innocent bystander." This mechanism is the most common form of drug-induced allergic cytopenia. The reactions are acute after minute doses. C3d can be detected on the cell surface [22, 23].

3. *"Autoimmune" type.* The drug changes first the cell surface, leading to the develop-

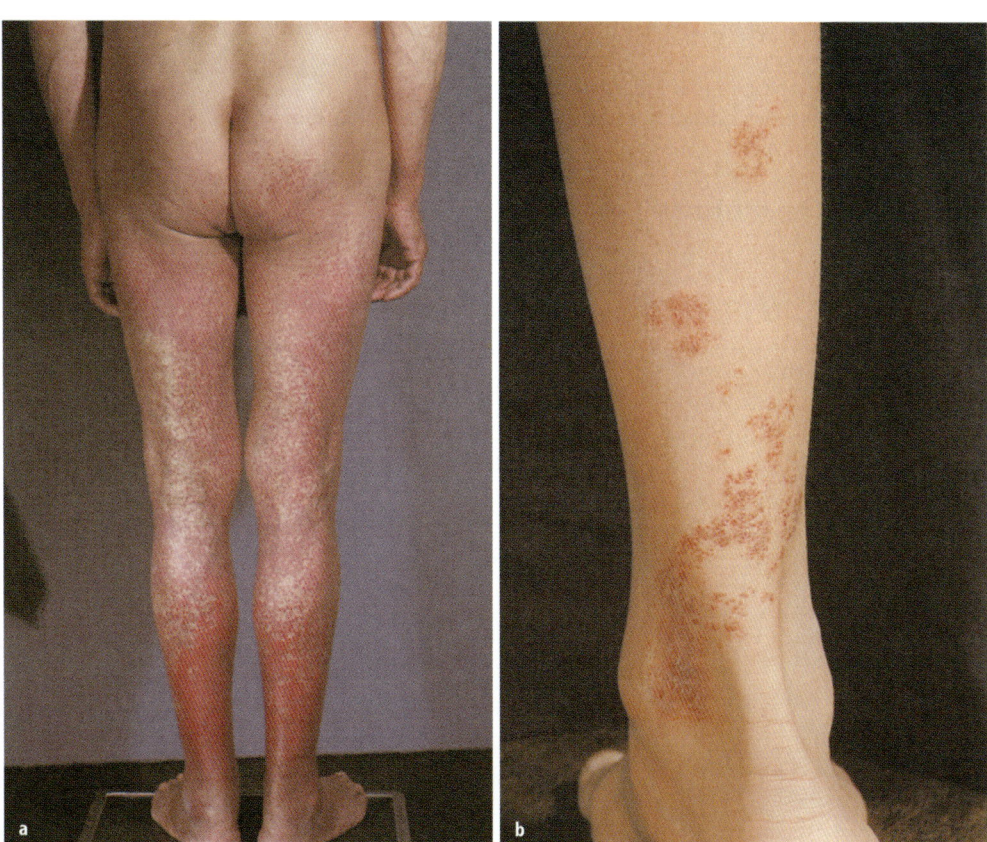

Fig. 5.22a,b. Clinical manifestations of allergic thrombocytopenic purpura

ment of a new "autoantigen." Autoimmune diseases of the blood may be triggered (e.g., hemolytic anemia by alphamethyldopa). Autoantibody formation continues after withdrawal of the drug and does not differ from idiopathic autoimmune hemolytic anemia of the heat type.

5.2.2 Allergic Diseases of the Blood

5.2.2.1 Allergic Hemolytic Anemia

The most important drugs eliciting different types of allergic hemolytic anemias are listed in Table 5.38. After high doses of penicillin (over 10 million U/day), slowly developing anemia of the hapten type occurs. The direct Coombs' test is positive. After withdrawal, hemoglobin normalizes. Antibodies (mostly IgG) do not react with normal erythrocytes. Quinine, chlorpromazine, and isoniazid are the most common elicitors of hemolytic anemia of the immune complex type.

Alpha-methyldopa, L-dopa, mefenamic acid, as well as methysergide may induce subacute heat-autoantibody-mediated anemia. After several months of treatment, 11% of patients develop a positive direct Coombs' test; only in 0.7% of patients does anemia develop [23].

A common diagnostic criterion is the occurrence of hemoglobinemia and hemoglobinuria, a hemoglobin decrease with normal MCHB, an increase in indirect bilirubin and a decrease in haptoglobin. In rare cases, renal insufficiency or diffuse intravascular coagulation can occur.

Pathophysiologically, mixed forms occur, e.g., after nomifensin or cianidanol [13, 22]. Withdrawal of the eliciting drug is the main therapy.

5.2.2.2 Allergic Agranulocytosis

Allergic agranulocytosis develops in highly acute form mostly via the hapten mechanism. A few days (in repeated treatments within hours) after intake of the eliciting drug (e.g., aminopyrine, metamizol, sulfonylurea, Table 5.39), leukocytes decrease, fever attacks occur, and putrid tonsillitis develops with glossitis, thrush, bronchitis and severe disease.

Differential diagnosis comprises toxic granulocytopenias due to bone marrow depression (e.g., cytostatics), which develop slowly over a subacute chronic stomatitis. A possible new type of drug reaction has been described as neutropenia after high toxic doses of penicillin (220–550 million U) [16].

Therapy consists in withdrawal of the drug, high-dose i.v. immunoglobulin, adequate antibiosis, possibly glucocorticosteroids, and intravenous G-CSF.

Table 5.38. Drugs eliciting allergic hemolytic anemia (selection)

Hapten type	
Penicillin	Rifampicin
Cephalosporin	Cisplatin
Immune complex type ("innocent bystander")	
Aminophenazone	Melphalan
Acetylsalicylic acid	Metamizol
Butizide	Paracetamol
Quinidine	Phenacetin
Quinine	Rifampicin
Chlorpromazine	Streptomycin
Ibuprofen	Salicylamide
Insulin	Sulfonamide
Isoniazid	Sulfonylurea
Autoimmune type	
Chlorpromazine	Latamoxef
Glafenin	Levodopa
Hydantoin	Mefenamic acid
Ibuprofen	Methysergide
Methyldopa	Procainamide

Table 5.39. Drugs eliciting allergic agranulocytosis (selection)

Aminophenazone	Methyldopa
Aminopyrine	Novobiocin
Aminosalicylic acid	Penicillins
Quinidine	Phenothiazines
Chloral hydrate	Phenylbutazone
Chlorpromazine	Procainamide
Diazepoxide	Propranolol
Ethacrynic acid	Mercury diuretics
Gold salts	Salazosulfapyridine
Hydantoin	Sulfonamide
Metamizol	Sulfonylurea
Methimazol	Thiouracil

5.2.2.3 Allergic Thrombocytopenia

The prototype of allergic hematologic disease is apronalid purpura, first described by Ackroyd [1] through an immune complex type reaction. Today, the most common elicitors are listed in Table 5.40. Figure 5.21 shows a typical course of a thrombocytopenia in allergy against quinine [20] in a mixed analgesic preparation. Clinically, apart from a non-inflammatory purpura (Fig. 5.22a,b), sweating attacks, dyspnea, fever with shivering, and mucosal bleeding together with lowered platelet counts are typical. The diagnosis can be confirmed in vitro using patients' serum together with the suspected drug and adding it to a platelet suspension and measuring changes in platelet function (e.g., aggregation, serotonin, or platelet factor 3 release) with the adequate controls.

Treatment consists of immediate withdrawal of the drug and high-dose glucocorticosteroids together with i.v. immunoglobulins (0.4 g/kg over 5 days) [14]. Sometimes, fresh blood transfusion may be indicated. Continuation of therapy with vital drugs under systemic glucocorticoids has been reported [28].

In differential diagnosis, post-transfusion purpura should be considered developing mostly in PL^{A1}-negative women 1 week after transfusion of PL^{A1}-positive blood occurring with high antibody titers against PL^{A1} [14, 26]. Equally important is the exclusion of idiopathic thrombocytopenic purpura (ITP), where serum does not induce platelet changes in normals. Therapeutically, glucocorticosteroids together with high-dose immunoglobulins are given.

Besides allergic and toxic mechanisms, also enzyme defects can induce bone marrow depression via an idiosyncrasy (see also "Pseudoallergic Reactions," Sect. 5.7.3). It has been attempted to measure this in vitro by the inhibitory effect of certain substances on bone marrow stem cells [9].

5.2.2.4 Heparin-Induced Thrombocytopenia

The heparin-induced thrombocytopenia (HIT) is of major practical importance. Two types are differentiated [2]:

HIT 1, spontaneously reversible via inhibition of platelet adenylate cyclase activity and without major complications.

HIT 2, which is more dangerous, developing after 5–14 days and occurring with thrombocytopenia, but at the same time increasing the risk of thrombosis and embolization. Pathophysiologically, IgG antibodies against a multimolecular complex consisting of heparin and platelet factor 4 cause HIT 2 [7, 21]. The size and degree of sulfatation of the heparin molecule seem to be crucial in the elicitation of HIT 2. The mechanism corresponds to an immune complex cytotoxic mechanism through an Fcγ RII activation.

The strong platelet-stimulating effect leads to microparticles from lysed platelets, which circulate in the blood and enhance thrombosis [21].

Immediate withdrawal of heparin is the first step of therapy! Changing to coumarin in the first few days is contraindicated since this will further increase risk of thrombosis. For therapy, low molecular and low sulfatized heparinoids may be tried such as danaparoid, recombinant hirudin or a synthetic thrombin inhibitor argatroban [18, 24].

Table 5.40. Drugs eliciting allergic thrombocytopenia (selection)

Alprenolol	Metamizol
Allylcarbamide (e.g., Sedormid)	Novobiocin
	Para-aminosalicylic acid (PAS)
Aminopyrine	
Acetacolamide	Penicillamine
Acetylsalicylic acid	Phenacetin
Carbamazepine	Phensuximide
Cephalotin	Phenylbutazone
Quinine and quinidine	Procainamide
Chloramphenicol	Reserpine
Chloroquine	Rifampicin
Chlorothiazide	Salicylamide
Digitoxin	Stibophen
Furosemide	Sulfonylurea
Gold salts	Tetracycline
Heparin	Thiazide
Hydantoin	Tolbutamide
Isoniazid	Trimethoprim
Levodopa	Valproate
Meprobamate	

5.2.2.5 Eosinophilia

After certain drugs (Table 5.41), blood eosinophilia, sometimes without incompatibility symptoms, develops possibly due to increased interleukin-5 production from T lymphocytes. The prognostic relevance is unclear; for safety reasons, sometimes withdrawal of the drug is recommended.

Table 5.41. Drugs inducing eosinophilia

Allopurinol	Isoniazid
Aminosalicylic acid	Kanamycin
Cephalosporins	Nalidixic acid
Chloral hydrate	Nitrofurantoin
Dacarbazine	Penicillamine
Digitalis	Rifampicin
Erythromycin	Sulfonamides

Eosinophilia Myalgia Syndrome. The pathogenesis of the eosinophilia myalgia syndrome (EMS) described in 1989 after intake of L-tryptophan for depression and sleeplessness is not clear. In epidemiological studies comparing different batches of the drug, an impurity (peak E) with 1.1 ethylidene-bis-tryptophan was determined as elicitor. Apart from scleroderma-like changes and neuropathy, signs of myositis and in 50% autoantibodies with extremely elevated eosinophil counts in the peripheral blood were observed (1,000–36,000/µl) [3, 27].

5.2.3 Allergic Cytotoxic Organopathies

5.2.3.1 Drug-Induced Hepatitis

After certain drugs, antibodies against liver cells and constituents (e.g., microsomes, cytochrome P450 isotypes) may develop with cytotoxic effects on hepatocytes detectable in vitro [4, 11, 12, 17]. Drugs under discussion are halothane, chlorpromazine, some anticonvulsants, thyreostatics, as well as rarely antibiotics (sulfanomides, erythromycin estolate) [6].

5.2.3.2 Drug-Induced Nephropathy

After certain drugs, acute tubular disturbance of the kidney, sometimes occurring with exanthematous drug eruptions, has been reported; the mechanisms are unclear. Apart from classic immune complex nephritis (serum nephritis) (see Sect. 5.3), specific antibodies against altered renal antigens such as tubular basement membrane constituents [8] have been reported. Rarely, an allergic basis of nephrotic syndrome (gold, penicillamine, captopril, lithium) with positive lymphocyte transformation has been reported (see also Sect. 5.7.4 on "Drug-Induced Exanthematous Eruptions").

References

1. Ackroyd JF (1952) Sedormid purpura: An immunological study of drug hypersensitivity. Progr Allergy 3:531
2. Aster RH (1995) Heparin-induced thrombocytopenia and thrombosis. N Engl J Med 332: 1374–1376
3. Belongia EA, Hedberg CW, Gleich GJ (1990) An investigation into the cause of the eosinophilia myalgia syndrome associated with tryptophan use. N Engl J Med 323:357–365
4. Berg PA, Becker EW (1995) The lymphocyte transformation test – a debated method for the evaluation of drug allergic hepatic injury. J Hepatol 22:115–118
5. Brendel W, Ring J (1980) Transplantationsimmunologie. In: Filipp G (ed) Allergologie. Banaschewski, Munich, p 436
6. Dukes MNG (1998) Drug-induced hepatic injury. Elsevier, Amsterdam
7. Greinacher A, Potzsch B, Amiral J, Dummel V, Eichner A, Mueller-Eckhardt C (1994) Heparin in associated thrombocytopenia: isolation of the antibody and characterization of a multimolecular PF4-heparin complex as the major antigen. Thromb Haemost 71:247–251
8. Jäger L, Merk HF (1996) Arzneimittel-Allergie. Gustav Fischer, Jena
9. Kelton JG, Huang AT, Mold N (1979) The use of in vitro techniques to study drug-induced pancytopenia. N Engl J Med 301:621
10. Landsteiner K (1901) Wien Klin Wochenschr 14: 1132
11. Manns M (1989) Autoantibodies and antigens in liver diseases – updated. J Hepatol 9:272–280
12. Maria VAJ, Pinto L, Victorino RMM (1994) Lymphocyte reactivity to ex-vivo drug antigens in drug-induced hepatitis. J Hepatol 21:151–158
13. Mueller-Eckhardt C (1988) Ex vivo drug antigens. Are drug-induced immunoreactions such as immunohemolytic anemia related to genetic control? In: Estabrook RW, Lindenlaub E, Oesch F, Weck AL de (eds) Toxicological and immunological aspects of drug metabolism and environmental chemicals. Schattauer, Stuttgart, pp 329–342

14. Mueller-Eckart C, Kuenzlen E, Thilo-Korner D, Pralle H (1983) High-dose intravenous immunoglobulin for post transfusion purpura. N Engl J Med 308:287
15. Mueller-Eckhardt C, Salama A (1987) Immunhämolytische Anämien durch Medikamente. Dtsch Ärztebl 84:232–234
16. Neftel KA, Wälti M, Spengler H, Felten A von, Weitzmann SA, Bürgi H, Weck AL de (1981) Neutropenia after penicillins: toxic or immune-mediated? Klin Wochenschr 59:877
17. Pessayre D (1995) Mecanisme de hepatites medicamenteuses Gastroenterol. Clin Biol 19:47–56
18. Pihusch R (1998) Die Heparin-induzierte Thrombozytopenie. Phlebologie 27:111–116
19. Plötz G, et al. Hypereosinophilie-Syndrom. Hautarzt
20. Raif W, Schubothe H (1979) Durch körperfremde Substanzen induzierte immunhämatologische Erkrankungen. Allergologie 2:192
21. Raskob GE, George JN (1997) Thrombotic complications of antithrombotic therapy: a paradox with implications for clinical practice. Ann Intern Med 127:839–841
22. Salama A, Mueller-Eckhardt C (1985) The role of metabolite-specific antibodies in nomifensine-dependent immune hemolytic anemia. N Engl J Med 313:469–474
23. Salama A, Mueller-Eckhardt C (1992) Humanemediated blood cell dyscrasias related to drugs. Semin Hematol 29:54–63
24. Schiele F, Vuillemenot A, Kramarz P, Kieffer Y, Anguenot T, Bernard Y, Bassand JP (1995) Use of recombinant hirudin as antithrombotic treatment in patients with heparin induced thrombocytopenia. Ann J Hematol 50:20–25
25. Shulman NR, Aster RH, Leitner A, Hiller MC (1961) Immunoreactions involving platelets. V. Posttransfusion purpura due to a complement-fixing antibody against a genetically controlled platelet antigen. J Clin Invest 40:1597
26. Shulman NR (1972) Immunologic reactions to drugs. N Engl J Med 286:508–512
27. Varga J, Uitto J, Jimenez SA (1992) The cause and pathogenesis of the eosinophilia-myalgia syndrome. Ann Int Med 116:140–147
28. Wanamaker WM, Wanamaker SJ, Celesia GG, et al. (1976) Thrombocytopenia associated with long-term levodopa therapy. J Am Med Assoc 235:2217
29. Zweiman B, Patten E (1982) Immunohematologic diseases. J Am Med Assoc 248:2677–2682

5.3 Allergic Diseases due to Immune Complexes

5.3.1 Immune Complex Anaphylaxis

Binding of antigen by specific antibodies leads to immune complexes which generally have a protective function leading to clearance of the antigen from the organism through activation of the mononuclear phagocyte system [31]. Furthermore, immune complexes may have a regulating function in immune response, especially complexes from anti-idiotype antibodies and antibodies against environmental antigens (network theory according to Jerne).

However, circulating immune complexes may induce disease, when by activation of complement or Fcγ receptors pathogenic reactions are triggered [17, 28].

In the sensitized organism (IgG or IgM antibodies) antigen administration (mostly parenterally) may induce anaphylactic immediate reactions clinically manifesting sometimes even more acutely and dramatically than IgE-mediated reactions and described under the term "immune complex anaphylaxis" [1, 20, 26]. Clinical examples are dextran anaphylaxis (see Sects. 5.1.4, 5.7).

5.3.2 Serum Sickness

Serum sickness was first described by von Pirquet and Schick, giving rise to the term "allergy" in the following year (see Chap. 1), and represents the prototype of immune complex disease [16]. This has been forgotten by some younger allergists. Within 7–14 days after antigen administration, circulating antigen antibody complexes [5, 12] lead to complement activation and activation of Fcγ receptors on inflammatory cells with release of mediators and proteases (Fig. 5.23) and clinical symptoms such as fever, urticaria, arthralgia, lymph node swelling, nephritis, endocarditis, and vasculitis [1, 6, 16]. In parallel with the decrease in concentration of free antigens and the increase in concentration of specific antibodies, the clinical symptoms occur in the phase of circulating immune complexes (Fig. 5.24). This principle was called "toxic body" by von Pirquet [16]. Crucial for the elicitation of serum sickness is the dose of antigen applied; after high doses of

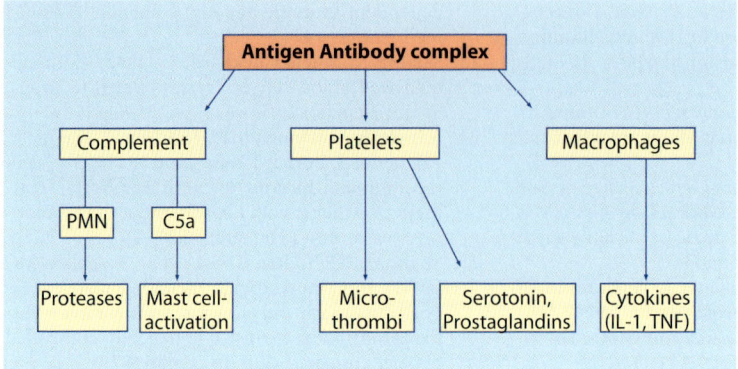

Fig. 5.23. Sequelae of the appearance of circulating immune complexes

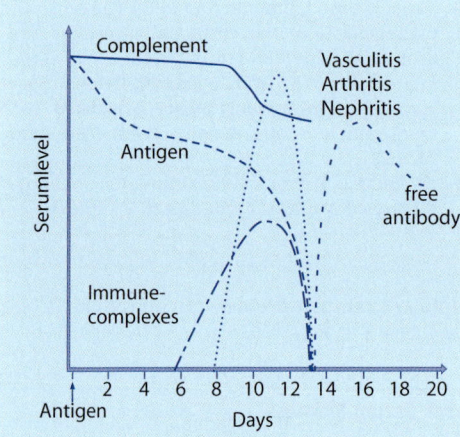

Fig. 5.24. Immunologic reaction in a patient with experimentally induced serum sickness (according to F. Dixon)

foreign serum in 80–100% of patients serum sickness can be expected.

Different types of immune complexes can be distinguished according to solubility ($<10^6$ D = soluble, $>10^6$ D = hardly soluble complexes). For the mechanism of complement activation, refer to Chap. 2, "Pathophysiology."

The detection of activated complement products, complement consumption, or circulating immune complexes has diagnostic relevance [12, 24, 30].

While serum sickness was a major problem at the beginning of the 20th century (animal sera as antitoxins), it has almost been forgotten in recent decades. However, today with the development of new biologicals of animal origin (monoclonal antibodies from the mouse) in diagnosis and therapy, new problems have arisen. Major elicitors are drugs, especially xenogeneic proteins (e.g., antitoxins or antilymphocyte antibodies) [18, 19, 25]. Similar symptoms, however, may be observed due to bacterial, viral or tumor antigens. Serum sickness after insect stings and allergen-specific immunotherapy has been reported [10].

Circulating immune complexes are detectable under physiological conditions in healthy individuals (background value of 10–20 μg/ml aggregated gammaglobulin). These clinically silent immune complexes may represent idiotype-anti-idiotype complexes, as shown in healthy volunteers with cytotoxic antibodies against melanocytes and anti-idiotypic antibodies [14].

Commercial plasma protein solutions (human serum albumin, but also unmodified gammaglobulin) contain a high percentage of aggregated proteins able to elicit serum sickness-like symptoms [19]. By separation of these aggregates, the immunogenicity of xenogeneic protein solutions can be decreased and the compatibility dramatically improved [19]. Induction of immunological tolerance has been demonstrated against xenogeneic antilymphocyte globulin successfully using highly purified monomeric xenogeneic IgG [18].

In serum sickness by animal sera (e.g., snake venom), horse IgG has stronger immunogenicity than horse albumin as demonstrated in immune elimination by accelerated elimination in sensitized organisms [12, 25].

After serum sickness has subsided, often positive rheuma factors can be demonstrated

(4–6 weeks), which, however, do not contain specific antigen in the cryoprecipitate possibly representing idiotype-anti-idiotype complexes.

The detection of antigen in the disease eliciting immune complexes would be of major diagnostic relevance; however, it is rarely achieved.

5.3.3 Allergic (Immune Complex) Vasculitis

Allergic (immune complex) vasculitis is elicited by an immunological type III reaction, when circulating immune complexes in mild antigen excess are not eliminated properly by the reticuloendothelial system and complement activation with local attraction and activation of neutrophil granulocytes occurs (experimental model of the Arthus phenomenon). Synonyms are "leukocytoclastic vasculitis," "anaphylactic purpura," "hypersensitivity angiitis," "arteriolitis allergica," and "vasculitis hyperergica." Histologically, a perivascular neutrophil infiltrate with occasional eosinophils and typical leukocytoclasia with nuclear fragments and fibrinoid degeneration of the vascular wall is typical (Fig. 5.25). In immunofluorescence or immune electron microscopy (Fig. 5.26), de-

Table 5.42. Classification of vasculitis according to pathophysiology (*ANCA*, antineutrophil cytoplasmic antibody)

Immune complex-mediated
- Purpura Schönlein-Henoch
- Urticaria vasculitis
- Immune complex vasculitis in infectious disease (viral, bacterial)
- Drug-induced vasculitis (e.g., sulfonamides)
- Paraneoplastic vasculitis
- Cryoglobulinemia
- Vasculitis in lupus erythematosus
- Rheumatoid vasculitis
- Serum sickness
- M. Behçet
- Erythema elevatum et diutinum

ANCA-associated/-mediated
- Wegener's granulomatosis
- Microscopic polyangiitis
- Churg-Strauss syndrome
- Some forms of drug-induced vasculitis (e.g., thiouracil)

Directly antibody-mediated
- Goodpasture's syndrome
- M. Kawasaki

Cell-mediated
- Transplant rejection
- Hemorrhagic pigmentary dermatoses
- Other forms of lymphocytic vasculitis

Unknown pathogenesis
- M. Horton
- Takayasu's arteriitis
- Polymyalgia rheumatica

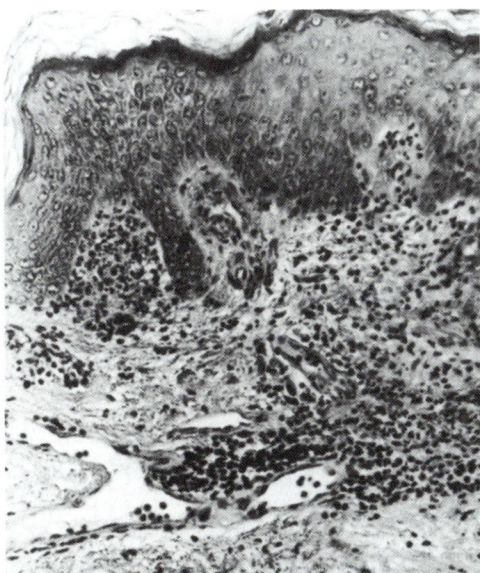

Fig. 5.25. Leukocytoclastic vasculitis. Postcapillary venules with infiltration of the vessel wall and perivascular infiltrate with neutrophils (1:650) (reprinted with the consent of Prof. Dr. H.H. Wolf [32])

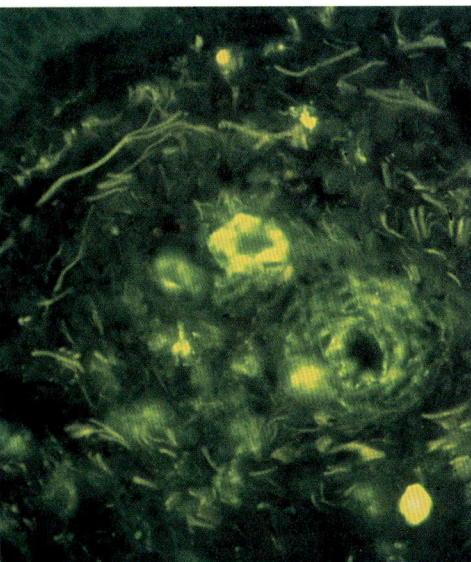

Fig. 5.26. Demonstration of C3 precipitates in the direct immunofluorescent antibody test performed on a patient with allergic vasculitis

posits of C3, IgG, and IgM can be found. Immune complex vasculitis should be differentiated from other forms of allergic vasculitis (e.g., with lymphocytic infiltrates – as in progressive pigmentary purpura) (Table 5.42) [3, 9, 12, 27].

Clinically, three types of allergic vasculitis can be distinguished [32]:

- Hemorrhagic type (corresponding to purpura Schönlein-Henoch) (Fig. 5.27)
- Papulonecrotic type with necrotizing ulcers and scarring (Figs. 5.28, 5.29)
- Polymorphic nodular type with urticarial, maculopapular, and nodular skin lesions

A special form is "urticaria vasculitis" with long-persisting (>24 h) wheals with sometimes preceding lupus erythematosus [12, 13, 27] (see Sect. 5.1.3 on "Urticaria").

The cardinal symptom is purpura (Fig. 5.27), characterized by erythrocyte extravasation, which does not disappear under pressure with the diascope. Punctual extravasations (petechia) or fluctuating hemorrhages (ecchymosis, suggillation) occur. A pathophysiological classification of inflammatory versus non-inflammatory purpura is helpful (Table 5.43). Platelet function is normal, and the Rumpel-Leede test is positive.

The exanthema is symmetrical and often pronounced in the lower extremity (hydrostat-

Table 5.43. Inflammatory and non-inflammatory purpura

Inflammatory
Neutrophils: allergic vasculitis
ANCA-associated vasculitis
Lymphocytes: progressive pigmentary purpura
Granulomatous: granulomatous vasculitis
Non-inflammatory
Coagulopathy
Thrombocytopenia
Atrophy (age, corticosteroids)
Vitamin deficiency (vitamin C, scurvy)

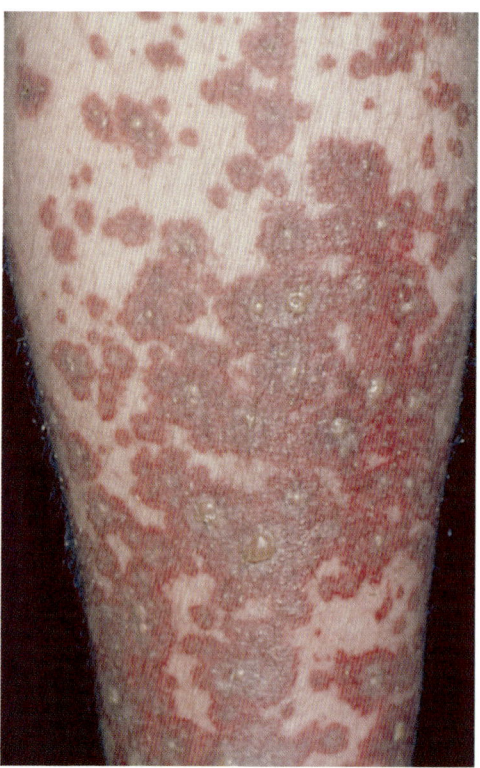

Fig. 5.27. Allergic vasculitis (hemorrhagic type)

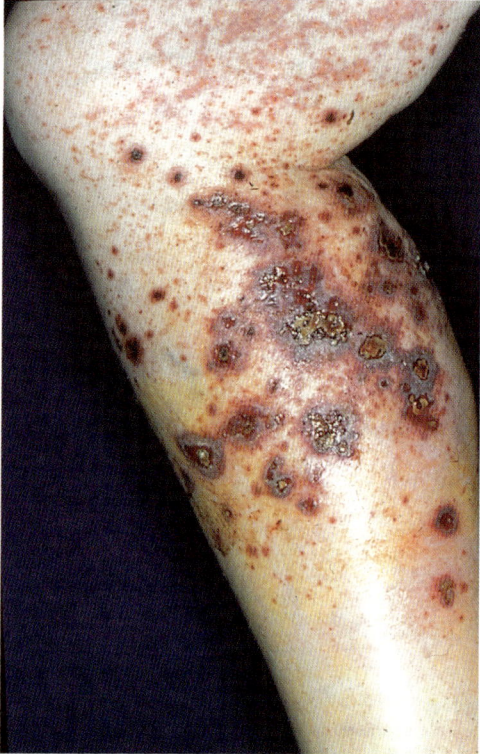

Fig. 5.28. Allergic vasculitis (papulonecrotic type)

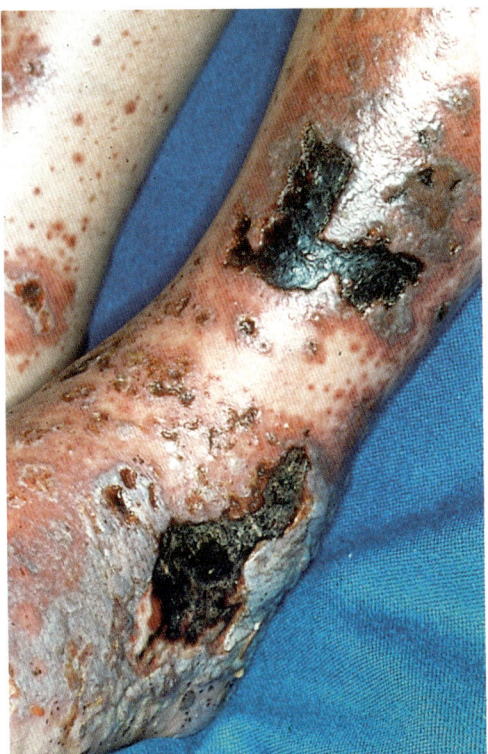

Fig. 5.29. Allergic vasculitis (necrotic type)

Table 5.44. Therapy of immune complex diseases

Antihistamines (H_1 and H_2 antagonists combined, serotonin antagonists?)
Mast cell stabilizers
Glucocorticosteroids
Inhibitors of neutrophil function (e.g., colchicine, dapsone, clofazemine)
Inhibitors of TNF, pentoxiphyllin, infliximab
Prostaglandin E_2?
Plasmapheresis
Cytostatics (cyclophosphamide, cyclosporin A)

ic pressure). Erythrocyte sedimentation is elevated, and circulating immune complexes can be detected in the serum. In many cases, systemic manifestations of other organs (kidney, lung, CNS, gastrointestinal tract, and heart) may occur. Eliciting antigens may be viruses (e.g., hepatitis B), bacteria (e.g., streptococci), parasites (e.g., schistosoma), tumors (such as paraneoplastic syndrome), foods [2, 7] or drugs.

Therapy. The avoidance of eliciting noxious agents as well as treatment of the underlying disease is vital (Table 5.44).

Symptomatically, glucocorticosteroids are used; however, their use is controversial. The anti-inflammatory effect may be beneficial; on the other hand, the vasoconstrictive effect and the immunosuppressive action may prolong the disease.

Antihistamines are recommended by some authors to decrease endothelial permeability.

Cytostatics (cyclophosphamide) can be used as well as immunosuppressives (cyclosporin). Agents with inhibitory effects on neutrophils are useful such as colchicine, dapsone, or clofazemine [8, 29].

Possible newer approaches comprise prostaglandin E_2 or TNF-inhibiting pentoxyphyllin or infliximab [33].

References

1. Becker EL, Austen KF (1966) Mechanisms of immunologic injury of rat peritoneal mast cells. I. The effect of phosphonate inhibitors on the homcytotropic antibody-mediated histamine release and the first component of rat complement. J Exp Med 124:379–395
2. Brostoff J, Challacombe SJ (eds) (1987) Food allergy and intolerance. Tindall, London
3. Bruckbauer HR, Ollert M, Ring J (1997) Vaskulitiden der Haut. Bay Int 17:166–179
4. Burden AD, Tillman DM, Foley P, Holme E (1996) IgA class anticardiolipin antibodies in cutaneous leukocytoclastic vasculitis. J Am Acad Dermatol 35:411–415
5. Cochrane CG, Koftler D (1973) Immune complex disease in experimental animals and man. Adv Immunol 16:185
6. Dixon FJ, Vasquez JJ, Weigle WO, Cochrane CG (1958) Pathogenesis of serum sickness. Arch Pathol 65:18
7. Eisenmann A, Ring J, von der Helm D, Meurer M, Braun-Falco O (1988) Vasculitis allergica durch Nahrungsmittelallergie. Hautarzt 39:318–321
8. Fauci AS (1979) Cyclophosphamide therapy of severe systemic necrotizing vasculitis. N Engl J Med 301:235
9. Gross WL, Schmitt WH, Lotti T (1995) ANCA-assoziierte Vaskulitiden. Hautarzt 46:511–524
10. Hunt HJ, Valentine MD, Sobotha AK, Junginger JW, Lichtenstein LM (1976) Serum sickness associated with nonvenom protein in mixed hyme-

noptera whole body extract. J Allergy Clin Immunol 57:246–254
11. Jenette CJ, Milling DM, Falk RJ (1994) Vasculitis affecting the skin. Arch Dermatol 130:899–906
12. Kohler PF (1983) Immune complexes and allergic disease. In: Middleton E, Ellis EF, Reed CE (eds) Allergy, principles and practice, 2nd edn. Mosby, St. Louis, pp 167–199
13. Meurer M (1981) Urticarial vasculitis. In: Ring J, Burg G (eds) New trends in allergy. Springer, Berlin Heidelberg New York, pp 148–151
14. Morgan AC Jr, Rossen R, Twomey JJ (1979) Naturally occurring circulating immune complexes: normal serum contains idiotype-anti-idiotype complexes dissociable by certain IgG antiglobulins. J Immunol 122:1672
15. Ollert, deleted in production
16. Pirquet C v, Schick B (1905) Die Serumkrankheit. Deutike, Leipzig
17. Ravetch JV (1994) Fc receptors: Rubor redux. Cell 78:533–560
18. Ring J, Seifert J, Lob G, Coulin K, Angstwurm H, Frick E, Brass B, Mertin I, Backmund H, Brendel W (1974) Intensive immunosuppression in the treatment of multiple sclerosis. Lancet II:1093
19. Ring J, Seifert J, Seiler F, Brendel W (1976) Improved compatibility of ALG therapy by application of aggregate free globulin. Int Arch Allergy Appl Immunol 52:227–234
20. Ring J (1978) Anaphylaktoide Reaktionen nach Infusion natürlicher und künstlicher Kolloide. Springer, Berlin Heidelberg New York
21. Ruzicka T, Burg G (1987) Effects of chronic intracutaneous administration of arachidonic acid and its metabolites. Induction of leukocytoclastic vasculitis by leukotriene B4 and 12-hydroxyeicosatetraenoic acid and its prevention by prostaglandin E2. J Invest Dermatol 88:120–123
22. Sais G, Vidaller A, Jucgla A, Gallardo F, Peyri J (1995) Colchicine in the treatment of cutaneous leukocytoclastic vasculitis. Results of a prospective, randomized controlled trial. Arch Dermatol 131:1399–1402
23. Scherer R, Wolff HH (1979) Vasculitis allergica. Allergologie 2:62
24. Sedlacek HH (1980) Pathophysiological aspects of immune complex diseases. Klin Wochenschr 58:543–593
25. Seifert J, Land W, Ring J, Lob G, Brendel W (1978) Antigen-Eliminationstechnik. Fortschr Med 96: 695–697
26. Smedegard G, Revenas B, Arfors KE (1979) Anaphylaxis in the monkey: hemodynamics and blood flow distribution. Acta Physiol Scand 106: 191–198
27. Soter NA, Austen KF, Gigli I (1974) Urticaria and arthralgias as manifestations of necrotizing angiitis (vasculitis). J Invest Dermatol 63:485–490
28. Sylvestre DL, Ravetch JV (1994) Fc receptors initiate the Arthus reaction: Redefining the inflammatory cascade. Science 265:1095–1098
29. Theissen U, Luger TA, Schwarz T (1996) Erfolgreiche topische Anwendung von Cyclosporin A bei Pyoderma gangraenosum. Hautarzt 47:132–135
30. Theofilopoulos AN, Dixon FJ (1980) Detection of immune complexes; techniques and implications. Hosp Pract 15:107
31. van Furth R, Cohn ZA, Hirsch JG, et al. (1972) The mononuclear phagocyte system: a new classification of macrophages, monocytes, and their precursor cells. Bull Wld Hlth Org 46:845
32. Wolff HH, Scherer R (1981) Allergic vasculitis. In: Ring J, Burg G (eds) New trends in allergy. Springer, Berlin Heidelberg New York, pp 140–147
33. Zhang Y, Ramos BF, Jakschik BA (1992) Neutrophil recruitment by tumor necrosis factor from mast cells in immune complex peritonitis. Science 258:1957–1959

5.4 Hypersensitivity Pneumonitis (Allergic Alveolitis)

5.4.1 Definition

Hypersensitivity pneumonitis (exogenous allergic alveolitis) (previously also classified under "pneumoconioses") represents an allergic disease of the alveoli and terminal bronchi against fine dusty, mostly organic material occurring with precipitating antibodies. Hypersensitivity pneumonitis has aspects of both type III and IV reactions with lymphocytic and granulomatous reactions. In 2% of airway diseases, hypersensitivity pneumonitis is not a rare disease [6, 7, 12, 13, 17, 34].

5.4.2 Clinical Symptoms and Diagnosis

The first description dates back to Ramazzini (1718) as pneumonia-like disease in merchants after contact with grain dust. As allergic disease, farmer's lung was classified by Pepys [24] and bagassosis by Salvaggio [28] in the 1960s after first reports by Gronemeyer in 1951.

An acute and chronic form are distinguished. In the acute form, 4–6 h after exposure dyspnea with tachypnea, coughing (some-

5.4 Hypersensitivity Pneumonitis (Allergic Alveolitis)

Table 5.45. Symptoms and signs of hypersensitivity pneumonitis

Common cold	91%
Dyspnea	85%
Cough	82%
Shivering	56%
Sputum expectoration	51%
Malaise	47%
Tightness of chest	42%
Weight loss	31%
Nightly sweating	29%
Headache	25%
Nausea	19%
Loss of appetite	18%
Rhinitis/pharyngitis	15%
Myalgia	14%
Vertigo	12%
Hemoptoe	8%
Auscultatory noises	73%
Fever	40%
Leukocytosis	76%
CRP elevation	72%
ESR elevation	46%

times itchy throat), fever, fatigue, myalgia, headache, tightness of the chest, as well as sputum (sometimes hemoptoe) develop. In the auscultation, a fine vesicular noise is heard, changing to rough basal noises and the typical end-expiratory rattling noise followed by fibrotic noises in inspiration (sclerosiphony) (Table 5.45).

Chest X-ray shows small patches of nodular shadows (1–3 mm) and milky opacification. Lung function shows restrictive ventilatory disturbance as well as disturbed diffusion capacity (diminished for CO_2). Decreased arterial oxygen concentrations are found, especially after exercise [34].

Blood count shows leukocytosis with deviation, sometimes eosinophilia. The differential diagnosis (Table 5.46) includes bronchial asthma as type I reaction (sometimes elicited by similar exposure) which can be excluded by precipitating antibodies and negative IgE as well as lung function (no obstructive ventilatory disturbance). The family history of atopy is negative. In the bronchial provocation test, the reaction occurs after 4–6 h as diffusion disturbance.

More difficult to diagnose are chronic courses characterized by dry coughing, general malaise, weight loss, sometimes increased ESR, leukocytosis and hypergammaglobulinemia. In the X-ray, signs of lung fibrosis are found. Patients are often treated for long periods as having "common cold, bronchitis, etc." Other differential diagnoses are listed in Table 5.47.

Table 5.47. Differential diagnoses of hypersensitivity pneumonitis

Toxic lung disease
Organic toxic alveolitis
("organic dust toxic syndrome," ODTS)
Byssinosis
Harvester's fever
Pig breeder's fever
Humidifier fever
Anorganic toxic alveolitis
Metal smoke fever
Polymer smoke fever
Silo worker's disease
Autoimmune alveolitis
Interstitial lung disease
e.g., sarcoidosis
Pneumoconioses (berylliosis, asbestosis, silicosis)

Table 5.46. Differential diagnosis between allergic bronchial asthma and hypersensitivity pneumonitis

Symptoms	Allergic asthma	Hypersensitivity pneumonitis
Symptoms	Wheezing, acute attacks	Dyspnea, fever, cough, general symptoms
Latency	<1 h	6–12 h
Duration (after exposure)	Mostly hours	Days
History of atopy	Positive	Negative
Chest X-ray, acute	Lung inflation	Infiltrates
Chronic	Emphysema	Fibrosis
Lung function	Obstructive diffusion disturbance	Restrictive diffusion disturbance
Skin test	Immediate reaction (20 min)	Type III reaction (8–24 h)
Serology	RAST+	Precipitating antibodies +
Bronchial provocation test[a]	Immediate reaction	Delayed reaction (4–12 h)

[a] Note the different parameters of lung function disturbance

	ODTS	HP
Exposure	Massive	Little to moderate
Selection	All exposed	Certain individuals
Course	1 day	Days to weeks
Chest X-ray	Negative	Infiltrates
IgG antibodies	±	++
Lung function	Normal to mild restriction	Strong restriction
BAL	3 d PMIV increased	Lymphocytosis

Table 5.48. Differential diagnosis between "organic dust toxic syndrome" (ODTS) and hypersensitivity pneumonitis (HP)

Table 5.49. Diagnostic criteria for hypersensitivity pneumonitis (German Society for Allergology and Clinical Immunology) [3]. For diagnosis of hypersensitivity pneumonitis, criteria 1–3 plus 1 additional criterion have to be positive

1. Allergen exposure
2. Symptoms of alveolitis
3. IgG/IgA antibodies
4. Pathologic lung function (diffusion, hypoxemia)
5. Typical chest X-ray infiltrates
6. Typical BAL findings
7. Positive bronchial provocation

Toxic irritative processes through endotoxins or other irritants in organic materials can induce bronchoalveolar diseases [7, 11, 13, 20, 21, 22, 27, 34, 38, 41] (Table 5.48): byssinosis in cotton wool workers, grain dust (harvesting dust) disease, flax or hemp workers lung. In these cases, no relevant sensitization can be demonstrated immunologically or in provocation tests. Silo workers disease through toxic effects of nitric gases, furrier's disease with foreign body granulomas around animal hair in lung tissue as well as autoimmune alveolitis (in lupus erythematodes or scleroderma) need to be differentiated (see the diagnostic criteria for hypersensitivity pneumonitis of the German Society of Allergology and Clinical Immunology as well as the German Society for Pneumology in Table 5.49).

5.4.3 Pathophysiology

There are three phases in the histological changes (Fig. 5.30): In the acute phase (4–30 h), perivascular infiltrates of neutrophil and eosinophil granulocytes predominate, which transmigrate through the alveolar walls (type III reaction). In the further course (30 h to weeks), mononuclear infiltrates (type IV reaction) with the beginnings of granuloma formation and multinuclear giant cells are observed (see Sect. 5.8).

In chronic conditions, fibrotic changes are typical.

During bronchoalveolar lavage, a decreased CD4/CD8 ratio with increased lymphocytes of the TH_1 secretion type is typical. Sometimes TH_2 can be found [4]. In direct immunofluorescence, deposits of immunoglobulins in alveolar walls have been observed [1, 6, 34].

In the blood, a high concentration of IgG antibodies (mostly as precipitins in immunodiffusion) against eliciting allergens can be detected. The immune complexes thus formed and deposited lead to activation of macrophages, maintaining further inflammatory processes. It is interesting that non-smokers have a higher incidence of hypersensitivity pneumonitis, possibly due to inhibition of macrophage functions in smokers [16, 39].

Antibodies may also be detected by complement fixation [30, 32, 34] or using indirect immunofluorescence (e.g., bird feathers) or enzyme or radioimmunoassays.

The interpretation of antibody results is difficult since they also may be found in healthy exposed individuals, although in lower concentrations. More detailed investigations (long-term follow-up) and accidental autopsies of possibly asymptomatic exposed persons have yielded evidence that in many cases a clinically latent, but minimal form of alveolitis may be present in these individuals.

In the skin test – sometimes after an immediate reaction – the occurrence of a papule after 6–12 h up to 24 h is characteristic (80% in hypersensitivity pneumonitis, 50% in exposed individuals with demonstrable antibody, 10% in non-exposed controls). Histologically, leu-

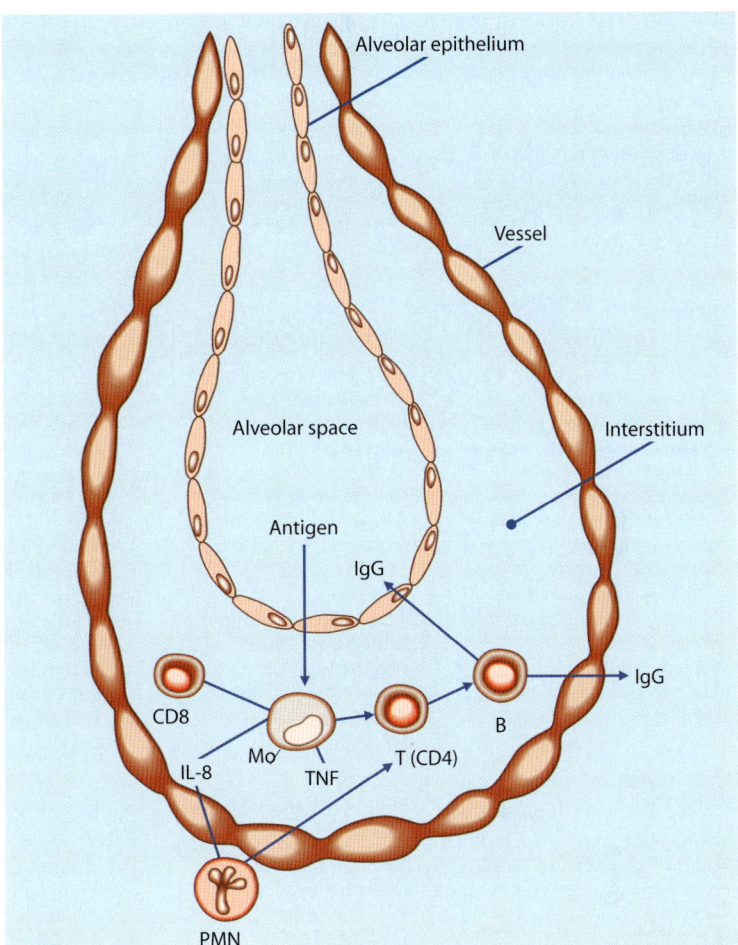

Fig. 5.30. Pathophysiology of exogenous allergic alveolitis

kocytoclastic vasculitis with immunoglobulin and complement deposits in direct immunofluorescence can be found. Unfortunately, skin tests are not often routinely performed since allergen extracts are poorly purified and standardized; false-positive reactions are common.

Bronchial provocation tests after exposure (mixing dust or using nebulizers) should be performed under inpatient conditions.

5.4.4 Allergens and Common Forms of Hypersensitivity Pneumonitis

Organic allergens of animal or plant origin, but also chemicals and drugs, are common elicitors of hypersensitivity pneumonitis (Table 5.50) [2, 8, 9, 10, 11, 19, 25, 28, 29, 31, 33, 34, 40].

The classic example of hypersensitivity pneumonitis is farmer's lung elicited by bacteria, especially thermophilic actinomycetes with spores between 0.8 and 2 µm in diameter, able to penetrate alveolar spaces. These microorganisms are especially dominant in moldy hay with high humidity and temperature (45%). One gram of moldy hay may contain 10^8 spores of *Micropolyspora faeni*. Farmer's lung is more common in humid regions in dairy farmers and late winter when the fresh hay has already been used.

In central Europe, hypersensitivity pneumonitis is common in bird breeders with antibodies against allergens in bird droppings (but also feathers, serum, and eggs), mostly gammaglobulins and albumin with cross-reactivi-

Table 5.50. Hypersensitivity pneumonitis: allergens and diseases (according to [34])

Allergen (most common)	Disease[a]	Allergen source
Bacteria		
Micropolyspora faeni, *Thermoactinomyces vulgaris*	Farmer's lung	Damp hay, grain
Thermoactinomyces sacchari	Humidifier lung	Humidifiers and air conditioners
"Multiple" microbial agents	Water vapor lung bagassosis	Moldy sugarcane
	Tobacco worker's lung	Tobacco leaves
		Fungal waste
		Moldy cotton
Enzymes		
Alcalase, maxatase	Washing powder lung	Enzymes from *B. subtilis*
Fungi		
Alternaria and others	Wood cutter's lung	Moldy wood
Alternaria	Paper worker's lung	Moldy paper mix
Cryptostoma corticale	Maplebark lung	Moldy maple bark
Penicillium frequentans	Cork worker's lung (suberosis)	Cork (Portugal)
Penicillium casei	Cheese washer's lung	Moist cheese storages
Penicillium brevicompactum	Tomato breeder's lung	Tomatoes
Aspergillus clavatus	Malt worker's lung	Malt in breweries
Aspergillus fumigatus	Espartosis	Fiber production from esparto grass
Streptomyces olivaceus	New Guinea lung	Straw roofs
Cephalosporium trochoderma	Textile worker's lung	Textile fibers
Botrytis cinerea	Winemaker's lung	Grapes
Various fungi	"Coptic lung"	Mummies
Pleurotus florida	Fungi worker's lung	Edible fungi (oyster mushroom)
Mixed fungi	Fruit farmer's lung	Fruit in cooling rooms
	Moldy lung	Organic waste, moldy cotton
Plant allergens		
Wood fiber	Wood dust alveolitis	Wood cutting dust
Animal allergens		
Bird dust (feathers, feces, egg)	Bird breeder's lung	Bird droppings, bed feathers
Bread beetle protein (*Sitoph. gran.*)	Bread beetle's lung	Grain and flour
Fish proteins	Fish flour lung	Miller's lung
Pig epithelium	Pig hair lung	Animal feeding
Rat serum antigens	Animal keepers	Rat urine
Pituitary extracts	Pituitary sniffer's lung	
Pancreatin	Pancreatin powder	Pharmaceutical industry
Silkworm proteins	Silk breeder's lung	Silkworm
Crustacea dust	Crustacean lung	Pearl oyster handling
Drugs		
Nitrofurantoin		
Hydrochlorothiazide		
Carbamazepine		
Amiodarone		
Phenytoin		
Gold salts		
Chemicals		
Isocyanates	Isocyanate alveolitis	Plastic production
Acid anhydrides	Chemicals	Plastic, glues
Silicon implants		

[a] The term "alveolitis" should be preferred to the common term "lung"

ties between various bird species (budgerigar, parrot, canary, etc.) [6, 34, 37]. The fine dust of dry pigeon feces seems to be especially allergenic. In Germany, there are an estimated 110,000 pigeon breeders. The prevalence of hypersensitivity pneumonitis is estimated at 0.2–10% of exposed individuals. In the United Kingdom, 12% of the population is supposed to keep birds (mostly budgerigars) without alarming figures of high prevalences of hypersensitivity pneumonitis. A study from the island of Gotland revealed among farmers a 10–100 times higher prevalence of IgE-mediated allergic diseases (especially against housedust and storage mites) than hypersensitivity pneumonitis [36].

In preparing lists of allergens and corresponding diseases, it has to be considered that not infrequently several allergens of various origin (bacteria, fungi, parasites) are involved together in the elicitation of the disease (e.g., humidifier lung) (Table 5.50).

Rare cases are observed under treatment with pituitary gland extracts, in the preparation of pancreatin, in fungi farming, under nitrofurantoin treatment (3 weeks after beginning), with ACE inhibitors, or with silicon implants.

Hypersensitivity pneumonitis can also occur in animals (e.g., horses) [33].

5.4.5 Allergic Bronchopulmonary Mycosis

The disease of allergic bronchopulmonary mycosis (mostly aspergillosis) needs to be distinguished from hypersensitivity pneumonitis; it develops mostly on the basis of a chronic bronchial asthma and consists of a combination of type I and III allergy together with intrabronchial colonization with molds. Relapsing lung infiltrates in patients with allergic bronchial asthma are characteristic [35]. In the diagnosis, precipitating antibodies together with specific IgE antibodies, dual skin reactions, as well as positive demonstration of molds in the sputum culture are relevant [34]. Other diseases due to aspergilli are aspergillus pneumonia as well as aspergilloma.

Besides allergic bronchopulmonary mycosis, there are true combinations of type I and III reactions such as exogenic allergic asthma and hypersensitivity pneumonitis through hay dust or isocyanates.

In this context, other forms of mold allergy together with an infection occurring in the paranasal sinuses should be mentioned such as the recently described "allergic fungal sinusitis" (see also Sect. 5.1.1 on "Rhinitis").

5.4.6 Therapy of Hypersensitivity Pneumonitis

Strict allergen avoidance is the primary commandment. Prophylactic measures include reduction of allergen concentrations through constructing better and drier storage rooms. With air masks, the amount of inhaled allergen can be reduced. The airstream helmet with an airflow passing through a filter can be used during work [18]. A new mask is the "Dust Master"; there are also half-masks (3M Co.). In highly sensitized individuals, a change of occupation or cessation of the exposed work is the only way.

Glucocorticosteroids may reduce the symptoms of hypersensitivity pneumonitis. Doses between 40 and 60 mg prednisolone (in children 0.2 mg/kg body wt.) are given; steroid medication is, however, no alternative to allergen avoidance!

For therapy control, measurement of vital capacity, diffusion capacity, and O_2 partial pressure under exercise are recommended.

The efficacy of cromoglycate is controversial. Allergen-specific immunotherapy in hypersensitivity pneumonitis is contraindicated. In severe cases, cytostatics and immunosuppressives are given [34, 42].

References

1. Allen DH, Basten A, Woolcock AJ (1977) Studies of cell and humoral immunity in birdbreeders hypersensitivity pneumonitis. Am Rev Resp Dis 115:45
2. Bäck O, Lindgren R, Wiman LG (1974) Nitrofurantoin induced pulmonary fibrosis and lupus syndrome. Lancet I:930
3. Bergmann KC, Costabel U, Knape H, Kroidl R, Müller-Wening D, Repp H, Rust M, Schwarz H, Sennekamp J (1990b) Empfehlungen zur Diagnosestellung einer exogen-allergischen Alveolitis. Allergologie 13:111
4. Boyd G, McSharry C, McLeod K, Sriram S, Boyd F (1999) Lymphocyte responses in pigeon breeders

with extrinsic allergic alveolitis/hypersensitivity pneumonitis (EAA/HP) are predominantly T helper 2-type. Am J Resp Crit Care Med 159:A742
5. Doerr W (1953) Pneumokoniose durch Getreidestaub. Virchows Arch Pathol Anat 324:263
6. Fink JN (1992) Hypersensitivity pneumonitis. Clinics in chest Medicine 13:303
7. Fruhmann G (1988b) Pneumokoniosen durch organisches Material. Deutsches Ärzteblatt 85:3170
8. Fuchs A, Liebetrau G (1989) Die Vogelhalterlunge – eine Form der exogen allergischen Alveolitis. Z Klein Med 44:1407
9. Heiner DC, Snears JW, Kniker WT (1962) Multiple precipitins to cow's milk in chronic respiratory disease. Am J Dis Child 103:634
10. Hinojosa M (2001) Stipatosis or hypersensitivity pneumonitis caused by esparto (*Stipa tenacissima*) fibers. J Invest Allergol Clin Immunol 11:67–72
11. Jelke G (1986) Krank durch Fortschritt. Expositionelle Besonderheiten bei der exogen-allergischen Alveolitis. Allergologie 9:137
12. Kroidl RF, Nowak D, Seysen U (1994b) Exogenallergische Alveolitis: Probleme und Fehler bei der Begutachtung. Allergologie 17:75
13. Malmberg P, Rask-Andersen A (1993b) Organic dust toxic syndrome. Semin Resp Med 14:38
14. Marinkovich VA (1975) Hypersensitivity alveolitis. J Am Med Assoc 231:944
15. McCarthy DS, Pepys J (1971) Allergic bronchopulmonary aspergillosis. Clinical immunology: 1. Clinical features, 2. Skin, nasal and bronchial tests. Clin Allergy 1:261, 415
16. McSharry C, Banham SW, Boyd G (1985) Effect of cigarette smoking on the antibody response to inhaled antigens and the prevalence of extrinsic allergic alveolitis among pigeon breeders. Clin Allergy 15:487
17. Molina C (1984) Immunopathologie bronchopulmonaire. Masson, Paris
18. Müller-Wening D, Repp H (1989b) Investigation on the protective value of breathing masks in farmer's lung using an inhalation provocation test. Chest 95:100
19. Murray MJ, et al. (1965) Pulmonary reactions simulating cardiac pulmonary edema caused by nitrofurantoin. N Engl J Med 273:1185
20. Newman-Taylor A, Pickering CAC, Turner-Warwick M, Pepys J (1978) Respiratory allergy to a factor humidifier contaminant presenting as pyrexia of undetermined origin. Br Med J:II
21. Olenchock SA, May JJ, Pratt DS, et al. (1990) Presence of endotoxin in different agricultural environments. Am J Industr Med 18:279
22. Parkers WR (1994) Occupational lung disorders. Butterworth, London
23. Patterson R (1978d) Studies of hypersensitivity lung disease with emphasis on a solid-phase radioimmunoassay as a potential diagnostic acid. J Allergy Clin Immunol 61:216
24. Pepys J (1994) Farmer lung's – a needle in a haystack, and Pandora's box. Allergy Clin Immunol News 6:68
25. Pepys I, Jenkins P, Festenstein G, Gregory P, Lacey M, Skinner F (1963) Farmer's lung. Thermophilic actinomycetes as a source of "farmer's lung hay" antigen. Lancet II:607
26. Raulf M, Liebers V, Steppert C, Baur X (1994) Increased gamma/delta positive T-cells in pneumonitis. Eur Respir J 7:140
27. Rylander R, Malmberg P (1992a) Non-infectious fever: inhalation fever or toxic alveolitis? Br J Industr Med 49:296
28. Salvaggio JE, Buechner HA, Seabury H (1966) Bagassosis I. Precipitins against extracts of crude bagasse in the serum of patients with bagassosis. Ann Intern Med 64:748
29. Sastre J, Ibanez MD, Lopez M, Lehrer SB (1990) Respiratory and immunological reactions among Shiitake (*Lentinus edodes*) mushroom workers. Clin Exp Allergy 20:13
30. Schatz M, Patterson R (1977) Immunopathogenesis of hypersensitivity pneumonitis. J Allergy Clin Immunol 60:27
31. Schulz KH, Felten G, Hausen BM, Noster U (1974) Allergy to spores of *Pleurotus Florida*. Lancet I:625
32. Schultze-Werninghaus G, Rust M (1988b) Asthma bronchiale und allergische Alveolitis durch Berufsallergene. Allergologie II:437
33. Seeliger HPR, Sühler H (1975) Farmerlunge beim Tier. Berl Münch Tierärztl Wochenschr 88:163
34. Sennekamp H-J (1998) Exogen allergische Alveolitis. Dustri, Munich
35. Slavin RG, Million L, Cherry J (1970) Allergic bronchopulmonary aspergillosis: characterization of antibodies and results of treatment. J Allergy Clin Immunol 46:150
36. van Hage-Hamsten M, Johansson SGO, Höglund S, Tüll P, Wirén A, Zetterström O (1985) Storage mite allergy is common in a farming population. Clin Allergy 15:555–564
37. Vogelmeier C, Krombach F, Münzing S, et al. (1993) Activation of blood neutrophils in acute episodes of farmer' lung. Am Rev Resp Dis 148:396
38. von Essen S, Robbins RA, Thompson AB (1990) Organic dust toxic syndrome. Clin Toxicol 28:389
39. Warren CPW (1977) Extrinsic allergic alveolitis: a disease commoner in non-smokers. Thorax 32:567–569
40. Weck AL de, Gutersohn J, Bütikofer E (1969) La maladie des laveurs de fromage ("Käsewascherkrankheit"): une forme particulière du syndrome du poumon de fermier. Schweiz Med Wochenschr 99:872
41. Westphal O, Lüderitz O (1961) Bacterial endotoxins. J Med Pharma Chem 4:497
42. Wild LG, Lopez M (2001) Hypersensitivity pneumonitis: A comprehensive review. J Invest Allergol Clin Immunol 11:3–15

5.5 Dermatitis/Eczema

5.5.1 Definition and Classification

The various forms of eczematous skin diseases are the most common skin diseases (approximately 5–10% of the population). The terms "dermatitis" and "eczema" are often used interchangeably to describe a disease best defined according to Miescher [42] (Table 5.51). Dermatitis/eczema is characterized by a strong itching sensation, a relapsing clinical course and a tendency to chronification.

The following different forms of eczematous diseases can be distinguished (Table 5.52). In the United States, the term "dermatitis" is often used identically to "eczema"; some want to stop using the term "eczema" [1]. The name "eczema" in its 1,400 years of history has served a useful life and is understood by lay people [2, 7, 49, 68]. The earliest definition by Aetius from Amida described something like "boiling, foaming" (*ekzeo* = I'm boiling) [2]. Interestingly, this idea illustrates very well the most modern pathophysiology of dermoepidermal inflammation with the subsequent intercellular edema formation (spongiosis).

The colorful spectrum of eczematous diseases may lead to confusion since definitions are given according to variable criteria (morphology, localization, route of contact, kinetics, etiology, or pathophysiology). It is most unfortunate that the term "contact dermatitis" only focuses on the route of elicitation and does not describe the actual difference in pathophysiology to atopic eczema, which also can be elicited by external contact (see below). Therefore the common classification as it is used in most textbooks (Table 5.52) is not very logical. Earlier the term "vulgar" eczema [28] was used for contact dermatitis; however, this is not an attractive diagnosis to give a patient today. Therefore one should focus on the different characteristics between "atopic eczema" and "contact dermatitis" both pathophysiologically and clinically (Table 5.53).

In the recent nomenclature consensus of the WAO, a new classification of "dermatitis" was proposed, restricting the term "eczema" to the forms of what has so far been called atopic eczema/dermatitis (Table 5.54). Thus only the allergic ("extrinsic" with IgE involvement) in contrast to the non-allergic ("intrinsic" without detection of IgE sensitization) variant should be named "atopic." The nummular form

Table 5.51. Definition of dermatitis/eczema

- Non-contagious epidermodermitis with typical clinical (itch, erythema, papule, seropapule, vesicle, desquamation, crusting, lichenification in the sense of synchronous or metachronous polymorphism) and
- dermatohistological (spongiosis, akanthosis, parakeratosis, lymphocytic infiltration into the epidermis) manifestation
- mostly on the basis of hypersensitivity

Table 5.52. Classification of dermatitis/eczema

Contact dermatitis
- Allergic
- Irritative-toxic

Atopic and non-atopic eczema
Seborrheic dermatitis
Nummular (microbial) dermatitis
Unclassified dermatitis

Table 5.53. Differences between contact dermatitis and atopic eczema

	Contact dermatitis	Atopic eczema
Genetic disposition	–	+
Elicitation (route)	Contact	?
Psychosomatic influence	–	++
Type of allergic reaction	IVa	I+IVb
Antibodies	–	IgE
T cells (elicitation)	TH1	TH2
Allergens	Haptens	Proteins
Amplifying cells	PMN?	EOS, mast cells
Role of allergens	Established	Controversial
Diagnosis	Patch test	Prick, specific IgE, atopy patch test

Table 5.54. Proposal of a new classification of dermatitis/eczema (according to WAO 2004; Chap. 1)

Dermatitis					
Eczema		Contact dermatitis		Other forms	
Atopic	Non-atopic	Irritative-toxic	Allergic	Nummular, seborrheic, etc.	

Table 5.55. Preferable characteristics of certain forms of dermatitis in various localizations (*AE*, atopic eczema; *CD*, contact dermatitis; *IT*, irritative-toxic dermatitis; *SD*, seborrheic dermatitis)

Body area	Most common form			Differential diagnosis
Dorsum of hands	CD	AE		
Palms/soles	AE	CD	IT	Tinea
Fingertips	AE	CD	IT	
Scalp	SD	CD	AE	Psoriasis
External ear	SD	CD		Psoriasis
Eyelid	AE	CD	SD	
Lips	AE	CD	IT	
Oral mucosa	IT	CD		
Mamilla	AE	CD		Morbus Paget, scabies
Anal	IT	CD	AE	Psoriasis
Genital	IT	AE		Scabies
Lower leg	CD	AE		Venous insufficiency ("stasis dermatitis"?)
Post-traumatic	IT	CE		

– also called "dysregulative microbial" [31] – is still not well understood in its pathophysiology. In childhood, it seems to be a variant of atopic eczema.

Whether seborrheic dermatitis [65], first defined by Unna, really represents this type of inflammation or rather a superficial skin infection (e.g., *P. ovale*) is under discussion [20].

Contact dermatitis and atopic eczema are the most common forms, followed by nummular, seborrheic and other forms of dermatitis.

One can also classify according to localization (e.g., hand, lower leg dermatitis) for practical reasons. The prevalence of certain forms differs according to localization (Table 5.55). The entity of "stasis dermatitis" is controversial.

Clinical subtypes are "dyshidrotic dermatitis" (pompholyx), which often turns – when in chronification – into "hyperkeratotic-rhagadiform dermatitis" [4, 17, 46, 58].

5.5.2 Contact Dermatitis

5.5.2.1 Pathophysiology

Contact dermatitis can be either due to toxic or to allergic mechanisms (Table 5.56). Acute toxic contact dermatitis ("irritant contact dermatitis") develops after irritation, usually showing sharp margins and no spreading phenomena. It occurs in any individual without a peculiar genetic disposition. Special forms are diaper dermatitis in infants and intertrigo. The chronic (cumulative-toxic) form develops more slowly in disposed individuals (frequently atopics) and is due to skin barrier disturbance; it occurs most commonly in house-

Table 5.56. Clinical and histological distinctions between irritative-toxic and allergic contact dermatitis

	Irritative-toxic	Allergic
Clinical characteristics		
Margin	Sharp	Spreading
Polymorphism	+	+++
Kinetic	Decrescendo	Crescendo
Pain	++	+/−
Itch	+	+++
Histology		
Spongiosis	0	+++
Exocytosis	++	++
Vesiculation	Non-spongiotic	Spongiotic
Keratinocyte necrosis	++	0
Eosinophils	0	+
Neutrophils	+	0
Mononuclear infiltrates	+	+
Edema	+	0

wives, hairdressers, metal workers, as well as health personnel. The most important noxious agents are: water, detergents, acids, alkali, solvents, secretions, mechanical factors, etc. A subtype can be classified as "exsiccation dermatitis" [8] after excessive washing.

Allergic contact dermatitis is due to an immunologic reaction of type IVa (sensitized T lymphocytes of TH1 type under IL-12 mediation) [3, 13, 14, 19, 20, 27, 34, 36, 60, 62, 64]. After skin contact, a specific hapten (e.g., chromate) is bound to an epidermal carrier protein, recognized by Langerhans cells [9, 19, 26, 27, 37, 38, 56, 61, 62] in the epidermis. Metal ions (e.g., nickel) have been reported as possibly leading to a structural alteration of the HLA-DR complex [34]. In the regional lymph nodes [61], antigen is presented to T lymphocytes, which then circulate in the orgnism and after renewed antigen contact migrate as specifically sensitized T cells to the skin using the skin homing receptor CLA (cutaneous lymphocyte antigen) and secrete or release certain cytokines [13, 36, 64]. Apart from Langerhans cells, other dendritic cells in the epidermis may be involved during inflammation and tolerance induction [6, 27].

So-called "group allergy" develops when different haptens are transformed by coupling to the carrier into identical substances. "Coupling allergy" describes the common phenomenon of concomitant allergic sensitizations against different substances in the same patient due to common occurrence of allergens in the environment.

The molecular characteristics of contact allergenicity are better understood than that of protein allergens. A crucial characteristic is the binding of the hapten to proteins [5, 39], which can occur through electrophil haptens (covalent binding with certain protein structures, e.g., benzochinone), nucleophil haptens (e.g., mercaptobenzothiazole), and lipophil haptens, which directly integrate within the cell membrane (e.g., urushiol from poison ivy).

Certain haptens only become immunologically active under UV influence (see Sect. 5.6 on "Photoallergy").

Most contact allergens also have a certain irritative potency.

5.5.2.2 Clinical Manifestations of Classic Contact Dermatitis

Usually in contact dermatitis, sensitization and elicitation occur through epidermal contact; but there are also systemically elicited forms ("hematogenous") where either sensitization or elicitation occur via systemic allergen administration [29, 35, 48] mostly via the gut. The most common elicitors of systemic contact dermatitis are drugs as well as foods and aromatic substances (flavors).

The clinical symptoms (Figs. 5.31–5.40) in the acute stage are of exsudative character (erythematous, vesicular, crusted), and in the chronic stage more infiltrative (papules, lichenification, hyperkeratosis).

The most common contact allergens (see Sect. 3.2.2) are *metals* (nickel, chromate, cobalt), *rubber accelerators* (used during vulcanization as antioxidants or stabilizers, not rubber proteins themselves!), *ointment vehicles* (e.g., lanolin, woolwax, emulsifiers, etc.), *epoxy resins* (solvents, hardeners in resins, sensitizing agents mostly are monomers and dimers, not

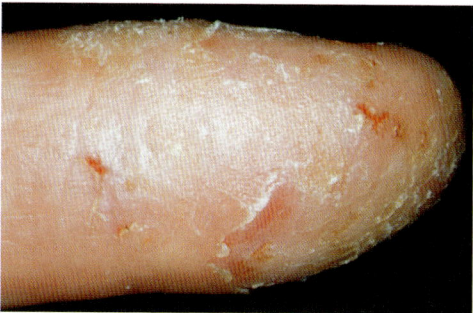

Fig. 5.31. Fingertip dermatitis seen in a dentist

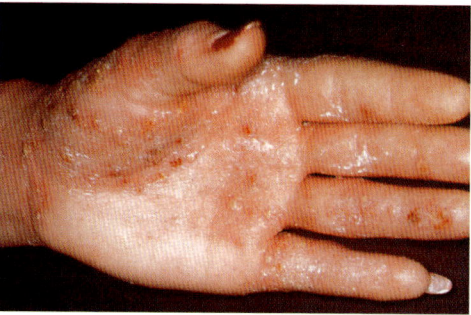

Fig. 5.32. Dyshidrotic hand dermatitis

5 Allergic Diseases (and Differential Diagnoses)

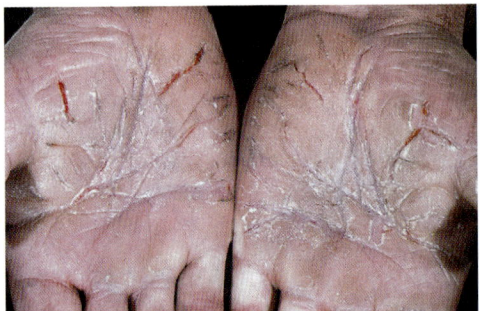

Fig. 5.33. Cumulative toxic hand dermatitis

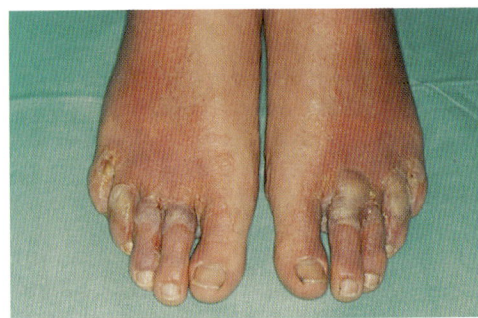

Fig. 5.34. Foot dermatitis (allergy to antimycotic medication)

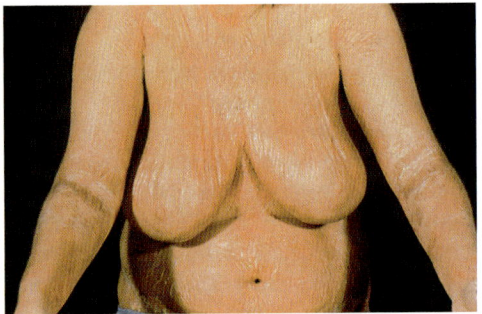

Fig. 5.35. Irritative contact dermatitis due to artificial application of a disinfectant

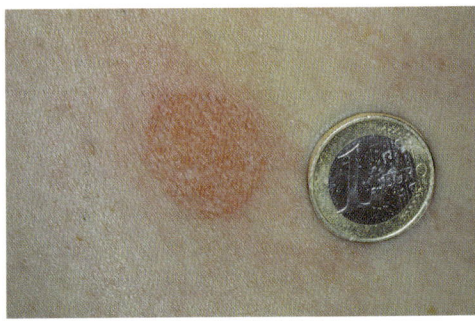

Fig. 5.36. Allergy to coins containing nickel

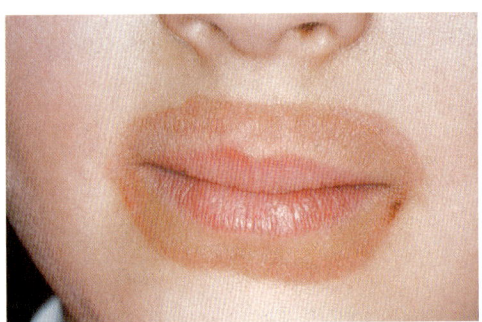

Fig. 5.37. Dermatitis caused by excessive licking of the lips

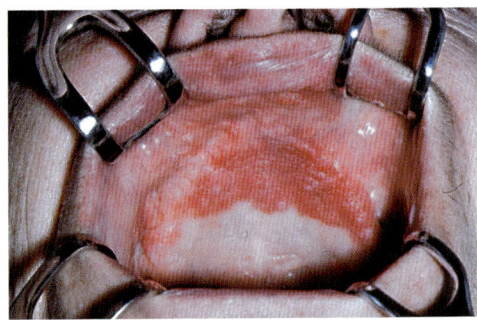

Fig. 5.38. Contact stomatitis

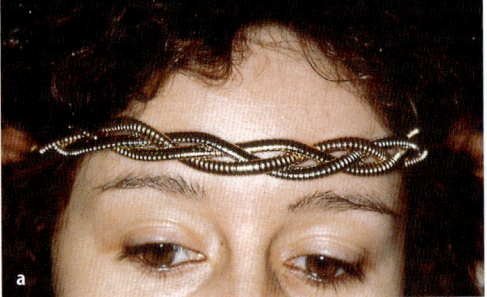

Fig. 5.39a,b. Nickel allergy (dermatitis caused by a headband)

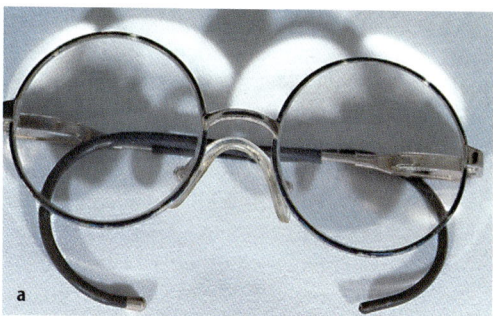
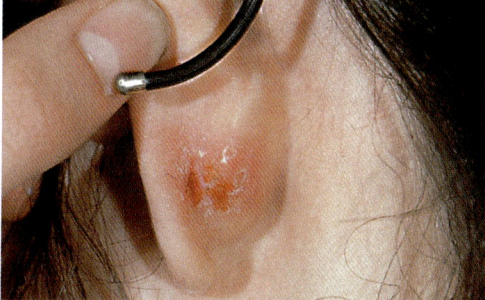

Fig. 5.40a,b. Nickel allergy (dermatitis caused by eyeglass frames)

the polymers), *disinfectants* (formaldehyde, parabens), *drugs* (there is a strong increase in iatrogenic sensitizations through rheuma and venous insufficiency ointments) as well as *plants*; the most common phytoallergens are sesquiterpenlactones from composites (= Asteraceae) such as chrysanthemum, arnica, chamomile, mugwort, as well as chinoid eczematogens from exotic woods [5, 30]. There is no allergen cross-reaction to the pollen of the respective plants!

Contact dermatitis can also be elicited via the air ("airborne contact dermatitis"), which often is confused with photoallergy.

5.5.2.3 The Patch Test

Since the first description of the patch test by J. Jadassohn in 1895 [33], the patch test is the classical method for diagnosis of contact dermatitis [4, 10, 15, 18, 20, 52, 55, 56]. The allergen is diluted properly (adequate concentrations have to be determined first in healthy volunteers in order to avoid toxic reactions) in an indifferent vehicle (mostly petrolatum) and fixed to a patch on the skin. Patches either are fixed in aluminum foil or aluminum chambers (Finn chambers). A new technique uses allergen-coated thin layer foils (TRUE test, thin layer rapid use epicutaneous test) [21]. After 1 or 2 days, the patch is removed. The test reaction is read after 24/48 and after 72 h and graded from 0 to +++ [0 = negative, (?) = questionable (erythema), + = weakly positive (erythema and infiltration, single papules), ++ = strongly positive (erythema, infiltrate, papules, and vesicles), +++ = very strongly positive (erythema,

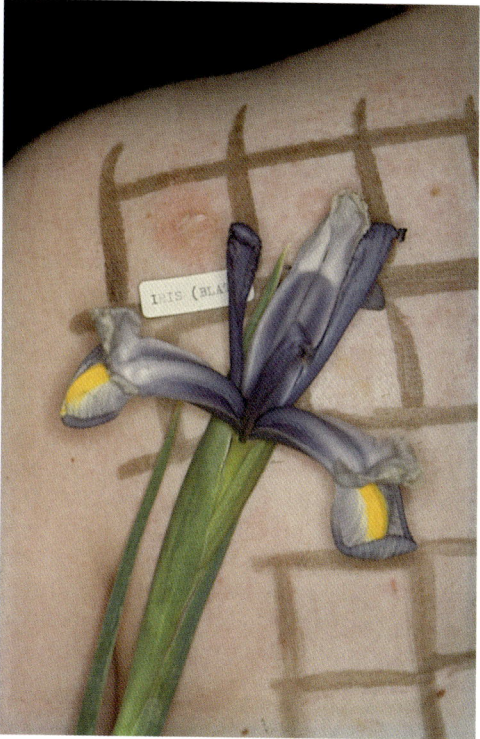

Fig. 5.41. Positive test reaction to phytoallergens (iris)

papules, confluent vesicles, erosion), IR = irritative reaction (Figs. 5.41, 5.42)]. In special cases, a third reading after 1 or 2 weeks may be indicated.

The open patch test (reading after 20 min) is used in the diagnosis of contact urticaria (see Sect. 5.1.3).

The "contact allergy time" (CAT) as the time interval needed to become sensitized against neoantigens through epidermal contact deter-

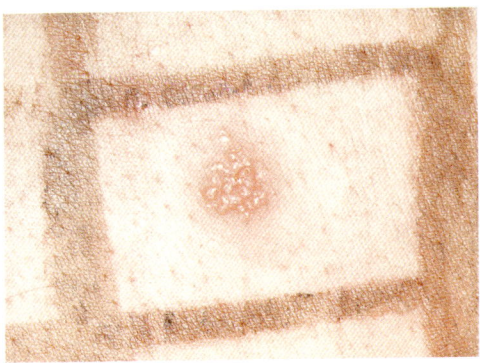

Fig. 5.42. Positive epidermal test

mines the afferent part of the cellular immune response quantitatively [11].

Allergic and toxic reactions can be distinguished: toxic reactions are sharply marginated, reach their maximum earlier (24–48 h) and are also positive in normal individuals (>20%). Besides toxic reactions, false-positive test results may occur through other factors of irritation such as adhesive tape irritation, too high concentrations, allergy against test materials, or concomitant to other very strong reactions ("angry back" or "excited skin syndrome") [12, 40, 42, 44]. Substances with a tendency to elicit false-positive reactions are: chromate, formaldehyde, thiomersal, and fragrance mix. Primary toxic substances may only be tested in very special cases with a clear-cut history (e.g., tear gas) and in high dilution.

False-negative test results occur under long-term glucocorticoid treatment or with too low concentrations (see Sect. 4.2). External steroid therapy should be stopped 1 week prior to patch tests. On the day of patch testing, no ointments at all should be applied. Antihistamines, beta-adrenergics, and xanthins do not influence patch test reactions. Strong UV radiation should be avoided 4 weeks prior to testing.

Even if carefully performed and read, the reproducibility of patch test reactions (especially of weakly positive reactions) remains unsatisfactory in some cases [23, 25, 55]. Unfortunately, there is no routine in vitro test for type IV allergies!

Positive patch test reactions should be evaluated regarding their relevance for the disease. This requires a high degree of expertise on the part of the physician and cooperation from the patient. Nevertheless, some test reactions remain unexplained when the substance is ubiquitous or when the occurrence is unrecognized.

In unclear cases, an epidermal provocation test (repeated open application test = ROAT) is used [32]: the substance suspected (e.g., cosmetic) is applied twice daily over 7 days into the elbow flexure, the volar forearm or the cheek. The open application avoids the risk of false-positive reactions.

When there are more than five positive test reactions – except group allergies – "angry back syndrome" should be suspected (see above). Substances should be retested in single small groups, especially in forensic, occupational situations or if lifesaving drugs are concerned [8, 59].

The selection of substances to be tested follows a careful history. There are standard selections through national or international contact dermatitis research groups (ICDRG) and additional specific "blocks" for special situations (occupation, localization, etc.) [4, 5, 8, 10, 18, 22, 23, 52, 55, 59].

Only clear-cut positive and well-defined allergens (no ointment mixtures!) should be documented in the allergy passport! Weakly positive or possibly irritative or "angry back"-induced test results should not be included because of potential lifelong and forensic consequences [8]. However, they should be recorded in the files.

Particular problems occur with questionable allergies against dental prosthetic materials where often psychosomatic influences play a role or against metal implant materials after orthopedic surgery (often positive nickel patch test reactions are not relevant for the implanted material situation) as well as against cosmetics due to the high number of possible substances (Table 5.57). Most common elicitors of cosmetic incompatibility are (in decreasing sequence): facial creams, antiperspirants/deodorants, eye make-up, nail cosmetics, hair colorings, soap [45]. The testing of individual products is crucial (Table 5.58). For the evaluation of positive patch test reactions, adequate controls are required.

Table 5.57. Possible ingredients of a simple "moisturizer cream" (*BHA*, butylhydroxyanisol)

Ingredient	Examples	Possible number of substances
Fat	Lanolin, paraffin	500
Polyalcohol	PEG	20
Emulsifier	Tween	1,000
Solvent	Alcohol, acetone	30
Thickening	Starch, traganth	30
"Moisturizer"	Mannit, inositol	50
Color	Azo dyes, pigments	500
Preservatives	Benzylalcohol, formaldehyde	150
Antioxidants	Tocopherol, BHA	40
Fragrance	Citronellal, eugenol	3,500
Sum		~6,000

Table 5.58. Recommended concentrations for patch testing of patient's cosmetics

Cream	Undiluted
Make-up	Undiluted
Mascara	Undiluted
Mascara (dry)	Undiluted
Lipstick	Undiluted
Perfume	20–100%
Deodorant	20–100%
Hairspray	20%
Hair coloring	10%
Hair bleaching	20% (separated!)
Nail polish	10%
Cold perm materials	2%
Toothpaste	2%
Soap	1%
Shampoo	1%

5.5.2.4 Therapy

Acute dermatitis is treated with moist cooling wraps, lotio alba and short-term topical glucocorticosteroids. For long-term success, allergen avoidance is crucial. Contact sensitization is lifelong in most cases.

Attempts to perform specific hyposensitization against contact allergens have been published (e.g., by oral administration) without convincing success for the clinical routine. Nevertheless, in many cases "hardening" occurs together with adequate skin care. Chronic forms of dermatitis with hyperkeratotic skin lesions require the use of keratolytics prior to glucocorticosteroids. They may be very therapy resistant. In severe cases of, e.g., dyshidrotic dermatitis, PUVA (psoralen plus UVA) therapy may be helpful.

The use of new topical immunosuppressants (tacrolimus or pimecrolimus) in these cases may be helpful.

References

1. Ackermann AB, Ragaz A (1982) A plea to expunge the word eczema from the lexicon of dermatology and dermatopathology. Am J Dermatopathol 4:315–326
2. Aetius von Amida (1549) Tetrabiblos (V.4, Sermo 1, Kap. 128). Froben, Basel, p 730
3. Akdis M, Klunker S, Schliz M, Blaser K, Akdis CA (2000) Expression cutaneous lymphocyte-associated antigen on human $CD4^+$ and $DC8^+$ Th2 cells. Eur J Immunol 30:3533–3541
4. Bandmann HJ, Dohn W (1967) Die Epicutantestung, 2nd edn. Bergmann, Munich
5. Benezra C (1986) Molecular recognition in allergic contact dermatitis. In: Ring J, Burg G (eds) New trends in allergy II. Springer, Berlin Heidelberg New York, pp 218–224
6. Bergstresser PR, Tigelaar RE, Dees JH, Streilein JW (1983) Thy-1 antigen-bearing dendritic cells populate murine epidermis. J Invest Dermatol 81:286
7. Bloch I (1911) Der älteste Gebrauch des Wortes "Eczema". Mh Prakt Dermatol 53:69–71
8. Borelli S (1980) Gewerbedermatosen, einschließlich Begutachtung. In: Korting GW (ed) Dermatologie in Praxis und Klinik, vol II. Thieme, Stuttgart
9. Braathen LR, Thorsby E (1983) Human epidermal Langerhans cells are more potent than blood monocytes in inducing some antigen-specific T cell-responses. Br J Dermatol 108:139–146
10. Brasch J, Geier J, Schnuch A (1998) Differenzierte Kontaktallergenlisten dienen der Qualitätsverbesserung. Hautarzt 49:184–191
11. Burg G, Przybilla B, Bogner J (1986) Contact – allergy time. In: Ring J, Burg G (eds) New trends in allergy II. Springer, Berlin Heidelberg New York, pp 230–239
12. Bruynzeel DP (1983) Angry back or excited skin syndrome. Thesis, Amsterdam
13. Cavani A, Albanesi C, Traidl C, Sebastiani S, Girolomoni G (2001) Effector and regulatory T cells in allergic contact dermatitis. Trends Immunol 22:118–120

14. Chase MW (1946) Inhibition of experimental drug allergy by prior feeding of the sensitizing agent. Proc Soc Exp Biol Med 61:257–259
15. Cronin E (1980) Contact dermatitis. Churchill Livingstone, Edinburgh
16. De Groot AC (1994) Patch testing. Elsevier, Amsterdam
17. Diepgen TL, Coenraads PJ (1999) The epidemiology of occupational contact dermatitis. Int Arch Occup Environ Health 72:496–506
18. Enders F, Przybilla B, Ring J (1988) Epikutantest mit einer Standardreihe. Ergebnisse bei 12 026 Patienten. Hautarzt 39:779–786
19. Enk AH, Angeloni VL, Udey MC, Katz SI (1993) An essential role for Langerhans cell-derived IL-1β in the initiation of primary immune responses in skin. J Immunol 150:3698–3703
20. Faergemann J (1993) *Pityrosporum ovale*-assoziierte Dermatosen. In: Braun-Falco O, Plewig GK, Meurer M (eds) Fortschritte prakt. Derm Venereol, vol 14. Springer, Berlin Heidelberg New York, pp 234–237
21. Fischer T, Bellberg K, Bruynzeel DP, Ducombs G, Hannuksela M, Lachapelle IM, Ring J, White IR, Wilkinson J (1988) European multicenter study of TRUE test. Contact Dermatol 19:91–97
22. Foussereau J, Benezra C, Maibach HI (1982) Occupational contact dermatitis, clinical and chemical aspects. Munksgaard, Copenhagen
23. Frosch P, Rustemeyer T, Schnuch A (1996) Kontaktdermatitis, parts I and II. Hautarzt 47:874–882, 945–961
24. Fuchs T, Aberer W (eds) (2004) Kontakteczema. Dustri, Deisenhofen (in press)
25. Gollhausen R, Ring J, Przybilla B (1987) Der iterative Test zur Unterscheidung kontaktallergischer oder irritativer Epikutantestreaktionen. Allergologie 10:427
26. Grabbe S, Kämpgen E, Schuler G (2000) Dentritic cells: multi-lineal and multi-functional. Immunol Today 21:431–433
27. Granstein RD, Askari M (1986) Cutaneous cells in activation of immunologic reactions: further characterization. J Invest Dermatol 87:141
28. Halter S (1959) Das vulgäre Eczema. In: Gottron A, Schönfeld W (eds) Dermatologie und Venerologie, vol III/1. Thieme, Stuttgart
29. Happle R (1994) Paraptisches Eczema. Hautarzt 45:1–3
30. Hausen B, Vieluf I (1998) Allergie-Pflanzen. Pflanzen-Allergene. Ecomed, Landsberg
31. Hornstein OP (1986) Anmerkungen und Vorschläge zur Definition und Klassifikation der Eczemakrankheiten. Z Hautkr 61:1281–1296
32. Hannuksela M, Salo H (1986) The repeated open application test (ROAT). Contact Dermatol 14:211–227
33. Jadassohn J (1895) Verhandl Dtsch Derm Gesellschaft 5. Kongreß 1896, p 103
34. Kapsenberg ML, Bos JD, Wierenga EA (1992) Cells in allergic responses to haptens and proteins. Springer Semin Immunopathol 13:303–314
35. Klaschka F (1987) Hämatogenes Kontakteczema durch Nahrungsmittel. Allergologie 10:93–97
36. Knop J, Malorny U, Macher E (1984) Induction of T effector and T suppressor lymphocytes in vitro by haptenized bone marrow-derived macrophages. Cell Immunol 88:411–420
37. Kripke ML, Munn CG, Jeevan A, Tang MM, Bucana C (1990) Evidence that cutaneous antigen-presenting cells migrate to regional lymph nodes during contact sensitization. J Immunol 145:2833–2842
38. Langerhans P (1868) Über die Nerven der menschlichen Haut. Virchows Arch A (Path Anat) 44:325
39. Lepoittevin J-P, Benezra C, Sigman CC, Baheri D, Fraginals R, Maibach HI (1995) Molecular aspects of allergic contact dermatitis. In: Rycroft RJG, Menné T, Frosch P (eds) Textbook of contact dermatitis. Springer, Berlin Heidelberg New York, pp 105–119
40. Luderschmidt C, Heilgemair G, Ring J, Burg G (1982) Polyvalente Kontaktallergie versus "Angry-back-Syndrom". Allergologie 5:262–268
41. Magnussen B, Kligman AM (1977) Usefulness of guinea pig tests for detection of contact sensitizers. In: Marzulli FN, Maibach HI (eds) Dermatotoxicology and pharmacology. Wiley, London, pp 551–560
42. Maibach HI (1981) The ESS, excited-skin-syndrome (alias the "angry-back"). In: Ring J, Burg G (eds) New trends in allergy. Springer, Berlin Heidelberg New York, pp 206–216
43. Miescher G (1962) In: Marchionini A (ed) Handbuch der Haut- und Geschlechtskrankheiten, supplementary vol 11/1. Springer, Berlin Heidelberg New York, p 1
44. Mitchell JC (1975) The angry back syndrome: eczema creates eczema. Contact Dermatol 1:193–194
45. Nater JP, De Groot AC (1983) Unwanted effects of cosmetics and drugs used in dermatology, 2nd edn. Elsevier, Amsterdam
46. Odia S, Vocks E, Rakoski J, Ring J (1996) Successful treatment of dyshidrotic hand eczema using tap water iontophoresis with pulsed direct current. Acta Derm Venereol 76:472–474
47. Rietschel RL, Fouler JF (2001) Fisher's contact dermatitis, 5th edn. Lippincott-Williams, Philadelphia
48. Ring J (ed) (1990) Endogenous and exogenous eczema. Semin Dermatol 9:195–246
49. Ring J ((1996) Zum Wandel des Eczema-Begriffes: Klassisches versus atopisches Eczema. Z Hautkr 10:752–756
50. Römpp H (1982) Chemielexikon, 8th edn. Franckh'sche Verlagshandlung, Stuttgart
51. Ross R, Gillitzer R, Kleinz J, Schwing H, Kleinert U, Förstermann AB, Reske-Kunz (1998) Involve-

ment of NO in contact hypersensitivity. Int Immunol 10:61–69
52. Rycroft RJG, Menné T, Frosch P (eds) (1995) Textbook of contact dermatitis. Springer, Berlin Heidelberg New York
53. Schäfer T, Böhler E, Ruhdorfer S, Weigl L, Wessner D, Filipiak B, Wichmann HE, Ring J (2004) Epidemiology of contact allergy in adults. Allergy (in press)
54. Schnuch A, Geier J, Uter W, et al. (1997) National rates and regional differences in sensitization to allergens of the standard series. Contact Dermatitis 37:200–209
55. Schnuch A, Aberer W, Agathos M, Brasch J, Frosch PJ, Fuchs T, Richter G (2001) Leitlinien der Deutschen Dermatologischen Gesellschaft (DDG) zur Durchführung des Epikutantests mit Kontaktallergenen. Hautarzt 52:864–866
56. Schulz KH, Fuchs T (1993) Der Epikutantest. Manuale allergologicum, IV, 4. Dustri, Deisenhofen, pp 1–39
57. Schuler G, Steinman RM (1985) Murine epidermal Langerhans cells mature into potent immuno-stimulatory dendritic cells in vitro. J Exp Med 161:526–546
58. Schwanitz HJ (1986) Das atopische Palmoplantareczema. Springer, Berlin Heidelberg New York
59. Schwanitz HJ, Szliska C (eds) (2001) Berufsdermatosen. Dustri, Munich
60. Scott P (1993) IL-12: initiation cytokine for cell-mediated immunity. Science 260:496–497
61. Silberberg I, Baer RI, Rosenthal SA (1974) The role of Langerhans cells in contact allergy. I. An ultrastructural study in actively induced contact dermatitis in guinea pigs. Acta Derm Venereol (Stockh) 54:321–331
62. Stingl G (1980) New aspects of Langerhans cell function. Int J Dermatol 19:189
63. Török I (1989) Eczema s betegsegek. Medicina, Budapest
64. Traidl C, Merk HF, Cavani A, Hunzelmann N (2000) New insights into the pathomechanisms of contact dermatitis by the use of transgenic mouse models. Skin Pharmacol Appl Skin Physiol 13:300–312
65. Unna PG (1887) Seborrhoeal eczema. J Cutan GU Dis 5:449–459
66. Uter W, Schnuch A, Geier J, et al. (1998) Epidemiology of contact dermatitis. The information network of Department of Dermatology (IVDK) in Germany. Eur J Dermatol 8:36–40
67. Willan (1808) On cutaneous diseases. Johnson, London

5.5.3 Atopic Eczema

Atopic eczema is one of the most common inflammatory skin diseases (found in 9–20% of German children!) with a chronic or relapsing course, and strong itching [20, 21, 30, 36, 40, 48, 49, 64, 68]. The multitude of names ("atopic dermatitis," "neurodermitis diffusa," "neurodermitis constitutionalis," "neurodermitis atopica," "prurigo Besnier," "endogenous eczema," "neurodermatitis," etc.) reflects the various pathophysiological concepts [5, 10, 20, 27, 40, 48, 49, 65, 68]. We prefer the term "atopic eczema" (or "atopic dermatitis") since it implies neither pathomechanisms (e.g., neurologic abnormalities) nor routes of contact (exogenous or endogenous), but focuses on the familial atopic trait.

5.5.3.1 Clinical Manifestation

Atopic eczema most often starts in childhood or adolescence; sometimes the first manifestation is cradle cap in infants (also called "crusta lactea" because of its similarity with burnt milk in a pan); it affects the face and extensor surfaces of infants, while later the large flexures, hands, and neck are most commonly involved. The eczema becomes drier with increasing age, the skin shows lichenification, and in adulthood excoriated nodules (prurigo-like) (Figs. 5.43–5.51) are common [30, 50]. Unfortunately, atopic eczema – contrary to common opinion – does not clear regularly before puberty, but two-thirds of affected children will also suffer from the disease as adults [26] (Fig. 5.52). Atopic eczema may also first appear in adulthood, sometimes even in elderly persons.

Atopic eczema occurs with so-called "stigmata" or "minimal variants" [30, 33, 38, 49, 52] (Table 5.59, Figs. 5.53, 5.54). There is still controversy regarding the primary skin lesion, which is described as erythema, flush, papule, seropapule, or vesicle. In the tradition of St. John or J.W. von Goethe and together with the French school [5], we say: "In the beginning there was the itch." In many cases all skin lesions can be explained as secondary reactions to the itch. In children undergoing oral provocation, I have often observed that they com-

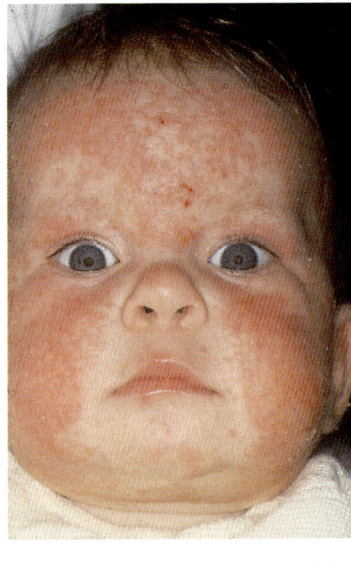
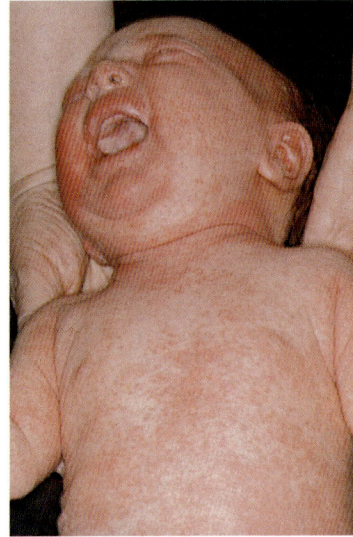

Fig. 5.43. (left) Atopic eczema in an infant ("cradle cap")

Fig. 5.44. (right). Atopic eczema in a newborn

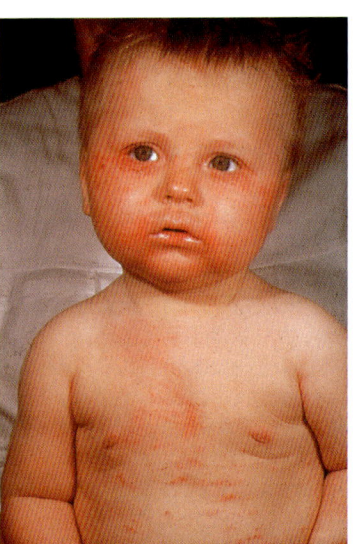
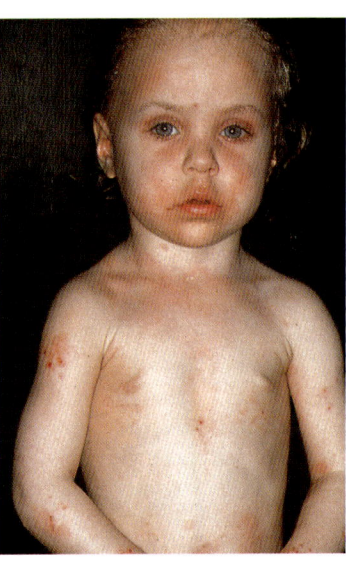

Fig. 5.45. (left) Atopic eczema in an older baby

Fig. 5.46. (right) Atopic eczema in a toddler

Table 5.59. Stigmata of atopic eczema

Sebostasis (dry skin)
Ichthyotic palms/soles
Linear grooves on the fingertips
Atopy lid fold (Dennie-Morgan)
Rarefication of lateral parts of eyebrows (Hertoghe)
Cap-like temporal hair growth (small distance between lateral eyebrow and temporal scalp hair)
Facial pallor with periorbital halo
White dermographism
Delayed blanch after acetylcholine

plain about itching without any visible skin lesion and start scratching, and only 15–20 min later do eczematous changes occur. For the diagnosis of atopic eczema, classically the criteria of Hanifin and Rajka [21] (Table 5.60) are cited, but are rarely used in practice.

5.5 Dermatitis/Eczema

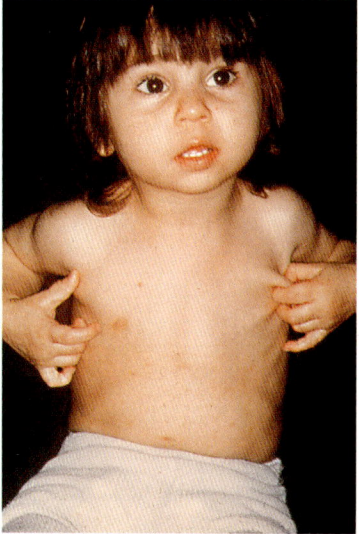
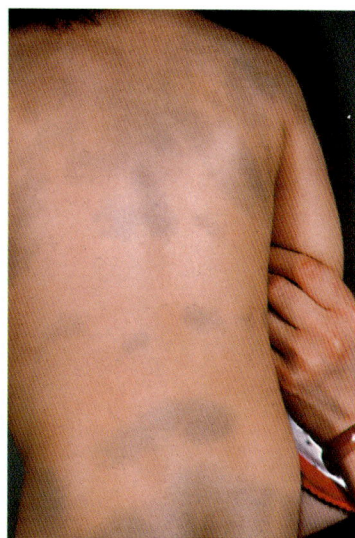

Fig. 5.47. (left) Itching as the primary symptom of atopic eczema

Fig. 5.48. (right) Atopic eczema on dark skin

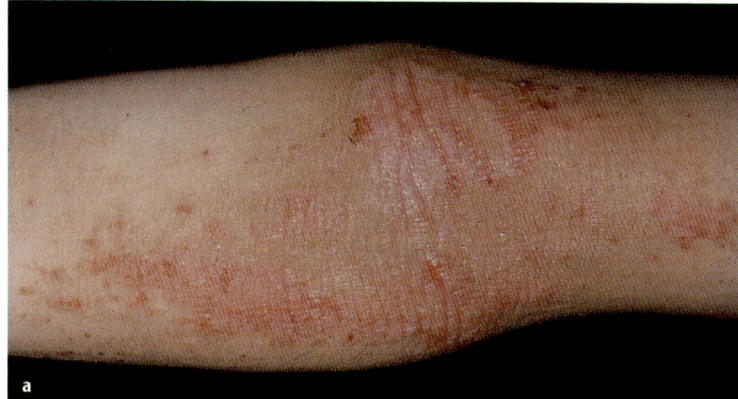
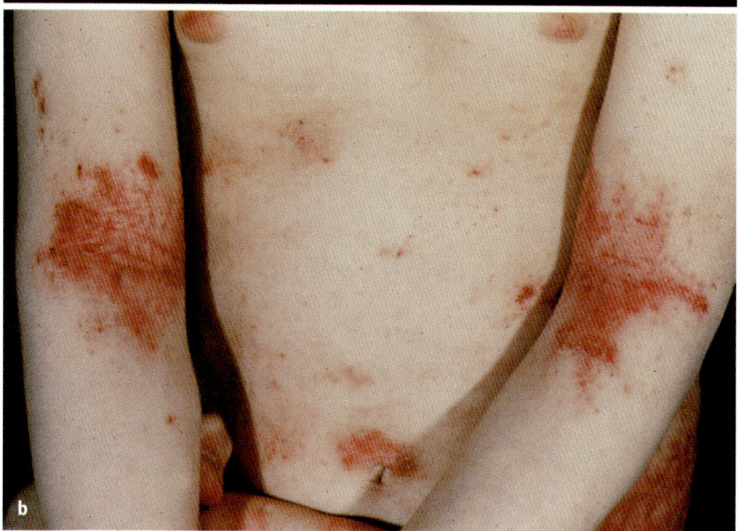

Fig. 49a,b. Elbow eczema

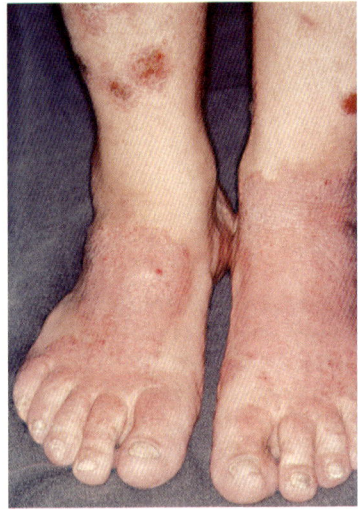
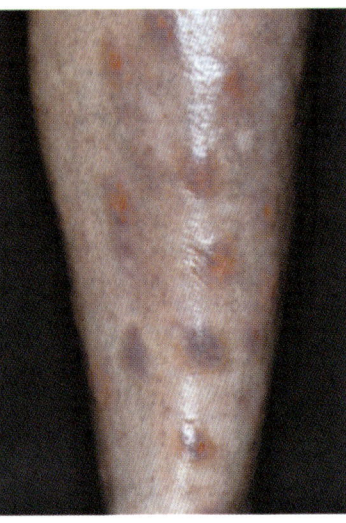

Fig. 5.50. (left) Atopic eczema on the lower legs and feet

Fig. 5.51. (right) Prurigo form of atopic eczema

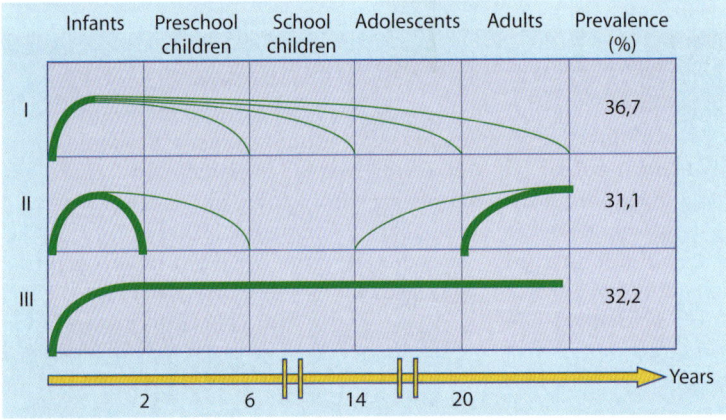

Fig. 5.52. Occurrence and course of atopic eczema at different ages (modified according to [26])

Table 5.60. Diagnosis of atopic eczema: criteria of Hanifin and Rajka [21] (three major and minor criteria each have to be positive)

Major criteria	Itch Typical morphology and distribution (lichenification in flexures of adults, face and extensor surfaces of children) Chronic relapsing eczema Personal and family history of atopy	**Minor criteria** *(cont.)*	Mamillar eczema Cheilitis Relapsing conjunctivitis Dennie-Morgan fold Keratoconus Subcapsular cataract Periocular halo Facial pallor Facial erythema Pityriasis alba Folding in the neck Itch when sweating Wool and solvent incompatibility Perifollicular accentuation Adverse food reactions Dependence of environmental and psychological factors White dermographism
Minor criteria	Sebostasis Ichthyosis Ichthyotic palm/sole Keratosis follicularis Type I sensitization (prick test) Elevated total serum IgE Early onset of disease Tendency to cutaneous infections (*Staph. aureus*, HSV) Tendency to unspecific hand and foot eczema		

Fig. 5.53. Ichthyosis hands as a stigma of atopic eczema

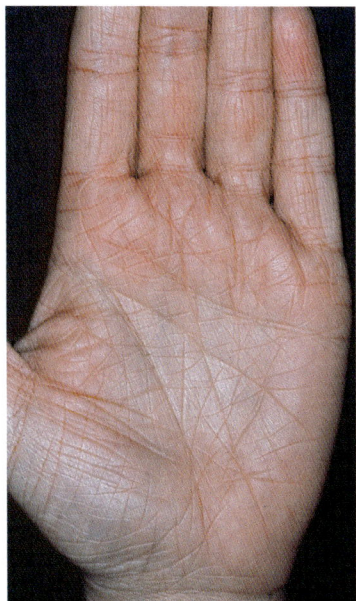
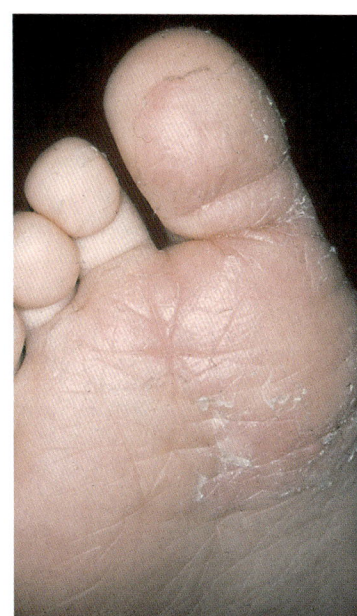

Fig. 5.54. Atopic "winter feet"

Table 5.61. Atopic eczema: diagnostic criteria (Ring 1982). With four or more positive findings, the diagnosis "atopic eczema" can be made (note that by this criterion, the diagnosis "atopic eczema" is possible without history or laboratory tests for atopy)

Eczema morphology (age-dependent)
Itch
Typical localization (age-dependent)
Atopy stigmata
Atopy in personal or family history
IgE sensitization

Table 5.62. Dermatohistopathology in atopic eczema

Acute
Acanthosis, hyperkeratosis, parakeratosis
Spongiosis, exocytosis, mild dermal lymphohistocytic infiltrate
Chronic-lichenified
Acanthosis, enlarged rete ridges, hyperkeratosis, parakeratosis, dense dermal infiltrate (mononuclear cells), increased mast cells, increase in capillaries and thickening of capillary walls, endothelial cell hyperplasia, fibrosis

Table 5.61 shows our diagnostic criteria from 1982: with four out of six positive parameters, the diagnosis atopic eczema can be made. Similarly in the 1990s, the "UK-refined criteria" [64] or the "Millennium criteria" [9] were developed.

Particular manifestations of eczema comprise so-called "sandbox dermatitis," "atopic winter feet," and "patchy lichenoid infiltrates" of Kitamura-Zazagawa-Takahashi and others [20, 22, 30, 38, 48, 49], some of them also included under minimal variants (for instance, infra-auricular fissures). For the determination of severity of actual eczematous skin lesions, the SCORAD (scoring system atopic dermatitis), developed by the European Task Force Atopic Dermatitis ETFAD [71], has proven valuable (Fig. 5.55).

In dermatohistology, patterns differ between acute and chronically lichenified lesions (Table 5.62) [59].

5.5.3.1.1 Genetics

Atopic eczema, allergic bronchial asthma, and allergic rhinoconjunctivitis are genetically closely linked [52]. Sixty percent of patients with eczema have other atopic diseases in their family history. The concordance rate of homozygous twins is 85% compared to 30% in heterozygous twins [54]. Inheritance is multifactorial: IgE formation in general (total IgE), the

5 Allergic Diseases (and Differential Diagnoses)

Patient: Name/Vorname   Geburtsdatum   Besuchsdatum

Eingesetztes topisches Steroid

(g)

Wirkstoff (Handelsname, Konzentration)   Menge/Monat   Anzahl der Erytheme/Monat

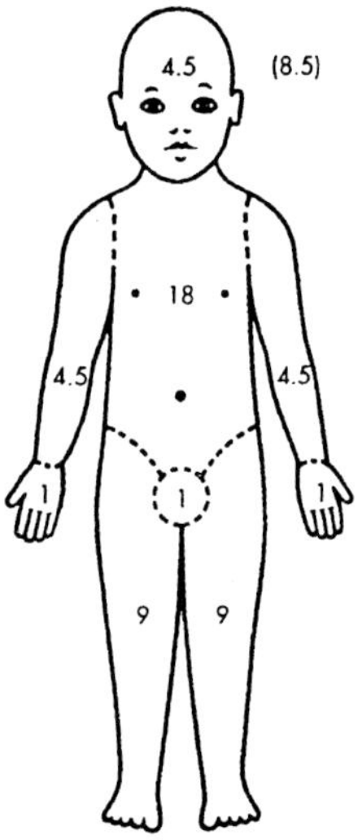

Ziffern in Klammern
für Kinder unter 2 Jahren

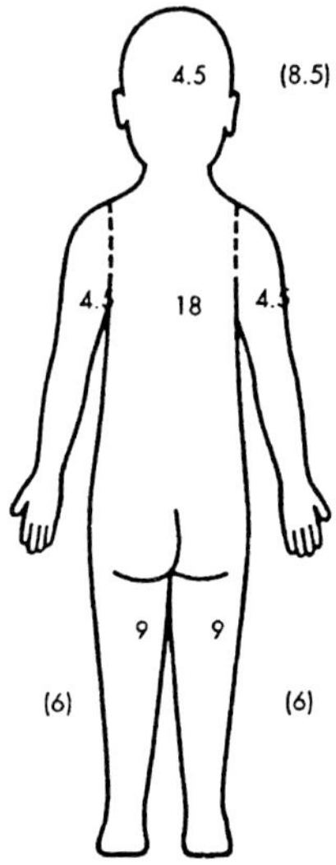

A: Ausmaß
Bitte geben Sie die Summe der
betroffenen Hautareale an.

B: Intensität

Bemessungswerte
Angaben zur Intensität (üblicherweise typische Stellen)   0 = keine   1 = leicht   2 = mäßig   3 = stark

Kriterien	*Intensität*	*Kriterien*	*Intensität*
Erythem		Exkoriation	
Ödem/Papelbildung		Lichenifikation	
Nässen/Krustenbildung		Trockenheit	
		Die Hauttrockenheit wird an nicht betroffenen Stellen bewertet	

C: Subjektive Symptome

Pruritus und Schlaflosigkeit   **SCORAD A/5+7B/2+C**

Visuelle Analog-Skala (Durchschnitt für die letzten drei Tage oder Nächte)

0 |||||||||||||||||||||||||||||||||||||||||||||||||||||||||||||||||||||||||||||||||||| 10
Pruritus (0–10)

0 |||||||||||||||||||||||||||||||||||||||||||||||||||||||||||||||||||||||||||||||||||| 10
Schlaflosigkeit (0–10)

Behandlung   Anmerkungen

Fig. 5.55. SCORAD (scoring for atopic dermatitis) index for assessing the severity of eczema

specificity of IgE antibodies and organ manifestations are influenced separately (see Sect. 3.1). There is no significant association between the diagnosis "atopic eczema" and HLA haplotypes [15].

5.5.3.2 Pathophysiology

5.5.3.2.1 Genetics

Recently, a close link of infantile atopic eczema with a gene on chromosome 3q21 was reported [31]. A second genome screen revealed an association with loci on chromosomes 1q21, 17q25, and 20p [15]. While the genes for the costimulatory CD80/86 molecules are found in the region of chromosome 3q21, the other loci do not reveal known relations to atopy. It is interesting that all four gene loci are also linked to psoriasis [15]. It may be speculated that these genes encode for general markers of skin inflammation independent of "atopy."

5.5.3.2.2 Increased IgE Production

Few diseases are characterized by elevated IgE values in the serum similarly to atopic eczema [36, 40, 42, 48, 49, 68]. These IgE antibodies are directed against environmental allergens, in central Europe in adults most commonly against cat epithelia, housedust mite, and grass pollen, in infants against hen's eggs and cow's milk. The evaluation of the relevance of IgE sensitization for the induction or elicitation of eczema may be difficult. It is achieved by careful history and provocation tests. The detection of IgE and IgE-receptors on epidermal Langerhans cells (Fig. 5.56) [6, 12, 55, 66] opens new perspectives for an understanding of the pathogenesis of atopic eczema (Table 5.63). Positive epidermal test reactions induced by typical aeroallergens (e.g., housedust mites) help to show the relevance of an IgE response for the eczematous skin lesions ("atopy patch test," APT) [16, 46] (Fig. 5.57). Compared to the prick test and RAST, the APT has a much higher specificity (Table 5.64).

There is no doubt that for a large group of eczema patients, IgE-mediated allergy plays a decisive role in the disease ("extrinsic" form). There are, however, (as in respiratory atopy) patients without IgE elevation or positive prick

Table 5.63. Langerhans cells, IgE and atopic eczema

IgE on Langerhans cells
IgE receptors [low- and high-affinity (CD23 and FcεR I) as well as IgE-binding protein]
Housedust mite allergen (Der p 1) next to IgE in doublestaining on Langerhans cell surface
Langerhans cells may present allergen via IgE
T-cell clones from atopy patch test reactions show TH2 characteristics and allergen specificity
Particularly increased expression of FcεR I in atopic eczema in lesional skin (contrary to contact dermatitis and other inflammatory skin diseases)

Table 5.64. Comparison of different allergy tests in atopic eczema (Darsow et al. [16])

Test	Sensitivity[a]	Specificity
Skin prick test	69–82%	44–53%
RAST	65–94%	42–64%
Atopy patch test	42–56%	69–92%

[a] Allergen-dependent (related to specific history)

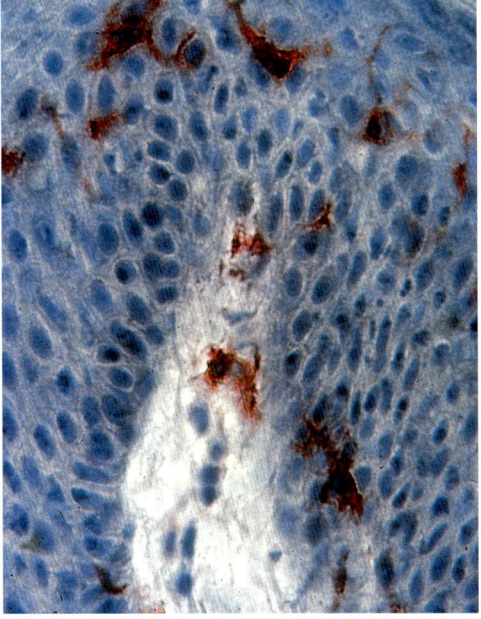

Fig. 5.56. IgE-positive Langerhans cells (reprinted by permission of T. Bieber)

test reactions ("intrinsic" form or "non-atopic" eczema) [69].

Recently, in very severe cases of atopic eczema, autoantibodies of IgE class against epider-

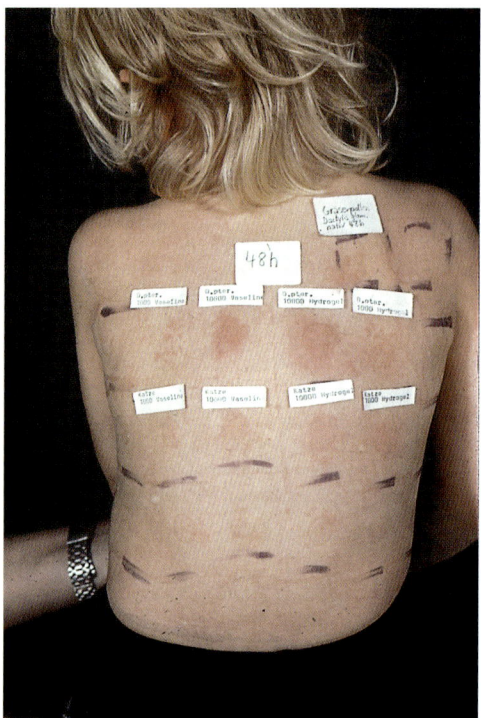

Fig. 5.57. Atopy patch test (APT)

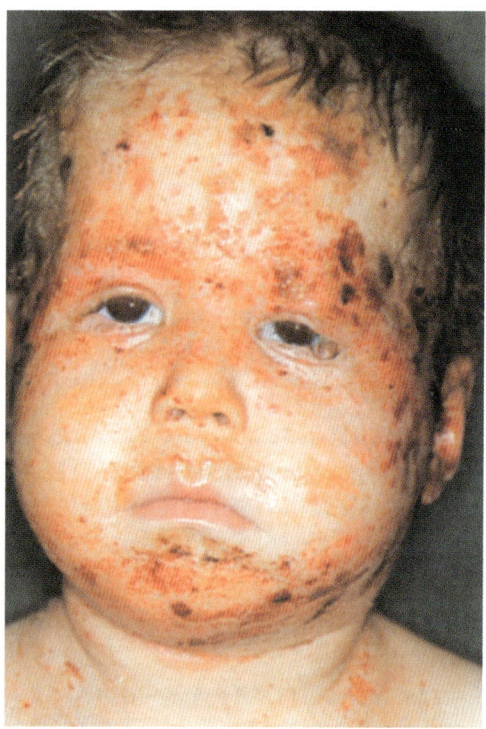

Fig. 5.58. Atopic eczema with massive superinfection by *Staphylococcus aureus*

mal proteins (Hom s 1) have been detected [60]; we see an increasing dynamic of eczema elicitation and maintenance via TH2 over TH1 to IgE autoantibodies, explaining the phenomena of chronification and resistance to therapy.

5.5.3.2.3 Disturbed T-Cell Regulation

Patients with eczema are often suffering from infections of fungal, bacterial, or viral origin (e.g., Kaposi's varicelliform eruption, or eczema herpeticum as well as increased staphylococcal colonization and infection of the skin; Fig. 5.58). Increased TH2 reaction occurs with decreased TH1 phenomena [14, 25, 53], which are most prominent in the so-called "hyper-IgE syndrome," which in its dermatological manifestation may be regarded as a maximal variant of atopic eczema [49].

Recent phenomena of spongiosis have been elucidated: activated CLA-positive T cells in the skin secrete beside other cytokines Fas-ligand, leading to apoptosis of keratinocytes and breaking up of intercellular E-cadherin junctions, while desmosomes stay intact and the inflammatory edema induces the picture of spongiosis [3, 58].

5.5.3.2.4 Autonomic Nervous System Dysregulation

Many patients show a dysbalance in autonomic nervous system reactivity [27], mostly in the sense of decreased β-adrenergic and increased α-adrenergic and cholinergic reactivity [3, 42] (see also "Stigmata"). In a Japanese study, patients with atopic eczema less frequently had hypertension than normals [Uehara, personal communication).

The imbalance of enhancing and inhibitory influences on mediator secretion can lead to an increased releasability of mediator secreting cells in atopic eczema. Patients with atopic eczema have increased plasma histamine levels as well as enhanced releasability of other mediators (e.g., leukotriene) [44]. These mediators not only have proinflammatory activity, but also – as histamine via histamine receptors on lymphocytes – regulatory effects in the immune response (see also Chap. 2), thus favoring IgE production and promoting a "circulus vitiosus" [42].

The well-known psychosomatic interactions fit into this concept very well [10, 18, 45]. Psychologic events may influence the disease positively and negatively through the action of nervous transmitters. In stress or anxiety, the same mediators are liberated as during itch or allergic inflammation (see Chap. 7, "Psyche and Allergy").

5.5.3.2.5 Dry Skin

The phenomenon of "dry skin" is complex in nature [7, 10, 11, 23] and describes at least three different dimensions ("rough" versus "smooth"; "fat" versus "lipid-poor"; "moist" versus "water-poor"); it can be better described as a barrier disturbance of the epidermis. In eczema, the following findings have been shown:

- Stratum corneum water content is not decreased
- Transepidermal water loss is increased
- Epidermal permeability is increased
- Skin roughness is increased
- Surface lipids are decreased
- Sebaceous glands are smaller
- Ceramide synthesis is altered
- Microscopically inflammatory reactions

Therefore, some authors regard "dryness" as a minimal inflammatory reaction [59] with the involvement of keratinocytes [19].

Previously, dryness was interpreted as decreased sebaceous gland activity ("sebostasis"); today alterations in intercellular lipid bilayer are seen as the basis of the epidermal barrier (the "bricks and mortar" model according to P. Elias). The chemical basis is a mixture of ceramides, which are decreased in atopic eczema and possibly qualitatively altered [7]. Ceramide synthesis follows a subtle balance of different enzymes such as sphingomyelinase, β-glucocerebrosidase, ceramidase, and sphingomyelindeacylase [23].

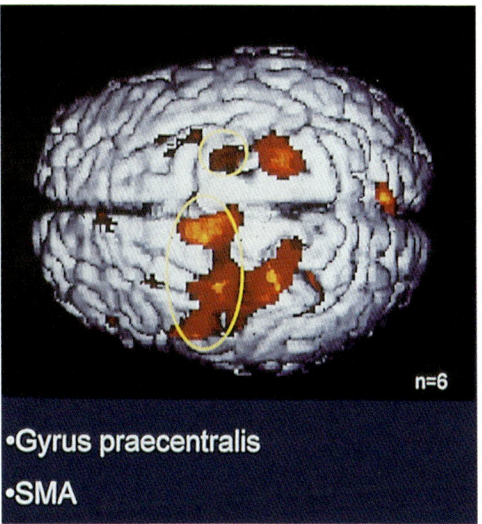

Fig. 5.59. Visualization of pruritus with the aid of positron emission tomography (PET). The *red areas* are significantly activated. Motor-associated areas are additionally marked (*yellow circles*). (From Darsow et al. [17])

5.5.3.2.6 Itch

Itch and dryness are closely related. Any skin exsiccated too much (e.g., by excessive showering) starts to itch and gives rise via scratching to eczematous lesions. On the basis of "hypersensitive" skin, patients react more strongly to a variety of stimuli and irritants (e.g., wool).

Recently, the itch sensation has been visualized with positron emission tomography (PET) [17] (Fig. 5.59). Atopic itch has several components, only some of them depending on skin inflammation.

5.5.3.3 Therapy

Individual treatment is the major principle, considering the patient's actual skin characteristics in the course of the disease [2, 11, 47]. There is no "miracle" pill or ointment, nor is there a general diet against atopic eczema! Monomania should be avoided; the disease is neither only allergic nor only sebostatic nor only psychologic in origin!

The basis of any therapeutic strategy is careful dermatologic basic skin care, especially during remission [11]. The individual selection of emollients (different for different body areas and different individuals) including bath or showering oils (a distinction should be made between emulsion and spreading type bath oils) is critical; avoid showering at too hot a temperature or for too long.

Acceptance by the patient is important; many patients do not like ointments which are too greasy although their skin looks very dry. Hydrophilic ointments (unguentum emulsificans aquosum) have been found helpful as basic vehicles.

Consistent avoidance of all eliciting factors detected during the diagnostic work-up is crucial (irritants, allergens, infection, food reactions) [36, 39, 47]. The inflamed skin manifesting as eczema is treated with anti-inflammatory drugs, preferably with topical glucocorticosteroids in the acute phase (see Sect. 5.5.4).

A new method of anti-inflammatory treatment of atopic eczema without glucocorticoids is available with the new topical immunosuppressives or calcineurin antagonists, which act topically. These substances (tacrolimus and pimecrolimus) inhibit like cyclosporin A activation of calcineurin phosphatase in T cells and also mast cells and basophil leukocytes by binding to a cytosolic immunophyllin (cyclophyllin, FK506 binding protein or macrophyllin 12). The intracellular signal transduction is thereby inhibited and the transcription of many proinflammatory cytokines is reduced [41, 57, 69]. (see also Sect. 6.3.2).

In contrast to glucocorticosteroids, these substances do not have atrophogenic effects in the skin. The two preparations available are tacrolimus in a relatively fatty ointment in 0.1% and 0.03% concentrations as well as the more aqueous cream pimecrolimus in a 1% cream. The place of these new compounds in the management of atopic eczema will be seen in the years to come.

For prophylaxis, avoidance of irritants and allergens (Table 5.65) also includes recommendations for breast feeding of the newborn infant, the use of encasings at home or rehabilitation under climatic therapy conditions (e.g., North Sea, high altitude in Davos, Switzerland) [10].

Frequent superinfections of the skin sometimes require antimicrobial therapy, best done with disinfectants (clioquinol, triclosan, gentian violet). In severe cases, systemic antibiotic or antimycotic (in head and neck dermatitis) treatment may help.

Table 5.65. Atopic eczema: irritants and elicitors

Physical	Mechanical stimuli, dryness, UV radiation, temperature
Chemical	Detergents, solvents, acids, alkali
Pharmacological	Vasoactive substances (alcohol, nicotine, amines)
Infectious	Superantigens
Psychological	Stress, emotional conflict

Wet wraps ("moist pyjamas"), cooling baths, topical steroids, lotio alba, and systemic antihistamines are used against severe itching (see Sect. 6.3.2 on "Pharmacotherapy").

The well-known psychosomatic interactions in atopic eczema sometimes require careful psychosomatic counseling of the patient and relatives [10, 18, 45].

UV therapy as adjuvant strategy has a good effect with different modalities, especially as long-wave UVA-1 [1, 28, 29].

Unsaturated fatty acids have been recommended as well as traditional Chinese herbs [2] or leukotriene antagonists [13].

The role of allergen-specific immunotherapy is controversial [70]; however, considering the new results with the atopy patch test and the clear-cut role of allergy in some patients, it should be investigated by control studies.

There is no need for desperation or pessimism when we look at the spectrum of therapeutic modalities available for atopic eczema (Fig. 5.60). All these treatment modalities require the active cooperation of the informed patient over months and years (Table 5.66). Therefore, "eczema school" programs have been developed, which after adequate training (eight atopic eczema academies in Germany) are offered in an interdisciplinary setting (allergy, dermatology, pediatrics, nutritionists, psychosomatics) for children, parents, and adults [18].

Table 5.66. Leaflet for patients with (atopic) eczema

- Your disease is based partly on inherited factors which can either lead to eczema, conjunctivitis, rhinitis, or bronchial asthma. This genetic predisposition, however, does not necessarily lead to disease. There is a genetic predisposition to increased hypersensitivity of skin and mucous membranes.
- In eczema, the skin is dry, looks rough, the hair sometimes looks rigid, a variety of factors from the environment (both irritant and allergic) can give rise to the development of eczematous skin lesions (red, itchy, sometimes oozing or crusted skin lesions), preferably on the big flexures elbow, knee, neck, hands, and face.
- The skin of patients with eczema (children and adults) needs constant care.

Skin care:
- Avoid too frequent bathing or showering (especially too hot or too foamy)!
- Use alkali-free soaps or syndets for cleaning your skin (mild products).
- When taking a bath or showering, restoration of the skin lipid is important. This can be done by adding a bath oil and/or by creaming after taking a bath or a shower with emollients (lotion, cream, etc.), especially on arms, legs, and hands.
- Take yourself time for skin care every morning and evening. Let the cream penetrate your skin (at least 5 min) before dressing. Don't change your ointments too often, stick to the products you tolerate. Thus, you can avoid additional allergies.

Clothing:
- Avoid wool or irritating textiles. Direct contact to the skin is best tolerated with cotton, silk, or linen.
- Wash underwear before first wearing, especially dark colored products.
- In changing T-shirts on your baby, watch the ears (avoid fissures under the earlobes!). Your favorite sweater may scratch your neck where there is no cotton underneath. Then use a silk scarf.
- During acute exacerbations, keep your baby dressed; an uncovered body surface starts itching and will be scratched.

Treatment of itch:
- The itch-scratch cycle deserves utmost attention. Often itch is the primary event inducing the new flare.
- Scratching often occurs as a reflex, it is not a matter of will. You should not forbid scratching! Rather treat the itch!
- Keep the nails cut short (scratching occurs also during sleep).
- Itch can be treated topically (anti-inflammatory creams, wet wraps, cooling procedures) or systemically (e.g., antihistamines; the sedating effect of old preparations may be helpful during night time). Topical therapy does less harm to the skin than pronounced scratching!
- Teachers and colleagues should know about the problem. People suffering from intense itch sometimes behave strangely (most of these children are not "hyperactive/hyperkinetic").

Allergen avoidance:
- According to the results of your allergy diagnosis, avoidance strategies should be implemented. These always have to be specific. Don't change your apartment into a prison-like environment with only glass and concrete. In housedust mite allergy, the bedroom and the mattress are most important and encasings are helpful.
- Some patients benefit from a longer stay in a different climate (sea level or high altitude; talk about this with your specialist).
- In high-risk families, pets should not be kept for allergy prevention. Tobacco smoke and indoor chemicals (cleaning, hobby activities) should be avoided.

Diet:
- There is no general anti-allergy diet. Patients with atopic eczema can principally eat what they want except for those foods detected as elicitors in careful allergy diagnosis including provocation tests. Positive skin prick or blood tests do not necessarily tell you whether this allergy is relevant for your skin disease. You may use these results as markers for self-observation.
- For allergy prevention, newborns from atopic parents should be breast-fed over 3–6 months; solid food should be only introduced after 6 months. If breastfeeding is not possible, use a hypoallergenic formula.
- Avoid ear-piercing in young children (nickel allergy!).
- If you are pollen-allergic wash your hair before going to bed.

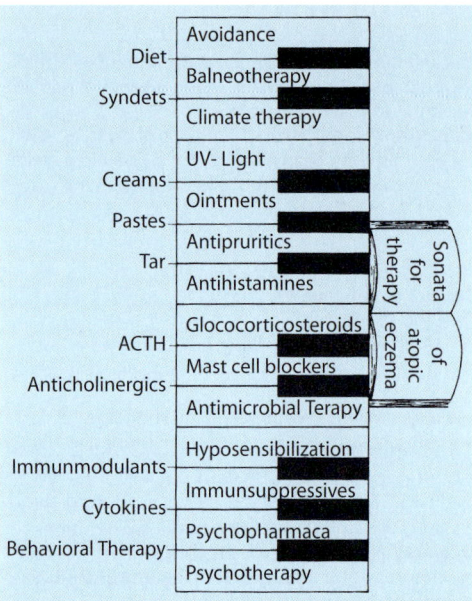

Fig. 5.60. "Therapeutic keyboard"

References

1. Abeck D, Schmidt T, Fesq H, Strom K, Mempel M, Brockow K, Ring J (2000) Long-term efficacy of medium-dose UVA1 phototherapy in atopic dermatitis. J Am Acad Dermatol 42:254–257
2. Abeck D, Ring J (eds) (2002) Atopisches Eczema (Neurodermitis) im Kindesalter. Steinkopff, Darmstadt
3. Akdis CA, Akdis M, Trautmann A, Blaser K (2000) Immune regulation in atopic dermatitis. Curr Opin Immunol 12:641–646
4. Atherton DJ (1981) Allergy and atopic eczema. Clin Exp Dermatol 6:317–325
5. Besnier E (1892) Premiere note et observations preliminaires pour servir d'introduction a l'etude des prurigos diathesiques (dermatites multiformes prurigineuses chroniques exacerbantes et paroxystiques, du type du prurigo de Hebra). Ann Derm Syph (Paris) 3,3:634–648
6. Bieber T (1994) FceR1 on human Langerhans cells: a receptor in search of new functions. Immunol Today 15:52–53
7. Bleck O, Abeck D, Ring J, Hoppe U, Vietzke J, Wolber R, Brandt O, Schreiner V (1999) Two ceramide subfractions detectable in Cer(AS) position by HPTLC in skin surface lipids on non-lesional skin of atopic eczema. J Invest Dermatol 113:894–900
8. Boguniewicz M, Leung DYM (1998) Atopic dermatitis: A question of balance. Arch Dermatol 134:870–871
9. Bos JD, Van Leent EJ, Sillevis Smitt JH (1998) The millennium criteria for the diagnosis of atopic dermatitis. Exp Dermatol 7:132–138
10. Borelli S, Schnyder UW (1962) Neurodermitis constitutionalis sive atopica, part II: Atiologie, Pathophysiologie, Pathogenese, Therapie. In: Miescher G, Storck H (eds) Entzündliche Dermatosen I. Handbuch der Haut- und Geschlechtskrankheiten [Suppl 11/1]. Springer, Berlin Heidelberg New York, pp 254–319
11. Braun-Falco O, Ring J (1984) Zur Therapie des atopischen Eczemas. Hautarzt 35:447–454
12. Bruynzeel-Koomen C, Van Wichen DF, Toonstra J, Berrens L, Bruynzeel PLB (1986) The presence of IgE molecules on epidermal Langerhans cells in patients with atopic dermatitis. Arch Dermatol Res 278:199–205
13. Carucci JA, Washenik K, Weinstein A, Shupack J, Cohen DE (1998) The leukotriene antagonist zafirlukast as a therapeutic agent for atopic dermatitis. Arch Dermatol 134:785–786
14. Cooper KD, Stevens SR (2001) T cells in atopic dermatitis. J Am Acad Dermatol 45:510–512
15. Cookson WO, Ubhi B, Lawrence R, Abecasis GR, Whalley AJ, Cox HE, et al. (2001) Genetic linkage of childhood atopic dermatitis to psoriasis susceptibility loci. Nat Genet 27:372–373
16. Darsow U, Vieluf D, Ring J for the APT Study Group (1999) Evaluating the relevance of aeroallergen sensitization in atopic eczema with the atopy patch test: a randomized, double-blind multicenter study. J Am Acad Dermatol 40:187–193
17. Darsow U, Drzezga A, Frisch M, Munz F, Weilke F, Bartenstein P, Schwaiger M, Ring J (2000) Processing of histamine-induced itch in the human cerebral cortex: a correlation analysis with dermal reactions. J Invest Dermatol 115:1029–1033
18. Fartasch M, Abeck D, Werfel T, Diepgen T, Schmid-Ott G, Ring J, Gieler U (2000) Aktueller Stand des interdisziplinären Modellprojektes "Neurodermitis-Schulung für Kinder und Jugendliche". Hautarzt 51:299–301
19. Giustizieri ML, Mascia F, Frezzolini A, De Pita O, Chinni LM, Gianetti A, Girolomoni G, Pastore S (2001) Keratinocytes from patients with atopic dermatitis and psoriasis show a distinct chemokine production profile in response to T cell-derived cytokines. J Allergy Clin Immunol 107:871–877
20. Hanifin JM (1982) Atopic dermatitis. J Am Acad Dermatol 8:1–13
21. Hanifin JM, Rajka G (1980) Diagnostic features of atopic dermatitis. Acta Derm Venereol 114:146–148
22. Herzberg J (1973) Wenig bekannte Formen der Neurodermitis. Hautarzt 24:407–501
23. Imokawa G (2001) Lipid abnormalities in atopic dermatitis. J Am Acad Dermatol 45:S29–32
24. Jakob T (2002) Mechanismen der Aktivierung und Mobilisation dentritischer Zellen in der

Haut. Habilitationsschrift, Technische Universität München
25. Jung T (2002) Zytokindysregulation bei atopischer Dermatitis. Dustri, Munich
26. Kissling S, Wüthrich B (1994) Dermatitis in young adults: personal follow-up 20 years after diagnosis in childhood. Hautarzt 45:368–371
27. Korting GW (1954) Zur Pathogenese des endogenen Eczemas. Thieme, Stuttgart
28. Kowalzick L, Kleinheinz A, Weichenthal M, Neuber K, Köhler I, et al. (1995) Low dose versus medium dose UVA1 treatment in severe atopic eczema. Acta Derm Venereol 75:43–45
29. Krutmann J, Czech W, Diepgen T, Niedner R, Kapp A, Schöpf E (1993) Highdose UVA1 therapy in the treatment of patients with atopic dermatitis. J Am Acad Dermatol 26:225–230
30. Kunz B, Ring J (1999) Clinic diagnostic features of atopic eczema. In: Oranje A, et al. (ed) Pediatric dermatology, vol 2. Blackwell, Oxford
31. Lee Y-A, Wahn U, Kehrt R, Tarani L, Businco L, Gustafsson D, Andersson F, Oranje AP, Wolkertstorfer A, Berg A v, Hoffmann U, Küster W, Wienke T, Rüschendorf F, Reis A (2000) A major susceptibility locus for atopic dermatitis maps to chromosome 3q21. Nature Genetics 26:470
32. Leung DYM (2001) Atopic dermatitis and the immune system: The role of superantigens and bacteria. J Am Acad Dermatol 45:S13–16
33. Leutgeb C, Bandmann HJ, Breit R (1972) Handlinienmuster, ichthyosis vulgaris und dermatitis atopica. Arch Derm Forsch 244:244–354
34. Neuber K (2002) Atopisches Eczema und *Staphylococcus aureus*. Dustri, Munich
35. Olesen AB (2001) Role of the early environment for expression of atopic dermatitis. J Am Acad Dermatol 45:37–40
36. Oranje AP (2000) Atopic dermatitis (AD): Evaluation and therapy. Pediatr Dermatol 17:75–83
37. Platts-Mills TAE, Mitchell EB, Rowntree S, Chapman MD, Wilkins SR (1983) The role of dust mite allergens in atopic dermatitis. Clin Exp Dermatol 8:233–247
38. Przybilla B, Ring J, Enders F, Winkelmann H (1991) Stigmata of atopic constitution in patients with atopic eczema or atopic respiratory disease. Acta Derm Venereol 71:407–410
39. Przybilla B, Eberlein-König B, Rueff F (1994) Practical management of atopic eczema. Lancet 343:1342–1346
40. Rajka G (1989) Essential aspects of atopic dermatitis. Springer, Berlin Heidelberg New York
41. Reitamo S, Rissanen J, Remitz A, Granlund H, Erkko P, Elg P, Autio P, Lauerma A (1998) Tacrolismus ointment does not affect collagen synthesis: results of a single-center randomized trial. J Invest Dermatol 111:396–398
42. Ring J (1979) Atopic dermatitis: a disease of general vasoactive mediator dysregulation. Int Arch Allergy Appl Immunol 59:233–239
43. Ring J (1991) Atopy: condition, disease, or syndrome? In: Ruzicka T, Ring J, Przybilla B (eds) Handbook of atopic eczema. Springer, Berlin Heidelberg New York, pp 3–8
44. Ring J, Bieber T, Vieluf D, et al. (1991) Atopic eczema. Langerhans cells and allergy. Int Arch Allergy Appl Immunol 94:194–201
45. Ring J, Schröpl F (1985) Das atopische Eczema. Medizinisches Hörspiel, Frankfurt (Audio-Kassette mit Begleitheft)
46. Ring J, Kunz B, Bieber T, Vieluf D, Przybilla B (1989) The "atopy patch test" with aeroallergens in atopic eczema. J Allerg Clin Immunol 82:195
47. Ring J, Brockow K, Abeck D (1996) The therapeutic concept of "patient management" in atopic eczema. Allergy 51:206–215
48. Ring J (ed) (1998) Neurodermitis. Ecomed, Landsberg
49. Ruzicka T, Ring J, Przybilla B (eds) (1991) Handbook of atopic eczema. Springer, Berlin Heidelberg New York
50. Saurat J-H (1985) Eczema in primary immunedeficiencies. Clues to the pathogenesis of atopic dermatitis with special reference to the Wiskott-Aldrich syndrome. Acta Derm Venereol (Stockh) 114:125–128
51. Schäfer T, Krämer U Vieluf D, Abeck D, Behrendt H, Ring J (2000) The excess of atopic eczema in East Germany is related to the intrinsic type. Br J Dermatol 143:992–998
52. Schnyder UW (1960) Neurodermitis, Asthma, Rhinitis, eine genetisch allergologische Studie. Karger, Basel
53. Schöpf E, Kapp A, Kim CW (1978) T-cell function in atopic dermatitis. Controlled examination of concanavalin A. Dose-response relations in cultured lymphocytes. Arch Dermatol Res 262:37 44
54. Schultz-Larsen F (1985) Atopic dermatitis. Etiological studies based on a twin population. Laegeforeningens, Copenhagen
55. Stingl G (2001) IgE-mediated, $Fc_\varepsilon RI$-dependent allergen presentation: A pathogenic factor in atopic dermatitis? J Am Acad Dermatol 45:S517–S520
56. Taieb A (1999) Hypothesis: from epidermal barrier dysfunction to atopic disorders. Contact Dermatitis 41:177–180
57. Thestrup-Pedersen K, Ring J (1999) Atopic dermatitis: summary of the 1st Georg Rajka Symposium 1998 and a literature review. Acta Derm Venerol 79:257–264
58. Trautmann A, Akdis M, Kleemann D, Altznauer F, Simon HU, Graeve T, Noll M, Brocker EB, Blase K, Akdis CA (2000) T cell-mediated Fas-induced keratinocyte apoptosis plays a key pathogenetic role in eczematous dermatitis. J Clin Invest 106:25–35
59. Uehara M (1985) Clinical and histological features of dry skin in atopic dermatitis. Acta Derm Venereol (Stockh) [Suppl] 114:8246
60. Valenta R, Seiberler S, Natter S, Mahler V, Mossabeb R, Ring J, Stingl G (2000) Autoallergy: A

pathogenetic factor in atopic dermatitis? J Allergy Clin Immunol 105:432–437
61. Wahlgren CF, Scheynius A, Hagermark O (1990) Antipruritic effect of oral cyclosporin A in atopic dermatitis. Acta Derm Venereol 70:323–329
62. Wakim M, Alazard M, Yajima A, Speights D, Saxon A, Stiehm E (1998) High dose intravenous immunoglobulin in atopic dermatitis and hyper-IgE syndrome. Ann Allergy Asthma Immunol 81:153–158
63. Werfel T (2000) Allergenspezifische T-Zell-Antwort bei Eczemakrankheiten. Dustri, Munich
64. Williams HC (ed) (2000) Atopic dermatitis. The epidemiology, causes and prevention of atopic eczema. Cambridge University Press, Cambridge
65. Wise F, Sulzberger MB (1933) Footnote on problem of eczema, neurodermatitis and lichenification. In: Wise F, Sulzberger MB (eds) The 1933 Year book of dermatology and syphilology. Year Book Publishers, Chicago, pp 38–39
66. Wollenberg A, Wen S, Bieber T (1999) Phenotyping of epidermal dendritic cells – clinical applications of a flow cytometric micromethod. Cytometry 37:147–155
67. Wright S, Burton JL (1982) Oral-evening-primrose-seed oil improves atopic eczema. Lancet 2:1120–1122
68. Wüthrich B (1975) Zur Immunpathologie der Neurodermitis constitutionalis. Huber, Bern
69. Wüthrich B (ed) (1999) The atopic syndrome in the third millennium. Karger, Basel
70. Zachariae H, Cramers M, Herlin T, Jensen J, Kragballe K, Ternowitz T, Thestrup-Pedersen K (1985) Non-specific immunotherapy and specific hyposensitization in severe atopic dermatitis. Acta Derm Venereol (Stockh) [Suppl] 114:48–54
71. Stalder R, Taieb A, et al. (1993) Consensus Report of the European Task Force on Atopic Dermatitis. Severity scoring of atopic dermatitis: the SCORAD index. Dermatology 186:23–31

5.5.4 Topical Glucocorticosteroid Therapy

Glucocorticosteroids have a central place in the treatment of inflammatory skin disease. They can be regarded as the greatest advance in topical dermatotherapy in the second half of the 20th century [28]. In Germany in the year 2001, there were 263 different preparations in various application forms including 70 combination preparations on the market (systemic substances not included).

5.5.4.1 Mechanisms of Action

Glucocorticosteroids have a variety of well-known effects due to control of synthesis of several enzymes at the chromosome level [2, 5, 9, 11]. The steroid is bound to a cytoplasmic receptor leading to a conformation change of the receptor complex [6], which then binds in the nucleus to chromatin and influences the transcription of messenger RNA. Steroids may both stimulate and inhibit transcription. The exact mechanisms are still not known; however, they enhance the activity of RNA polymerases at certain positions in the chromatin [2].

Glucocorticoids have a variety of metabolic effects; the best known (hence the name!) affects the glucose metabolism with the mobilization of muscular glycogen and neoglycogenesis from amino acids. This protein catabolism with a negative nitrogen balance maybe plays a role in the well-known immunosuppression and affects wound healing. In fatty tissue, lipolysis is enhanced, and in the kidney a mild mineralocorticoid effect exists, although it is $1,000\times$ weaker than aldosterone. In some tissues, glucocorticoids induce involution, especially in lymphatic tissues, the bone and the skin, most likely due to inhibition of DNA synthesis.

Furthermore, gestagenic effects (such as progesterone) have been described as well as psychic alterations (depression, sleeplessness, euphoria, alteration in behavior, and others).

In the skin, glucocorticosteroids inhibit the proliferation of epidermal, inflammatory, and lipid cells, the synthesis of collagen tissue, the liberation of mediators from mast cells, and pigment formation by melanocytes. They normalize altered cornification of epidermis cells, inhibit migration of inflammatory cells, and induce vasoconstriction [5] (Table 5.67).

The anti-inflammatory effect is of particular interest in dermatology, affecting almost all kinds of inflammation (infectious, allergic, physical, chemical, etc.). Apart from formation of lipocortin, inhibition of phospholipase plays a role which in the cell membrane is important in the formation of arachidonic acid from phospholipids. From arachidonic acid, highly active prostaglandins and leukotrienes are formed [2, 4, 6]. The anti-inflammatory effect

5.5 Dermatitis/Eczema

Table 5.67. Action of glucocorticosteroids on skin cells

Cells	Effects
Keratinocytes	Inhibition of proliferation
	Normalization of keratinization
Fibroblasts	Inhibition of collagen and proteoglycan synthesis
Lymphocytes	Inhibition of proliferation and cytokine secretion
Granulocytes	Inhibition of chemotaxis and activation
Mast cells/basophils	Inhibition of liberation of vasoactive mediators
Vascular system	Vasoconstriction
Melanocytes	Inhibition of pigment formation
Fatty tissue	Inhibition of proliferation

can be shown as inhibitory function on various cells (neutrophils, macrophages, lymphocytes) with additional vasoconstriction.

Pharmacologic effects of glucocorticosteroids depend on specific structures in the molecule (Fig. 5.61), the introduction of a fluor atom in position 9α increases the biological activity, and substitution in position 6α increases antiinflammatory effects. Esterification, acetonide formation as well as introduction of methyl or halogen groups in positions 16–21 lead to a variety of topically effective steroid preparations, which have been tested in various experimental systems (e.g., vasoconstriction assay) [1].

Table 5.68 shows the most common topical glucocorticoids, roughly classified according to pharmacologic potency.

New developments with fewer side effects include prednicarbate, methylprednisolonaceponide, and mometasone furoate.

For therapeutic efficacy, dermal resorption of the applied substance is necessary; this can be influenced by certain factors, such as:

- Stratum corneum thickness (tape stripping)
- Age (infant skin has higher permeability)
- Blood flow (increased skin blood flow increases resorption)
- Hydration (occlusion increases permeation by a factor of 10!) (Table 5.69)

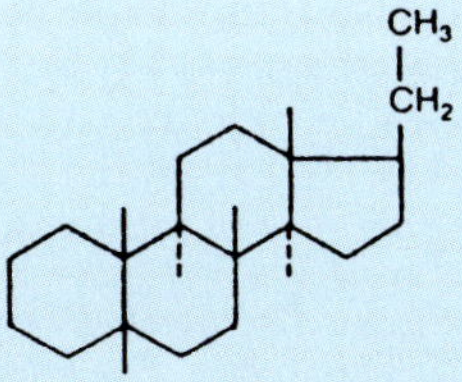

a) Pregnane

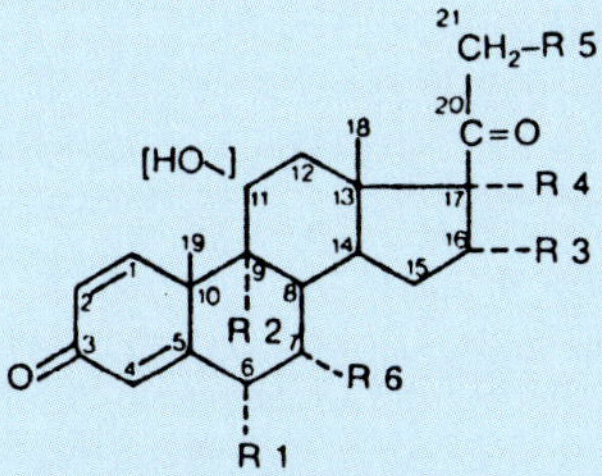

b) Structure of natural and synthetic Glucocorticosteroides

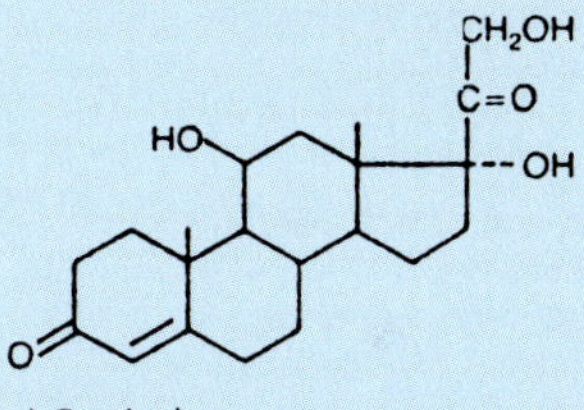

c) Cortisol

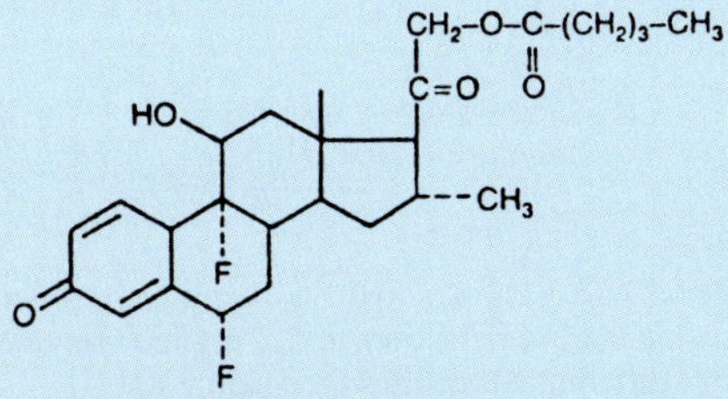

d) Diflucortolon-21-valerate

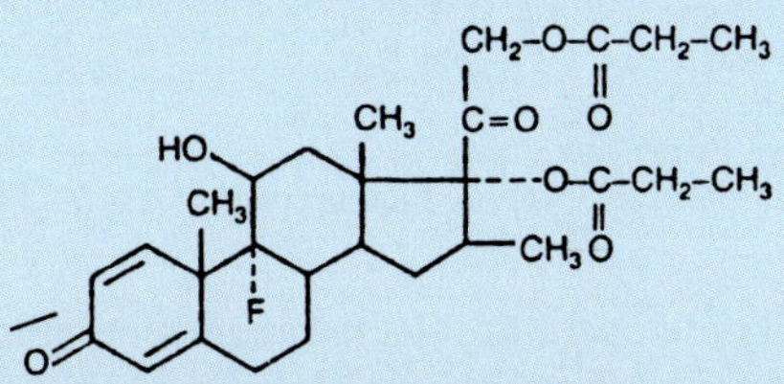

e) Betamethasone-17,21-dipropionate

Fig. 5.61. Natural and synthetic glucocorticosteroids as pregnane derivatives [21]

Table 5.68. Topical glucocorticosteroids of different potency (arbitrary selection) (according to [9, 17, 21])

Potency (group)	Substance
I =	Non-halogenated glucocorticosteroids Hydrocortisone Hydrocortisone-17-butyrate Hydrocortisone acetate Desonid Hydrocortisone buteprate Methylprednisolone aceponide Prednisolone Prednicarbate
II =	Weakly fluorinated glucocorticosteroids Alclomethasone Clobetasol butyrate Fluocortin butylester
III =	Moderate glucocorticosteroids Betamethasone-17-valerate Betamethasone-17-benzoate Betamethasone-17-pentanoate Desoximethasone Mometasone fuorate Triamcinolone-16–17-acetonide Flumethasone-21-pivalate Fludroxycortide Fluticasone-17-propionate Dexamethasone
IV =	Strong glucocorticosteroids Betamethasone-17–21-dipropionate Fluocinolone acetonide Diflorasone-17–21-diacetate Diflucortolone-21-valerate
V =	Very strong glucocorticosteroids Amcinonide Fluocinonide Halcinonide Clobetasol-17-propionate

Table 5.69. Excretion of hydrocortisone into the urine after local administration of 5.2 mg/cm^2 in acetone under different conditions (according to [7])

	% of dose applied
Normal skin	0.46
Under occlusion	4.48
After corneal stripping	0.91
After corneal stripping plus occlusion	14.91

- Skin temperature (increasing temperature increases permeation, part of the occlusion effect)
- Influence of vehicle (optimal solution of the effective agent, but not too high an affinity to the vehicle)
- Interaction of drugs (e.g., addition of 3% salicylic acid enhances the steroid penetration)
- Skin metabolism (biotransformation by oxidation, methylation, sulfatation, glucuronidation, etc.). Fluocortin butylester is hydrolyzed in the skin to the inactive steroid acid, leading to decreased efficacy, but also fewer side effects.

5.5.4.2 Practical Application of Topical Glucocorticoids

Topical glucocorticosteroids have to be indicated. They can suppress inflammation, but rarely are curative, which has to be considered in chronic disease.

If there is an indication for topical glucocorticosteroid therapy, the weakest effective preparation should be selected in order to avoid side effects. Maximally, apply twice daily, generally once daily (depot in the stratum corneum). Occlusion should never be longer than 12 h to avoid side effects!

After 1 week of therapy, the situation should be monitored by a physician (sometimes even daily). If there is no immediate rapid response within a week, the patient should consult a dermatologist.

Long-term steroid therapy never should be stopped abruptly (rebound phenomenon), slow dose reduction can be done either by changing to a less potent product or, preferably, by interval therapy (3 days steroid, 4 days vehicle only) [3, 10, 12, 13, 14]. Tachyphylaxis phenomena have been observed and may be overcome by changing the product.

With regard to epidermal proliferation kinetics (with a minimum at 6.00 p.m. in the daily rhythm), some authors recommend the application of topical steroids in the evening; we follow the individual itch intensity.

Crucial in the selection of topical steroid preparations is the vehicle [3]. Figure 5.62 shows a rough schedule of critical criteria (clinical course, skin type, body area for the selection of the vehicle) [21]. In chronic inflammation, fatty preparations are preferred while acute lesions should be treated with solutions and cooling wraps. In intertrigenous areas,

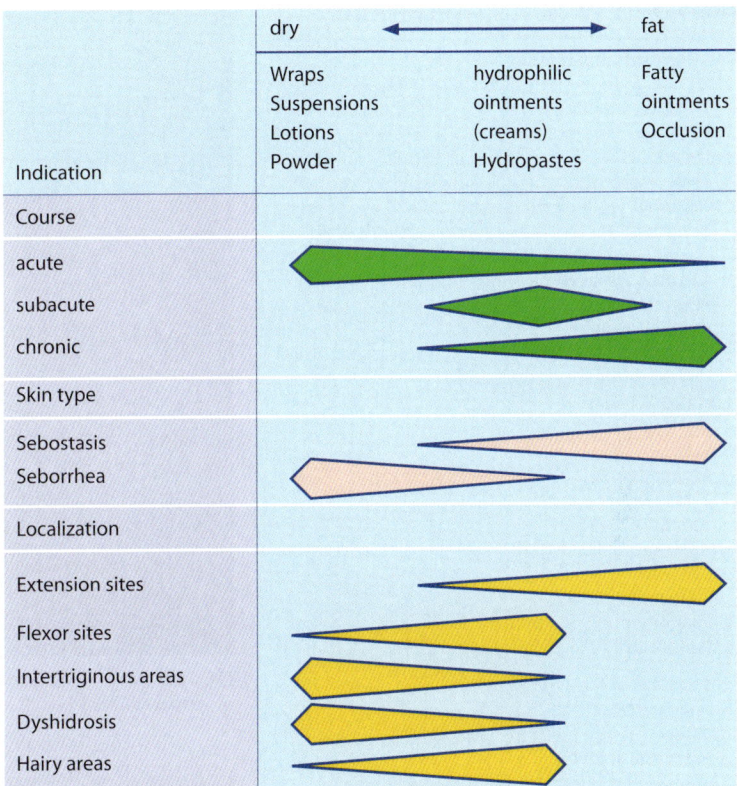

Fig. 5.62. Application forms of topical therapy. Guidelines for selecting the proper application form for topical glucocorticoid therapy according to the clinical course and the location and condition of the affected skin area

greasy ointments need to be avoided, whereas on the extensor surfaces and in chronic lesions they are indicated.

Corticoid preparations are available in all forms: greasy ointment (no water), water in oil ointments, oil in water (creams), lotio (suspension mixtures), lotion (milk), gel, paste (powder in ointment), alcoholic solutions (tinctura), plasters, sprays, foams, etc. The vehicles comprise substances of mineral (petrolatum, paraffin), animal (wool wax alcohols), plant (oils, wax, starch), and synthetic origin (propylene glycol) together with emulsifiers, preservatives, fragrances, etc. These constituents are important for potential contact allergy.

Combination preparations of glucocorticoids with antibiotics or antimycotics should be considered critically and only in occasional cases are they indicated. The "ex iuvantibus" practice often prevents correct diagnosis.

For individual prescriptions of mixtures, the galenic compatibility has to be considered to avoid instability of emulsions, loss of efficacy, and incompatibilities between substances. Many companies offer the vehicle ointment alone in addition to the steroid-containing compound.

5.5.4.3 Side Effects of Topical Glucocorticosteroids

The most relevant side effects of topical steroid therapy are listed in Table 5.70. The risk of systemic steroid therapy generally is much higher. However, sometimes after very intense topical steroid application (especially under occlusion) systemic side effects may occur [5, 9, 11, 16, 17, 21].

Almost all undesired side effects of corticoids are somehow related to the desired pharmacological effect and therefore in most cases dose dependent. Disturbance of ostiofollicular keratinization leads to comedo formation and steroid acne. Inhibition of proliferation and regeneration of the epidermis induces thinning and atrophy. The degeneration of collagen and

Table 5.70. Side effects of glucocorticosteroids

Systemic administration
Endocrinology
Diabetes mellitus
Catabolic metabolism
Osteoporosis
Hyperlipidemia
Alkalosis (sodium retention potassium excretion)
Suppression of pituitary gland (growth suppression in children)
Cushing's syndrome
Hypertension
Immune system
Inhibition of lymphocyte and granulocyte function, immunosuppression
Gastrointestinal
Peptic ulcer
Neurological
Myopathy
Neuropathy
Psychic alteration
Ophthalmological
Cataract
Glaucoma
Thromboembolic complication
Anaphylactoid reaction (very rare)
Topical application on skin
Striae distensae
Atrophy
Fatty tissue atrophy
Embolia cutis (after i.m. crystal suspension)
Increased photosensitivity
Pseudo-anetoderma
Cutis punctata linearis colli
Teleangiectasias
Rubeosis steroidica
Pigment changes
Perioral rosacea-like dermatitis
Granuloma gluteale infantum
Hypertrichosis
Purpura and ecchymosis
Acne
Hair loss
Infection
Disturbance of wound healing
Contact allergy

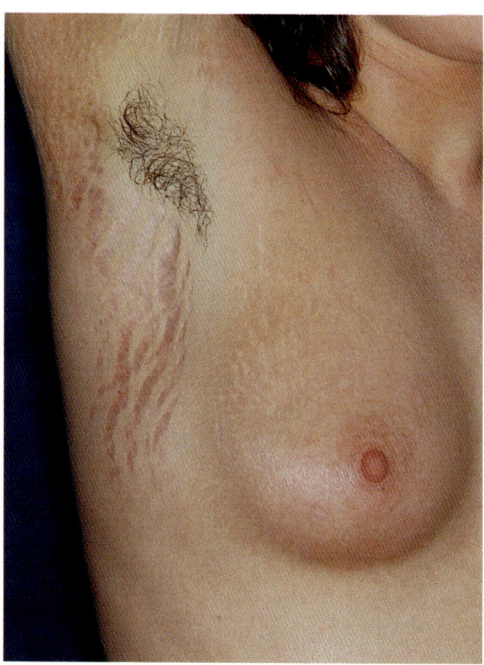

Fig. 5.63. Striae distensae after long-term application of glucocorticoids

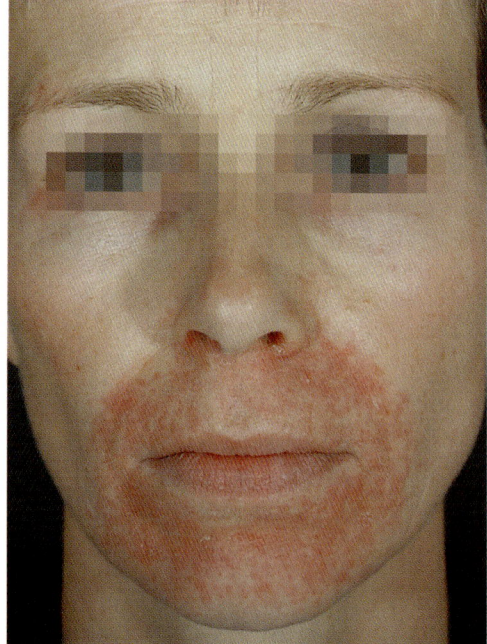

Fig. 5.64. Rosacea-like perioral dermatitis appearing in a patient who had used a fluoridated topical glucocorticoid preparation for several weeks

elastic fibers (also vessels) leads to senile elastosis, teleangiectasia, purpura, ecchymosis and striae distensae (Fig. 5.63).

A special form of topical corticoid side effect is the so-called perioral rosacea-like dermatitis, developing after long-term application of mostly fluorinated glucocorticoids (especially in atopics) and mostly in the face; it manifests as fine sharp papules and occasional pustules (Fig. 5.64). The indication for steroid treatment mostly remains trivial or unknown. The anti-inflammatory effect of the steroid induces improvement again and again, but is followed by heavy rebounds after withdrawal. Therefore, the patient will never learn the causal interactions. Only authoritative guidance of the patient can break this vicious cycle (I tell my patients: "Your skin is addicted to cortisone and we have to perform withdrawal!").

There are also allergic reactions (contact allergy) to cortisone preparations, mostly against constituents of the vehicle, but also against the steroid molecule itself.

After intramuscular application of corticoid crystal suspensions, partly irreversible local reactions may occur (embolia cutis, lipid or muscular atrophy) (Figs. 5.65, 5.66).

Practical Conclusions. Glucocorticosteroids are, even if applied topically, very active drugs, the use of which should be well indicated; it requires experience of skin diseases and steroid actions and side effects. The good doctor uses as little cortisone as necessary and as much indifferent vehicle therapy (emollients, lotio alba, paste, etc.) as possible!

References

1. Alpermann HG, Sandow J, Vogel HG (1982) Tierexperimentelle Untersuchungen zur topischen und systemischen Wirksamkeit von Prednisolon-17-ethylcarbonat-21-propionat. Arzneimittelforschung/Drug Res 32:633
2. Barnes PJ, Adcock I (1993) Anti-inflammatory actions of steroids: molecular mechanisms. Trends Pharmacol Sci 14:436–440
3. Braun-Falco O, Ring J (1984) Zur Therapie des atopischen Ekzems. Hautarzt 35:447–454
4. Carnuccui R, di Rosa M, Guerrasio B, Iuvone T, Sautebin L (1987) Vasocortin: a new glucocorticoid-induced anti-inflammatory protein. Br J Pharmacol 90:443–445
5. Claman WN (1984) Antiinflammatory effects of corticosteroids Immunol. Allergy Practice 4: 317–329
6. Clark CR (1985) Intracellular localisation of steroid receptors. In: Sluyser M (ed) Interaction of steroid hormone receptors with DNA. Ellis Horwood, Chichester, pp 7–56
7. Flower RJ, Rothwell NJ (1994) Lipocortin-I: cellular mechanisms and clinical relevance. Trends Pharmacol Sci 15:71–76

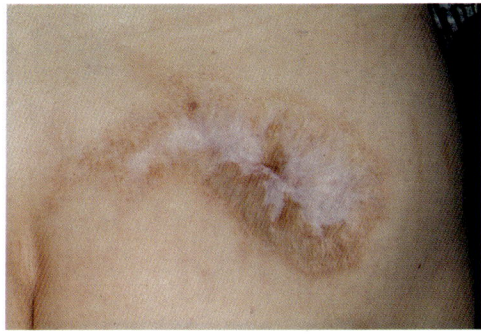

Fig. 5.65. Lipoatrophy occurring after the intramuscular administration of a glucocorticoid crystalline suspension

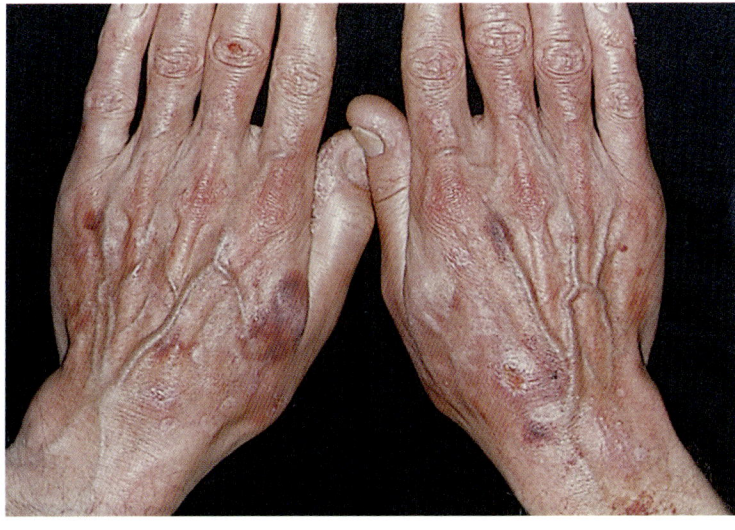

Fig. 5.66. Cutaneous atrophy following long-term treatment with a topical glucocorticoid

8. Guin JD (1984) Contact sensitivity to topical corticosteroids. J Am Acad Dermatol 10:773–782
9. Hatz II (1998) Kortison und Kortikoide. Deutscher Apothekerverlag, Stuttgart
10. Hornstein OP, Nürnberg E (eds) (1985) Externe Therapie von Hautkrankheiten. Pharmazeutische und medizinische Praxis. Thieme, Stuttgart
11. Kaiser H (1977) Cortisonderivate in Klinik und Praxis. Thieme, Stuttgart
12. Kligman AM (1986) Topical steroids: Perspectives and retrospectives. In: Ring J, Burg G (eds) New trends in allergy. II. Springer, Berlin Heidelberg New York, pp 342–352
13. Lubach D, Kietzmann M (1992) Dermatokortikoide – Pharmakologie und Therapie. In: Marghescu S, Wolff HH, Zaun H (eds) Kohlhammer, Freiburg
14. Maibach H, Stougthon RB (1973) Topical corticosteroids. Med Clin N Am 57:1253
15. Marghescu S (1983) Externe Kortikoidtherapie: Kontinuierliche versus diskontinuierliche Anwendung. Hautarzt 34:114–117
16. Miyachi Y (1982) Adrenal axis suppression caused by a small dose of a potent topical corticosteroid. Arch Dermatol 118:451
17. Niedner R, Ziegenmeyer J (eds) (1992) Dermatika – Therapeutischer Einsatz, Pharmakologie und Pharmazie. Wiss Verlagsgesellsch, Stuttgart
18. Poulsen J, Rorsman H (1980) Ranking of glucocorticoid creams and ointments. Acta Derm Venereol 60:57
19. Ponec M, Kempanaar SA, DeKloet ER (1981) Corticosteroids and cultured human epidermal keratinocytes. J Invest Dermatol 76:211–214
20. Przybilla B, Ring J (1983) Äußerliche Behandlung mit Glukokortikosteroiden. Med Monatsschr Pharm 6:192–205
21. Ring J, Fröhlich HH (1985) Wirkstoffe in der dermatologischen Therapie, 2nd edn. Springer, Berlin Heidelberg New York
22. Schaefer H, Zesch A, Schalla W, Stüttgen G (1980) Pharmakokinetik externer Glucocorticoide. Allergologie 3:194
23. Schell H, Hornstein OP (1980) Endogener Kortisolrhythmus und Epidermisproliferation. Akt Derm 6:27–33
24. Schleimer RP (1993) An overview of glucocorticoid anti-inflammatory actions. Eur J Clin Pharmacol 45 [Suppl]:1
25. Schmutzler W (1999) Antiallergische und antientzündliche Pharmakotherapie. In: Heppt W, Renz H, Röcken M (eds) Allergologie. Springer, Berlin Heidelberg New York, pp 160–174
26. Schöpf E (1972) Nebenwirkungen externer Corticoidtherapie. Hautarzt 23:295
27. Schöpf E (1980) Kortikosteroide in der Dermatologie. Allergologie 3:306
28. Sulzberger MB, Witten VH (1952) The effect of topically applied compound F in selected dermatoses. J Invest Dermatol 19:101
29. Wendt H, Frosch PJ (1982) Klinisch-pharmakologische Modelle zur Prüfung von Corticoidexterna. Karger, Basel
30. Wilckens T (1995) Glucocorticoids and immune function: hormonal dysfunction. Trends Pharmacol Sci 16:193–197

5.6 Photoallergy/Photosensitization

5.6.1 Classification

Incompatibility reactions in connection with exposure to UV light represent a special type of photobiologic reaction. In the following the term "light" is used for "non-ionizing electromagnetic radiation" in general. When light reaches the skin, part of the energy is reflected, another part affecting the organism after absorption to body constituents [3, 8, 16, 17, 42]. Substances increasing the sensitivity against light are called "photosensitizers" (Table 5.71).

Photosensitization can be either phototoxic or photoallergic in nature [8, 17, 24, 38].

Phototoxic effects occur through formation of pyrimidine adducts within the DNA, leading to cross-links within the double-helix (e.g.,

Table 5.71. Terminology of photobiologic reactions

Photobiologic reaction	Effect of light[a] on biological systems
Light incompatibility	Reaction after light exposure
Photosensitization	Increased sensitivity to light by defined endogenous or exogenous substances
Photosensitizer	Substance inducing photosensitization
Photoallergic reaction	Immunologically mediated photosensitization
Phototoxic reaction	Non-immunologic photosensitization
Photohypersensitivity	Increased sensitivity against light exposure
Photodermatosis	Skin disease provoked or aggravated by light

[a] "Light" in this context means "non-ionizing electromagnetic radiation"

Table 5.72. Differential diagnosis of phototoxic and photoallergic reactions

Phototoxic	Photoallergic
Mechanism:	
Direct cell damage	Immunologic sensitization
Manifestation after first contact:	
Yes	No
"Flare up" of earlier involved skin areas:	
No	Yes
Morphology:	
Erythema:	
+++	+
Edema:	
+–+++	+++
Papules/papulovesicles:	
+/–	++
Vesiculation:	
++–+++	+
Spreading phenomena:	
–	++
Margination of skin lesions:	
Sharp	Not sharp
Dermatohistology:	
"Sunburn cells" in epidermis:	
+	–
Spongiosis:	
–	+
Kinetics:	
Decrescendo	Crescendo

Table 5.73. Classification of photohypersensitivity diseases

Photoallergic reactions
Photoallergic contact dermatitis
Persistent light reaction (?) (chronic actinic dermatitis)

Possibly photoallergic reactions
Light-urticaria (solar urticaria)
Polymorphic light eruption

Phototoxic reactions
Acute and chronic light damage
Phototoxic dermatitis
Metabolic diseases (porphyria, Hartnup-syndrome, etc.)
(Questionable: hydroa vacciniforme, Mallorca acne)

Light-provoked dermatoses
Lupus erythematosus
Morbus Darier (dyskeratosis follicularis)
Porokeratosis
Herpes simplex
Lichen planus
Psoriasis
Atopic eczema (?)
Pityriasis rubra pilaris

psoralen phototoxicity) or via oxygen radicals affecting cell membranes [8, 15, 42].

Photoallergic reactions are due to immunological sensitization directed against a new photoallergen induced by action of UV radiation. Theoretically, phototoxic and photoallergic reactions can be well differentiated (Table 5.72), although in individual patients this may be difficult in practice.

5.6.2 Clinical Manifestations of Photohypersensitivity

Photohypersensitivity reactions should be distinguished from well-known adverse reactions induced by UV radiation, either acutely (sunburn) or chronically (atrophy, elastosis, carcinogenesis), which occur dose dependently in all individuals with normal sensitivity. Hypersensitivity against UV light may occur in metabolic disturbances or enyzme defects (e.g., various forms of porphyria) with endogenous photosensitizers or contact with exogenous photosensitizers (e.g., weeds in dermatitis pratensis or drugs).

Photoallergic reactions manifest mostly as photoallergic contact dermatitis. Photohypersensitivity reactions with an unknown elicitor (Table 5.73) comprise some forms of solar urticaria and so-called polymorphic light eruption (lay people often call it "sun allergy"), which differs from patient to patient in morphology, but is rather monomorphous in the individual patient [2, 3, 13, 24, 28, 36].

Photoallergic contact dermatitis is a relatively common form of photohypersensitivity (Fig. 5.67). Some patients under the combined influence of light and photoallergen develop a chronification, the so-called persistent light reaction, occurring with thickened erythematous lichenoid plaques and a strong itching or burning pain. Persistent light reaction is characterized by a general increase in photosensitivity in different parts of the UV spectrum. Persistent light reaction can further develop into chronic actinic dermatitis ("actinic reticuloid"), which may sometimes turn into cutaneous lymphoma [8, 17, 24].

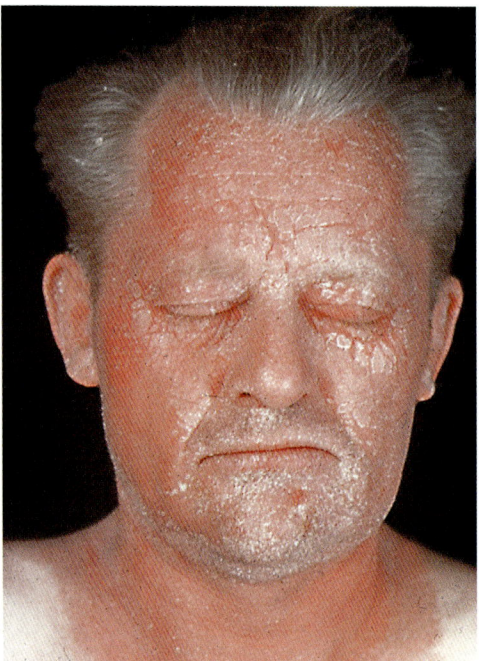

Fig. 5.67. Photoallergic contact eczema

In patients with *persistent light reaction* the minimal erythema dose (MED) is generally decreased, mostly in the UVB but also in the UVA range. Rarely there is also hypersensitivity against visible light. These patients develop inflammatory skin lesions after exposure to light, independent of allergen contact.

In the rare *solar urticaria*, UV radiation (mostly UVA) is the elicitor. The detection of the eliciting wavelength is important. In photoprovocation tests 0.2–5.0 J/cm² UVA will elicit reactions within 10–20 min. Anaphylactic shock in the solarium has been described. By pretreatment with other wavelengths hardening may be achieved [12, 32, 34].

In *polymorphic light eruption* photoprovocation may be possible in previously involved, but at the time of testing symptom-free, skin areas not exposed to light. This has to be done on three subsequent days with doses of 3×60–100 J/cm² UVA or UVA1, or 3×1.5× MED UVB or UVA+UVB.

The very rare disease of hydroa vacciniformia can sometimes be treated with UVA; the cause is unknown, vitamin B deficiency has been discussed.

Suspected systemic photosensitization may be detected by measuring the MED during a systemic administration (oral or parenteral) of a suspected agent, UV irradiation and demonstration of increased photosensitivity [1, 9, 25].

5.6.3 Photosensitizers

Photosensitizing agents are widely distributed in nature. They are found in tar (polyaromatic hydrocarbons, acridine derivatives) or colorings (eosin, fluorescein, methylene blue).

Many plants contain photosensitizers (Table 5.74), giving rise to phototoxic reactions after epidermal contact or after oral intake [26, 43]. The furocoumarins contained in many etheric oils or fragrances in cosmetics (Breloque dermatitis) are also the active agents in the elicitation of meadow grass dermatitis (dermatitis pratensis) [21, 26] (Fig. 5.68). Chlorophyll derivatives have been described as inductors of photodermatoses [18].

Various drugs (mostly after systemic administration) act as photosensitizers (Table 5.75). Photosensitizers eliciting clear-cut allergic reactions are also called "photoallergens." In the office the distinction is often difficult, since many photoallergens also have phototoxic potential.

Recently non-steroidal anti-inflammatory drugs have been shown to act as photosensitizers, especially the propionic acid derivatives (Fig. 5.69) [25, 32, 35, 39].

Table 5.74. Photosensitizors from plants

Umbelliferae
Heracleum, Angelica, Daucus carota (carrot), *Ammi majus, Apium graveolens* (celery), *Pastinaca*

Rutaceae
Citrus bergamia (bergamot), *Citrus sinensis* (orange), *Ruta graveolens, Dictamnus albus*

Moraceae
Ficus carica (fig)

Leguminosae
Psoralea corylifolia

Rosaceae

Compositae

5.6 Photoallergy/Photosensitization

Table 5.75. Photosensitizers in drugs and cosmetics (examples)

Disinfectants (e.g., halogenated salicylanilides, hexachlorophen, chlorhexidine, bithionol)
Antimycotics (buclosamide)
Chemotherapeutics (sulfonamides, tetracyclines, nalidixic acid, quinolones)
Sedatives (phenothiazine)
Diuretics (hydrochlorothiazide, furosemide)
Non-steroidal anti-inflammatory drugs (e.g., ibuprofen, ketoprofen, piroxicam, diclofenac)
Antiarrhythmics (quinidine, amiodarone)
Fragrances (musk ambrette, 6-methylcoumarin)
Sunscreen substances (e.g., para-aminobenzoic acid, benzophenones, isopropyldibenzoylmethane)
Antidiabetics (sulfonyl urea)

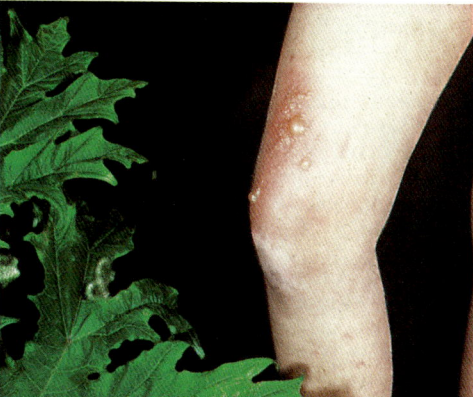

Fig. 5.68. Meadow grass dermatitis caused by furocoumarins – in this case by contact with the giant hogweed (*Heracleum mantegazzianum*)

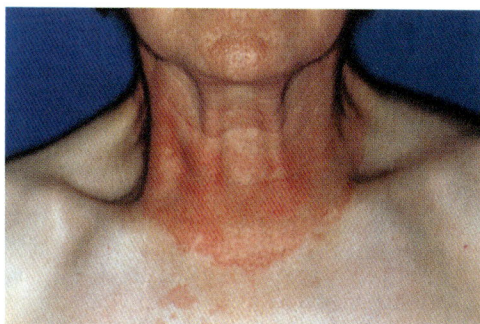

Fig. 5.69. Light-induced drug exanthema following the administration of carprofen

5.6.4 Diagnosis

In the diagnosis of photoallergic or phototoxic reactions, not only the *eliciting substance* but also the *eliciting wavelength* has to be determined [33]. Most of the eliciting wavelengths in photohypersensitivity are found in the UVA range, but sometimes also in the UVB range or visible light. With a clear-cut history and negative test results different wavelengths should be used. There is no general concordance between the absorption spectrum of a substance and the eliciting wavelength of the adverse reaction. UV radiation penetrates through certain textiles; affection of covered body areas does not exclude photosensitization.

A variety of genuine skin diseases can be provoked by light which are not currently understood pathophysiologically [24, 28].

Photo-patch Test. The most important technique with which to diagnose photoallergic reactions is the photo-patch test [14, 19, 23, 24, 30], when two samples each of the suspected substance are applied to the back skin. After 24 h the patch over one testblock is removed and the skin radiated with 10 J/cm^2 (when radiated with UVB with the half minimal erythema doses). After 48 and 72 h both testblocks are read. Under certain conditions a late reading after 3 weeks (labeling of test areas with a polaroid camera) is recommended.

For quantitative analysis photo-patch-threshold testing can be performed and the series of substances is irradiated with increasing doses (geometric increase) of UV. For differentiation of phototoxic and photoallergic test reactions dermatohistology is sometimes required.

Photo-prick Test. Concordant with the photo-patch test, other skin test procedures can be performed with and without irradiation (e.g., in solar urticaria).

Systemic Photo-provocation Test. For evaluation of the clinical relevance of a positive photo-patch-test reaction against drugs or foods, a systemic photo-provocation test can be performed [9, 25, 30]. Before and after systemic administration of the suspected substance various areas are irradiated at different time intervals (e.g., 50 J/cm^2 UVA).

5.6.5 Prophylaxis and Therapy

Information from the patient and recommendations for careful sun exposure are the basis of any treatment. Avoidance of elicitation agents is crucial. In patients with unknown photosensitizers the selection of the sunscreen is very important. Most of the commercial sunscreens describe the sun protection factor for UVB radiation only (rarely also for UVA), which, however, is the decisive wavelength for most patients with photosensitization. One should know that many of the common light filter substances in sunscreens can act as photoallergens [38, 39].

In patients with polymorphic light eruption as well as chronic photoallergic contact dermatitis with transition to persistent light reaction, PUVA therapy as well as UVA1 or small spectrum UVB (311 nm) can be used as conditioning [13, 15, 28]. In experimental models inhibitory effects of UV radiation on allergy-relevant reactions have been demonstrated [3, 6, 22, 32].

Prior to the production of new substances as drugs or cosmetics, screening tests for possible photosensitizing properties should be performed. There are various in vivo (guinea pig, rat, mice) and in vitro procedures (*Candida albicans* inhibition test, photohemolysis test) [5, 12, 14]. We have detected the photosensitizing properties of non-steroidal anti-inflammatory drugs using a photo-basophil-histamine-release test [31, 35].

References

1. Bergner T, Przybilla B (1992) Photosensitization caused by ibuprofen. J Am Acad Dermatol 26:114–116
2. Breit R (1987) Rötung und Bräunung der Haut durch UVA. Zuckschnverdt, Munich
3. Eberlein-König B, Fesq H, Abeck D, Przybilla B, Placzek M, Ring J (2000) Systemic vitamin C and vitamin E do not prevent photoprovocation test reactions in polymorphous light eruption. Photodermatol Photoimmunol Photomed 16:50–52
4. Epstein S (1939) Photoallergy and primary photosensitivity to sulfanilamide. J Invest Dermatol 2:43–51
5. Ferguson J, Johnson BE (1993) Clinical and laboratory studies of the photosensitizing potential of norfloxacin, a 4-quinolone broad-spectrum antibiotic. Br J Dermatol 128:185–195
6. Fjellner B (1981) Experimental and clinical pruritus. Studies on some putative peripheral mediators. The influence of ultraviolet light and transcutaneous nerve stimulation. Thesis, Stockholm
7. Fotiades J, Soter NA, Lim HW (1995) Results of evaluation of 203 patients for photosensitivity in a 7.3-year period. J Am Acad Dermatol 33: 597–602
8. Frain-Bell W (1986) Cutaneous photobiology. Oxford University Press, New York
9. Galosi A, Przybilla B, Ring J, Dorn M (1984) Systemische Photoprovokation mit Surgam. Allergologie 7:143–144
10. Gigli I, Lim HW (1981) Release of proinflammatory peptides by complement in porphyrin-induced photosensitivity. In: Ring J, Burg G (eds) New trends in allergy. Springer, Berlin Heidelberg New York, p 5848
11. Gollhausen R, Przybilla B, Galosi A, Köhler K, Ring J (1987) Environmental influences of UVB erythema. Photodermatology 4:148–153
12. Hasei K, Ichihashi M (1982) Solar urticaria. Determinations of action and inhibition spectra. Arch Dermatol 118:346–350
13. Hölzle E, Plewig G, Kries R v, Lehmann P (1987) Polymorphous light eruption. J Invest Dermatol 88:32–38
14. Hölzle E, Neumann N, Hausen B, Przybilla B, Schauder S, Hönigsmann H, Bircher A, Plewig G (1991) Photopatch testing: The 5-year experience of the German, Austrian and Swiss photopatch test group. J Am Acad Dermatol 25:59–68
15. Hönigsmann H, Stingl G (eds) (1986) Therapeutic photomedicine. Karger, Basel
16. Horio T (1975) Chlorpromazine photoallergy. Arch Dermatol 111:1469–1471
17. Ippen H (1973) Photochemie der Haut. In: Herrmann F, Oppen H, Schaefer H, Stüttgen G (eds) Biochemie der Haut. Thieme, Stuttgart, p 146
18. Jitsukawa K, Suizu R, Hidano A (1984) Chlorella photosensitization, a new phytophotodermatosis. Int J Dermatol 23:263
19. Jung EG (1981) Die belichtete Epikutantestung. Akt Derm 7:163–165
20. Jung EG, Hardmeier T (1967) Zur Histologie der photoallergischen Testreaktion. Dermatologica 135:243–252
21. Kavli G, Volden G (1984) Phytophotodermatitis. Photodermatology 1:65–75
22. Kripke ML (1986) Photoimmunology, the first decade. Curr Probl Dermatol 15:164–175
23. Lehmann P (1990) Die Deutschsprachige Arbeitsgemeinschaft Photopatch-Test (DAPT). Hautarzt 41:295–297

24. Lischka G, Jung EG (1982) Lichtkrankheiten der Haut, 2nd edn. Perimed, Erlangen
25. Ljunggren B, Bjellerup M (1986) Systemic drug photosensitivity. Photodermatology 3:26–35
26. Ljunggren B (1990) Severe phototoxic burn following celery ingestion. Arch Dermatol 126: 1334–1336
27. Maurer T (1983) Contact and photocontact allergens. A manual of predictive test methods. Dekker, New York
28. Plewig G, Hölzle E, Roser-Maaß E, Hofmann C (1985) Photoallergy. In: Ring J, Burg G (eds) New trends in allergy. Springer, Berlin Heidelberg New York, pp 152–169
29. Przybilla B, Ring J, Schwab U, Galosi A, Dorn M, Braun-Falco O (1987) Photosensibilisierende Eigenschaften nicht-steroidaler Antirheumatika im Photopatch-Test. Hautarzt 38:18–25
30. Przybilla B (1987) Phototestungen bei Lichtdermatosen. Hautarzt 38:S23–S28
31. Przybilla B, Schwab-Przybilla U, Ruzicka T, Ring J (1987) Phototoxicity of non-steroidal antiinflammatory drugs demonstrated in vitro by a photobasophil-histamine-release test. Photodermatology 4:73–78
32. Przybilla B, Ring J, Eberlein B (1988) Inhibition of in vitro basophil histamine release by UVA irradiation. J Allergy Clin Immunol 83:302
33. Przybilla B, Bergner T (1992) Diagnostik von lichtallergischen Exanthemen im erscheinungsfreien Intervall. Hautarzt 43:100–101
34. Przybilla B, Eberlein-König B (2000) Photoprovokationstests. In: Przybilla B, Bergmann K, Ring J (eds) Praktische allergologische Diagnostik. Steinkopff, Darmstadt
35. Ring J, Przybilla B, Ruzicka T (1987) Nonsteroidal antiinflammatory drugs induce UV-dependent histamine and leukotriene release from peripheral human leukocytes. Int Arch Allergy Appl Immunol 82:344–346
36. Ring J, Przybilla B (1990) UV irradiation and allergy. Allergologie 12(Suppl EAACI):75–79
37. Ruzicka T, Walter JF, Printz MP (1983) Changes in arachidonic acid metabolism in ultraviolet irradiated hairless mouse skin. J Invest Dermatol 81:300–303
38. Schauder S, Ippen H (1986) Photoallergic and allergic contact dermatitis from dibenzoylmethanes. Photodermatology 3:140–147
39. Schauder S, Schrader A, Ippen H (1996) Göttinger Liste 1996. Sonnenschutzkosmetik in Deutschland, 4th edn. Blackwell, Berlin
40. Schmidt T, Abeck D, Ring J (1998) Photoallergic contact dermatitis due to combined UVB-(4-methylbenzylidene camphor/octyl methoxy-cinnamate) and UVA-(benzophenone-3/butyl-methoxy-dibenzoylmethane) absorber. Dermatology 196:354–357
41. Schulz KH, Wiskemann K, Wolf K (1956) Klinische und experimentelle Untersuchungen über die photodynamische Wirksamkeit von Phenotiazinderivaten, insbesondere Megaphen. Arch Klin Exp Dermatol 202:285–298
42. Terui T, Okuyama R, Tagami H (2001) Molecular events occurring behind ultraviolet-induced skin inflammation. Curr Opin Allergy Clin Immunol 1:461–467
43. Wessner D, Hofmann H, Ring J (1999) Phytophotodermatitis due to *Ruta graveolens* applied as protection against evil spells. Contact Dermatitis 41:232–233
44. Wucherpfennig V (1931) Biologie und praktische Verwendbarkeit der Erythemschwelle des UV. Strahlentherapie 40:201–243

5.7 Adverse Drug Reactions

5.7.1 Drug Allergy: General Procedures

5.7.1.1 Classification

Adverse drug reactions are unexpected undesired reactions to drugs in normal doses [26] and represent an increasing problem in clinical medicine. Approximately 3–5% of hospitalizations are due to drug reactions [39], and 10–15% of hospitalized patients suffer from adverse drug reactions during their hospital stay.

Drug allergies are a serious problem: 0.32% of hospital patients die from adverse drug reactions in the United States, corresponding to 106,000 estimated fatalities in 1994 (the fourth commonest cause of death in the United States) [4, 31].

Apart from severe bullous reactions (Lyell's syndrome, etc.) (see Sect. 5.7.3), the vasculitic "hypersensitivity syndrome" as well as organ damage to liver, lung, or kidney, anaphylactoid reactions are the most dangerous and most frequently lethal adverse drug reactions. A study from the United Kingdom reported a marked increase in prevalence of anaphylactic reactions leading to hospitalization (1:10,000 in 1995) [42]. In a hit list of elicitors of fatal anaphylactic reactions, anesthetics, relaxants, antibiotics, and radiographic contrast media are on top.

The frequency of fatal drug allergy is estimated to be 1:10,000 [56]; for most drugs allergy prevalences are lower (0.1–1%). Some groups of drugs, however, have a higher risk (over 2%), e.g., foreign proteins (xenogeneic protein, allergen extracts, organ extracts, vaccines, transfusions, enzymes, and hormones) and antibiotics (penicillin, ampicillin, sulfonamides, erythromycin). It is unlikely that there are drugs which under guarantee will never elicit an allergy! Anaphylactoid reactions to corticosteroids have been reported. Precise studies to compare the prevalences of side effects are difficult to perform. The term "frequent" implies different aspects such as an actual increased prevalence of side reactions (relative percentage) as well as an absolutely increased usage of the drug (absolute numbers).

The classification of adverse drug reactions can be done according to clinical symptoms (e.g., anaphylactoid reaction, fever, exanthematous eruption, organ disease) and suggested or proven pathomechanism time course kinetics (acute 0–60 min, subacute 1–24 h, delayed or accelerated for more than 24 h) (according to [23]).

5.7.1.2 Pathophysiology

Drug allergies can be classified like all other allergic diseases (modified classification of Coombs and Gell) (Table 5.76). In order to elicit an allergy, the drug has to be immunogenic; this holds true for proteins and peptides (>7 amino acids). Low molecular drugs are haptens and need binding to body carrier proteins to gain immunogenicity. The chemical basis of sensitization is known for very few drugs; for penicillin, we know the critical antigenic determinants: the penicilloyl group as "major determinant" (that is most frequent, not most dangerous!) and the "minor determinants" (less frequent) of penicillenate and penicillamine [62]. Similar molecules can show "cross-reactions"; small molecules can elicit a reaction when they have capacity for at least divalent binding to the antibody molecule.

Metabolism of drugs is important for the induction of incompatibility reactions. In the balance between activation and detoxification, disturbances may be crucial, involving especially the enzymes of the cytochrome P450 system as well as N-acetyltransferase (NAT) [34, 35]. In cutaneous drug reactions, keratinocytes also play a role with metabolizing enzymes [45].

For the frequency of sensitization, the route of administration is essential: the risk of allergy induction increases in the following sequence: oral, intravenous, intramuscular, subcutaneous, and topical.

Table 5.76. Drug allergy: different pathomechanisms

Mechanism (type)	Symptoms	Example
I (IgE)	Anaphylaxis	Penicillin, allergen extracts, insulin
II (Cytotoxic)	Agranulocytosis Anemia Thrombocytopenia	Metamizol Penicillin, cephalosporin Carbamazepine
III (Immune complex)	Anaphylaxis Serum sickness Vasculitis Alveolitis	Xenogeneic serum, dextran Xenogeneic serum, penicillin Allopurinol, phenylbutazone Pituitary extracts, nitrofurantoin
IV (Cell mediated)	Eczema (also systemic!) Photoallergy (Fixed drug eruption) (Maculopapular) (Toxic epidermal necrolysis)	Antibiotics, disinfectants Halogenated salicylanilides, nalidixic acid Barbiturates, quinine Penicillin, gold, barbiturates, β-blockers Sulfonamides, NSAIDs, allopurinol
V (Granulomatous)	Granuloma	Allergen extracts, soluble collagen
VI (Neutralizing/stimulating)	(Drug-induced LE?) Insulin resistance	Hydralazine, procainamide Anti-insulin IgG antibodies

5.7.1.3 Risk Factors

The risk of a drug allergy depends both on the characteristics of the substance and on the patient (Table 5.77). Risk factors from the patient can be seen in underlying diseases (immunodeficiency, infectious disease, metabolic defects such as decreased or slow acetylators). Whether drug allergies are more frequent in atopics is controversial. Most studies have not differentiated according to reaction types and have given controversial results. There is evidence that IgE-mediated reactions may be more frequent in atopics compared to normals.

Table 5.77. Risk factors for drug allergy

1. Risk factors from the drug
Duration of administration
Frequency of administration
Dose
Route of administration
Dose of reactive metabolites
2. Risk factors from the patient
Underlying disease (immunodeficiency, metabolic disturbance)
Age
Genetic disposition (polymorphisms, HLA)
Atopy (?)
Previous incompatibility of the same drug

With increasing age and more frequent underlying diseases, the intensity of clinical symptoms of drug reactions is also increasing.

5.7.1.4 General Diagnosis of Drug Allergy

The diagnosis of adverse drug reactions follows the same principles used for classical allergy diagnosis:

- History and clinical symptoms
- Skin test
- In vitro diagnostics
- Provocation test

5.7.1.4.1 History and Clinical Symptoms

History is the most important part of allergy diagnosis! In most cases of adverse drug reactions, however, the allergist has not seen the clinical symptoms of the incompatibility reaction himself and needs information from the patient or from colleagues (questionnaires have proven useful). Therefore, every physician should carefully document all the symptoms together with the suspected drug when there is a suspicion of adverse drug reaction. It is not enough to write down the general class of drug (e.g., "penicillin" is often used as a wide term for any antibiotic), but the individual substance, the brand name, the producer, the formula, the batch number (especially in intravenous solutions and biologicals) should be recorded. If possible, single substances of combination drugs should be documented since the drug content may change over the years under the same brand name (Table 5.78). The allergist also needs the "physician's desk reference" from previous years!

Sometimes the intensity of a reaction can be evaluated from the treatment given. The time course is especially important; some patients suffer from a mild anaphylactic reaction, which only becomes serious after administration of epinephrine. In anesthesia-related complications, the anesthesia protocol is of the utmost importance for allergy diagnosis.

According to clinical symptoms, rough information for suspected pathomechanisms can be found with large overlaps. No single symptom is characteristic for a certain pathomechanism (urticaria can be induced by IgE antibodies, but also by immune complex reactions, or pseudo-allergic reactions).

Sometimes fever reactions occur together with other complaints in the sense of serum sickness; however, they can also be due to toxic

Table 5.78. Important information from the history of adverse drug reactions

Substance	Effective agents, additives Brand name, producer Administration formula, batch number Possible incompatibilities
Reaction type	Clinical symptoms Time course (in surgery also anesthesia protocol!) Severity
Therapeutic procedures performed	

effects. Hematologic complications are common in cytotoxic reactions (e.g., allergic agranulocytosis) (see Sect. 5.2). Central nervous symptoms (cramps, paresthesia, cognitive failure) are seen in pseudo-allergic reactions (e.g., with local anesthetics).

In the literature, a hypersensitivity syndrome is described as a very severe drug reaction with sepsis-like symptoms, high fever with or without skin involvement and frequent hypereosinophilia in the peripheral blood. Anticonvulsants as elicitors are known. The mechanism of these reactions – in earlier textbooks also called "drug fever" – is not clear. Lymphocyte transformation tests may be helpful [5].

5.7.1.4.2 Skin Test

Two to 3 weeks after remission of symptoms or withdrawal of systemic glucocorticoid or antihistamine therapy, skin tests should be performed, if possible not later than after 3 months. Certain drugs able to inhibit skin reactions should be withdrawn (see Sect. 4.2). Skin tests stay positive over longer periods of time compared to in vitro tests. However, they also bear the risk of systemic reactions. Fatalities after simple scratch tests in highly sensitized patients have been reported [14].

The general problem of all drug allergy tests is the haptenic nature of the low molecular substances which have to bind in the body to proteins to gain antigenic properties. Therefore, real progress in the field of drug allergy is only possible when haptens can be coupled to high molecular carriers, for instance penicillin to penicilloyl polylysine (PPL) [62].

Prior to testing of unknown substances, concentrations used need to be evaluated carefully [51] in order to avoid toxic reactions. The choice of solvent in water-insoluble drugs is important. Drug test solutions should be freshly made up more often than allergen extracts. Positive test reactions should be evaluated together with controls in healthy volunteers (in order to exclude irritative reactions).

Patch tests with topical preparations must include vehicles and other ingredients. In positive reactions the single substances need to be tested in adequate concentrations; this is only possible with confidential cooperation from the pharmaceutical industry (confidentiality agreement!) and the informed patient.

In pseudo-allergic reactions skin tests are usually negative; they should, however, be performed in order to detect rare true allergies and in order to avoid dramatic immediate type reactions.

5.7.1.4.3 In Vitro Diagnosis

The development of reliable in vitro tests for allergy diagnosis of adverse drug reaction is a major endeavor in research in order to save patients from having to undergo unnecessary provocation tests. Unfortunately, only for a few drugs (e.g., penicillin) are standardized RAST procedures available for routine diagnosis.

Besides RAST, IgE-mediated reactions may be detected by in vitro histamine release, sulfidoleukotriene formation (CAST-ELISA) [63] or basophil activation (CD63) from peripheral leukocytes after stimulation with the suspect drug. In these tests, the problem of hapten coupling to protein is inherent.

The diagnosis of non-IgE-mediated reactions requires the measurement of other antibody classes, e.g., with passive hemagglutination, immunodiffusion, or specific RIA or EIA assays. Immune complex anaphylaxis due to dextran is mediated by high titers of specific IgG antibodies against dextran (see Sect. 5.3). In this model, the importance of time points for taking blood samples for investigation has been elucidated. The highest antibody titers were found in serum samples drawn prior to the administrations of the drug [46]; immediately after the clinical reaction, antibody titers were markedly reduced or not measurable; only after several days or weeks were antibodies again increased. The retrospective asservation of samples (laboratory or blood bank) may be decisive for final diagnosis!

Some authors recommend the lymphocyte transformation test (LTT) as an in vitro test for adverse drug reactions [5, 40, 53]. In our experience, the LTT can be helpful in the diagnosis of cell-mediated reactions while immediate-type reactions only rarely show reliable results.

A major difficulty of all cellular procedures is the high variance of the test results. In adverse drug reactions, the problem of standardization (vehicle, concentration, metabolites, controls) causes difficulty; many procedures (e.g., use of liver microsomes) [34] are not available for routine tests and are only possible in specialized laboratories.

5.7.1.4.4 Provocation Test

The provocation test, e.g., the exposure of the patient to the specific relevant substance under controlled conditions, often remains the only reliable method in the diagnosis of adverse drug reactions; this holds especially true for pseudo-allergic reactions [43, 48].

Prior to the provocation test, the other diagnostic procedures need to be performed in order to gain information about the intensity of the patient's sensitization. Any provocation test bears a certain risk and has to be performed with the utmost caution (sometimes under inpatient conditions).

In the diagnosis of adverse drug reactions, oral provocation is the commonest test. The oral provocation test (OPT) should not only include the suspected agent from the patient's history but also a selection of standard substances as possible alternatives. The recommendation of an alternative drug on the basis of the literature only without actual proof of tolerability in an OPT may be dangerous [43, 48].

For example, we have observed several – sometimes severe – anaphylactoid reactions after administration of acetaminophen in patients with a history of anaphylaxis to analgesics.

The evaluation of OPT results can sometimes be difficult, especially with regard to the "allergy passport" (Table 5.79). In contrast to the procedure for contact allergy and patch test results (only clear-cut positive patch test reactions are recorded in the allergy passport!), we also document the so-called "allergy suspicion" in adverse drug reactions (Table 5.80). However, in the allergy passport, both test results and diagnostic considerations should be documented (e.g., "suspicion by history," "skin test positive," "RAST positive") [60]. So-called prophetic testings (without a history of adverse reactions) are rarely indicated.

The most common mistakes in the diagnosis of adverse drug reactions are listed in Table 5.81.

Table 5.79. Documentation for an "allergy passport"

Criteria for registration of a substance:
- The substance can be avoided
- The clinical relevant sensitization usually persists over longer periods
- High allergenic potency
- Risk of systemic reactions (anaphylaxis)
- Alternative drug tested in provocation tests
- The allergy passport should contain the following information:
- Location and date, name of the allergist
- Clinical symptomatology and severity of the adverse reaction
- Eliciting substance
- Information regarding the diagnostic test procedures
- Tested alternatives (e.g., information regarding the dose tolerated in OPT)

Table 5.81. Common mistakes in the diagnosis of adverse drug reactions

- Insufficient history
- Wrong substance tested
- Wrong test procedure
- Wrong interpretation of skin test reactions (especially intradermal)
- Insufficient precautions for skin tests and provocation tests
- Wrong interpretation of psychic factors (under- and overestimation)
- Inadequate allergy passport
- Testing under therapy with antiallergic drugs

Table 5.80. Allergy diagnosis in adverse drug reaction: Score for inclusion in allergy passport (together with B. Przybilla). 0–1 point = no allergy passport, 2 points = "allergy suspicion," 3 or more points = allergy passport necessary

Criterion	Score points		
	0	1	2
Clinical symptoms (history)	Negative	Doubtful	Clear-cut
Provocation test	Negative	Doubtful	Clear-cut
Skin test (epidermal)	Negative or	(+)	+
Skin test (cutaneous)[a]	Negative or (+)	+	++

[a] A positive in vitro test may replace a positive cutaneous skin test

Often doctors advise the patient with adverse drug reactions: "Just don't take this drug any more." This advice is as intelligent as the recommendation for a patient with abdominal pain: "Don't press on it again!"

5.7.1.5 Hyposensitization in Drug Allergy

In spite of multiple alternative substances, it may occur that the patient is allergic to a life-saving drug and the possibility of hyposensitization should be discussed. This has been done successfully for various drugs although the mechanism of this "hyposensitization" (also called "adaptive deactivation" or "tolerance induction") is by no means clear.

Principally, one has to distinguish between anaphylactic reactions and cutaneous drug eruptions. The best experiences date from immediate reactions to penicillin, antibiotics and insulin (Table 5.82). Hyposensitization can be performed orally or intravenously. In patients with anaphylaxis, the dose increase is done at 15–30 min intervals. According to the severity of the history, 0.1–1‰ of a usual dose is the starting dose. Tables 5.82 and 5.83 show successful schedules for penicillin and insulin. "Hyposensitization" in cutaneous drug eruptions usually does not induce lasting tolerance. After renewed administration, the drug has to be carefully started with a low dose.

Contraindications for drug hyposensitizations comprise severe and life-threatening conditions without adequate possible therapy such as severe bullous skin diseases (Stevens-Johnson syndrome, Lyell's syndrome, necrotic vasculitis), severe organopathies (hepatitis, nephritis), as well as cytotoxic reactions (agranulocytosis, thrombocytopenia, anemia). Maybe this should be reconsidered after future studies using granulocyte colony-stimulating factor (G-CSF) or erythropoietin as emergency treatment.

Severe underlying diseases may also represent a contraindication. In suspected IgE-mediated allergy, beta-blocking agents and angiotensin-converting enzyme inhibitors should be withdrawn prior to hyposensitization.

Table 5.83. Successful hyposensitization in drug eruptions

Antibiotics	Virostatiics
Penicillin	Zidovudine
Ciprofloxacin	Nevirapine
Ethambutol	
Rifampicin	**Anticonvulsives**
	Carbamazepine
Sulfonamides	Phenobarbital
Cotrimoxazole	
Sulfadiazine	**Cytostatics**
Dapsone	Azathioprine
	6-Mercaptopurine
Antimycotics	Carboplatin
Itraconazole	
	Other
Antiparasitics	Allopurinol
Pyrimethamine	Insulin

5.7.1.6 Adverse Reactions to Special Drugs

5.7.1.6.1 Penicillin and Betalactam Antibiotics

Penicillin allergy may manifest in many reaction types (I–V). The prevalence of all reactions is between 5% and 10% [16]. The incidence of anaphylactic reactions is approximately 1%, of lethal cases 1:50,000. Regarding the common use of penicillin (80 million penicillin administrations per year in the United States), this is a great practical problem: 32 of 43 fatal anaphylactic reactions in the US army were penicillin mediated (see Sect. 5.1.4). Attempted suicide through the elicitation of anaphylaxis by a penicillin-allergic individual has been reported [55]. Often penicillin allergy is observed after the first therapeutic administration of penicillin; here sensitization may have occurred unnoticed via food (cow's milk, chicken, etc.), conjunctival prophylaxis at birth or penicillin-containing wound ointments. A

Table 5.82. Schedule for hyposensitization in penicillin allergy (oral)

Steps	Dose (units)	Steps	Dose (units)
1	100	9	24,000
2	200	10	48,000
3	400	11	80,000
4	800	12	160,000
5	1,600	13	320,000
6	3,200	14	640,000
7	6,400	15	1,000,000
8	12,000		

positive reaction against Penicillium notatum in the standard allergy test is not of relevance for penicillin allergy!

The skin test (always begin with a prick or scratch!) is performed with penicilloyl polylysin (PPL) in a concentration of 50 nM/ml to 500 nM/ml (major determinant) as well as penicillin G (200,000 U/ml), benzylpenicillin or benzylpenicillenate (10^{-2} mM] (minor determinants).

If negative, intradermal tests are started: PPL 25–250 nM/ml, penicillin G 10–1,000 U/ml.

The frequency of positive skin test reactions in patients with a history of penicillin allergy is approximately 30%. Negative skin tests do not exclude penicillin allergy; positive tests do not 100% predict adverse reactions at the next penicillin administration! However, the risk of penicillin allergy in patients with a positive skin test is significantly higher (30%), while provocation tests in patients with a negative skin test in spite of a positive history have only shown 3% positive reactions [20]. The experience with RAST is similar: a positive RAST does not necessarily imply adverse reactions, and negative RASTs do not exclude allergy [29]. In the single patient, the synopsis of skin test, in vitro test results, and history should be evaluated in a risk-benefit consideration towards the desired therapeutic effect. Penicillin allergy is not life-long. Skin test studies in penicillin-allergic patients show that allergy to penicillin G as well as PPL decreases over the years.

Penicillin and cephalosporins of the first generation have shown a cross-reactivity of 10%; this does not hold true for the newer cephalosporins (third generation].

β-Lactam antibiotics (penicillin and cephalosporin) differ by various side chains of the β-lactam ring structure whereby cephalosporins have an additional substitution at the 3-position of the dihydrothiazine ring.

While 10 years ago the most frequent IgE-mediated sensitizations were due to the penicilloyl group, in recent years the spectrum has changed towards an increasing number of reactions to minor determinants and amoxicillin [34].

If penicillin treatment is life-saving, hyposensitization can be attempted with slowly increasing doses with the utmost caution [54]. Fortunately, penicillin can be replaced for most indications by alternative antibiotics. Very special indications remain: streptococcal endocarditis, life-threatening *Pseudomonas* infection, sepsis with serratia or neurosyphilis.

5.7.1.6.2 Analgesics

Anaphylactoid reactions after analgesics represent the major problem in allergy due to the wide use of these drugs. They may be elicited via different mechanisms: opiates are direct histamine liberators. The most commonly used agents in "mild" analgesics are salicylates, para-aminophenol derivatives, pyrazolones, as well as other contents like vitamins or codeine [28, 43, 59]. Combination drugs are commonly used in many countries as well. The identification of the eliciting substance is the major aim of allergy diagnosis. Skin test procedures have limited sensitivity. However, strongly positive (+++) prick reactions often have diagnostic relevance. Intradermal reactions are more difficult to evaluate; adequate controls are crucial! Positive skin test reactions after codeine- or opioid-containing analgesics are a sequel of direct histamine liberation. Rarely, IgE-mediated reactions against opiates have been reported (e.g., morphine) [19].

The relevance of positive prick tests increases with increasing severity of the anaphylactoid reaction in history. Twenty-five percent of patients with grade III anaphylactic reactions (shock) had positive prick test reactions in our study, while in patients with skin symptoms only (grade I) there were positive skin tests in only 7% [43].

For most cases, OPTs are required for final diagnosis to avoid life-threatening reactions in the future and offer tolerable alternatives. OPT has to be performed under emergency conditions. A slow increase in dose from 10% via 50% to 100% of a usual single dose of a substance has been proven useful; in very severe reactions (e.g., propyphenazone anaphylaxis) starting with 1% or 2.5% of a single dose is recommended. Provocation tests have to be performed blinded and placebo controlled in order to avoid psychosomatic interactions. The results of OPT with analgesics show characteristic reaction patterns: 40% of our patients reacted to acetylsalicylic acid with concomitant reactions to other analgesics. These patients had negative skin tests and possible pseudo-allergic mechanisms. In contrast, 50% of patients only reacted to pyrazolone compounds, with occasional positive skin reactions suggesting allergic mechanisms. It was interesting that there was no cross-reaction between different pyrazolones such as metamizol (dipyrone) and propyphenazone [43]. Eight percent of our patients also reacted to para-aminophenol derivatives such as acetaminophen. *The common practice of avoiding OPTs and just recommending acetaminophen as alternative is not justified.*

We use a standard block of analgesics for OPT comprising acetylsalicylic acid (ASA), acetaminophen, dipyrone, propyphenazone, tramadol, ibuprofen, and sometimes nefopam or dextropropoxyphen. For the special problem of ASA idiosyncrasy, see Sect. 5.7.3.

It should be stressed that with other substances suspected in a mixed preparation these also have to be tested including also additives.

5.7.1.6.3 Insulin

With increasing purity of insulin preparations, the previously frequent incompatibility reactions have become rare. Insulin of different species shows pronounced cross-reactivity. Even after the introduction of recombinant human insulin, allergic reactions have been observed. The unusual route of administration (subcutaneous), possible impurities, additives (depot substances such as protamine, zinc, preservatives such as surfen, phenolcresol, or glycerin acetate), as well as unphysiological molecular structures (aggregates of insulin) have been discussed [57]. A genetic association with HLA-D 3 has been suggested.

Interestingly, some patients with type I diabetes have insulin autoantibodies, without ever having been treated with insulin, persisting for years and sometimes occurring with antibodies against cytoplasmic island cell antigens [57].

The clinical symptoms of insulin allergy vary; there are many different types of allergic reactions to insulin. Granulomatous reactions in patients allergic to surfen at the injection site need to be mentioned. Maybe the lipatrophy sometimes observed after insulin injection is also immunologically mediated [18, 57].

Almost half of patients under insulin treatment form antibodies of IgE and IgG class against insulin without clinical incompatibility. Sometimes high titers of neutralizing IgG antibodies against insulin give rise to insulin resistance [18], a phenomenon that may be classified under type VI reactions (see Table 5.76).

Anaphylactic reactions to insulin represent the major problem; for diagnosis, skin tests (start with 0.01 U in a prick or 0.0001 U intradermally) as well as RAST and histamine release are used.

When insulin allergy is diagnosed, the indication for insulin therapy should be evaluated. If this is given, hyposensitization under inpatient conditions can be attempted (see above). If the patient has received insulin within the previous 24 h, the dose is reduced to one-tenth of the last dose and increased daily by 5 U.

If the last insulin injection dates back further, hyposensitization with human recombinant insulin is performed as rush hyposensitization (Table 5.84). The starting dose represents 1/100 of the last positive prick test concentration.

5.7.1.6.4 Heparin

Heparin and heparinoids are glucosaminoglycans (molecular weight 3,000 to 40,000) and are

Table 5.84. Schedule of rush hyposensitization in insulin allergy

Day	Dose	Administration	Day	Dose	Administration
1	0.0001	i.c.	4	8.0	s.c.
	0.001	i.c.		12.0	s.c.
	0.01	i.c.		16.0	s.c.
2	0.1	i.c.	5	20.0	s.c.
	0.5	i.c.	6	25.0	s.c.
	1.0	i.c.	7	30.0	s.c.
3	2.0	s.c.			
	4.0	s.c.			
	6.0	s.c.			

used for anticoagulation. Mostly, they are prepared from mucosa of pig intestine or beef lung. Allergic reactions against heparin may be mediated via different mechanisms (type I to type IV). Anaphylactic reactions are rare but have been reported (cited by Zürcher and Krebs; Sect. 5.7.3). Cytotoxic reactions in the sense of heparin-induced thrombocytopenia have been covered in Sect. 5.2.

More frequent are local reactions manifesting either as the Arthus reaction with leukocytoclastic vasculitis or as a recently more commonly occurring indurating dermatitis type IV reaction [33, 37]. Apart from the exclusion of allergic sensitization against xenogeneic animal proteins, testing is done by prick and intradermal tests as well as subcutaneous provocation testing. There are considerable cross-reactions, sometimes also with low molecular heparinoids, which should always be tested as possible alternatives.

In some cases, recombinant hirudin (Lepirudin) can be recommended after negative provocation testing in patients with severe heparin allergy and contraindication for coumarin derivatives.

5.7.1.7 Rare Drug Reactions

With the new development of recombinant drugs and gene technology, also new side effects of drugs should be expected such as against:

- Recombinant drugs
- Monoclonal antibodies (even if hybrids with human immunoglobulin form large parts of the protein and mouse sequences are only small)
- Reactions against viral vectors during gene therapy

In the United States, a fatal case in a gene therapy study with adenovirus as the vector has been brought to public attention. The precise mechanisms are not clear; overstimulation of the innate immune system with massive secretion of various cytokines, especially interleukin-6 and TNF, leading to shock lung [acute respiratory distress syndrome (ARDS) and multiorgan failure] have been discussed.

5.7.1.8 HIV Infection and Drug Allergy

Adverse drug reactions are a major problem for HIV patients, especially exanthematous drug eruptions, which are a hundred times more frequent in HIV patients than in the general population [11]. Maculopapulous eruptions, unspecific "hypersensitivity syndrome" and rare complications such as "metabolic lipodystrophy syndrome" have been observed under combined highly active antiretroviral therapy (HAART) [38].

While previously sulfonamides and other antimicrobials were the most frequent eliciting agents of adverse drug reactions, recently nucleoside reverse transcriptase inhibitors (e.g., abacavir), non-nucleoside reverse transcriptase inhibitors (e.g., delavirdin, efavirenz, nevirapine, etc.) as well as protease inhibitors (like amprenavir) have become common [38]. The reasons for the increased prevalence of exanthematous drug eruptions in HIV infections are not clear. Besides the immanent challenge due to the multiple pharmacotherapy with drugs to be taken continuously, the use of very different and new substances with ill-defined side reactions needs to be discussed. Also rather high doses and possible metabolic interactions may be considered as well as the general situation of an overstimulated immune system with upregulation of co-stimulatory molecules, cell surface receptors, and cytokine secretion.

References

1. Aberer W, Kränke B (1997) Überempfindlichkeitsreaktionen auf Impfstoffe. Allergologie 20:407–411
2. Adkinson NF (1998) Drug allergy. In: Middleton E, Reed CE, Ellis EF, Adkinson NF, Yunginger JW, Busse WW (eds) Allergy: principles and practice. CV Mosby, St. Louis, pp 1212–1224
3. Baldo BA (2000) Diagnosis of allergy to penicillins and cephalosporins. Structural and immunochemical considerations. Allergy Clin Immunol Int 12:206–212
4. Bates DW, Cullen DJ, Laird N, et al. (1995) Incidence of adverse drug events and potential adverse drug events. JAMA 274:29–34
5. Berg PA, Daniel PT, Brattig N (1987) Immunologie und Nachweis medikamentöser Allergien. In: Fuchs E, Schulz KH (eds) Manuale allergologicum IV, 11. Dustri, München-Deisenhofen, pp 1–13
6. Bircher AJ (1996) Arzneimittelallergie und Haut. Thieme, Stuttgart
7. Bircher AJ (2001) Hyposensibilisierung bei Arzneimittelallergie. In: Ring J, Darsow U (eds) Allergie 2000. Dustri, München-Deisenhofen, pp 219–228
8. Brockow K, Romano A, Blanca M, Ring J, Pichler W, Demoly P (2002) General considerations for skin test procedures in the diagnosis of drug hypersensitivity. Allergy 57:45–51
9. Classen DC, Pestotnik SL, Evans RS, Burke JP (1991) Computerized surveillance of adverse drug events in hospital patients. JAMA 266:2847–2851
10. Coleman JW, Blanca M (1998) Mechanisms of drug allergy. Immunol Today 19:196–198
11. Demoly P, Bousquet J (2001) Epidemiology of drug allergy. Curr Opin Allergy Clin Immunol 1:305–310
12. Demoly P, et al. (2004) Provocative testing. Allergy (in press)
13. DeShazo RD, Kemp SF (1997) Allergic reactions to drugs and biologic agents. JAMA 278:1895–1906
14. Dogliotti M (1968) An instance of fatal reaction to the penicillin scratch test. Dermatologica 136:489–496
15. Eapen SS, Connor EL, Gern JE (2000) Insulin desensitization with insulin lispro and an insulin pump in a 5-year-old child. Ann Allergy Asthma Immunol 85:395–397
16. Eichler G, Merk HF (1997) Unerwünschte Arzneimittelreaktionen durch Antibiotika. Allergologie 20:368–374
17. Fam AG, Dunne SM, Iazzetta J, Paton TW (2001) Efficacy and safety of desensitization to allopurinol following cutaneous reactions. Arthritis Rheum 44:231–238
18. Federlin K (1974) Insulinallergie. Dtsch Med Wochenschr 99:535–537
19. Fisher MM, Baldo BA (2000) Immunoassays in the diagnosis of anaphylaxis to neuromuscular blocking drugs: the value of morphine for the detection of IgE antibodies in allergic subjects. Anaesth Intens Care 28:167–170
20. Gadde J, Spence M. Wheeler B, Adkinson NF (1993) Clinical experience with penicillin skin testing in a large inner-city STD clinic. JAMA 270:2456–2463
21. Gall H, Merk H, Scherb W, Sterry W (1994) Antikonvulsiva-Hypersensitivitätssyndrom auf Carbamazepin. Hautarzt 45:494–498
22. Hedin H, Richter W, Ring J (1976) Dextran-induced anaphylactoid reactions in man: role of dextran reactive antibodies. Int Arch Allergy Appl Immunol 52:145–152
23. Hoigné R (1965) Arzneimittel-Allergien. Klinische und serologisch-experimentelle Untersuchungen. Huber, Bern
24. Hoigné R, Schlumberger HP, Vervloet D, Zoppi M (1993) Epidemiology of allergic drug reactions. In: Burr ML (ed) Epidemiology of clinical allergy. Monogr Allergy 31. Karger, Basel, pp 147–170
25. Jäger L, Merk HF (1996) Arzneimittel-Allergie. Gustav Fischer, Jena
26. Karch FE, Lasagna L (1975) Adverse drug reactions. A critical review. JAMA 234:1236–1241
27. Kelkar PS, Li JT-C (2001) Cephalosporin allergy. N Engl J Med 345:804–811
28. Kleinhans D (1985) Reaktionen vom Soforttyp auf Analgetika-Wirkstoffe. Allergie und Intoleranz. Allergologie 8:254–259
29. Kraft D, Wide L (1976) Clinical patterns and results of radioallergosorbent test (RAST) and skin tests in penicillin allergy. Br J Dermatol 94:593–601
30. Lasagna L (1986) The placebo effect. J Allergy Clin Immunol 78:161–165
31. Lazarou J, Pomeranz BH, Corey PN (1998) Incidence of adverse drug reactions in hospitalized patients. A meta-analysis of prospective studies. JAMA 279:1200–1205
32. Maucher OM, Fuchs A (1983) Kontakturtikaria im Epikutantest bei Pyrazolonallergie. Hautarzt 34:383–386
33. Menzel SH, Vente C, Fuchs T (1997) Heparin-Allergie. Allergo J 6:372–376
34. Merk H (1989) Arzneimittelallergie: Einfluß des Fremdstoff-Metabolismus. Allergologie 12:171–173
35. Merk HF (1998) Skin metabolism. In: Lepoittevin JP, Basketter DA, Goossens KA, Karlberg AT (eds) Allergic contact dermatitis. Springer, Berlin Heidelberg New York, pp 68–80
36. Moneret-Vautrin D, Laxenaire MC (1993) The risk of allergy related to general anaesthesia. Clin Exp Allergy 23:629–633
37. O'Donnell BF, Tan CY (1993) Delayed hypersensitivity reaction to heparin. Br J Dermatol 129:634–636

38. Pallela FJ, Delaney KM, Moorman AC, et al. (1998) Declining morbidity and mortality among patients with advanced human immunodeficiency virus infection. HIV Outpatient Study Investigators. N Engl J Med 338:853–860
39. Parker CW (1975) Drug allergy. N Engl J Med 292:511–521
40. Pichler WJ (1993) Diagnostische Möglichkeiten bei Medikamentenallergien. Schweiz Med Wochenschr 123:1183–1192
41. Pichler WJ, Yawalkar N (2000) Allergic reactions to drugs: involvement of T cells. Thorax 55 [Suppl 2]:S61–S65
42. Pouyanne P, Haramburu F, Imbs JL, Bégaud B (2000) Admissions to hospital caused by adverse drug reactions: cross incidence study. Br Med J 320:1036
43. Przybilla B, Bonnländer AR, Ring J (1986) Anaphylactoid reactions to mild analgesics. In: Ring J, Burg G (eds) New trends in allergy. II. Springer, Berlin Heidelberg New York, pp 262–271
44. Przybilla B, Fuchs T, Ippen H, et al. (1991) Empfehlungen für die Aufklärung von Überempfindlichkeitsreaktionen auf Arzneimittel. Allergologie 14:58–60
45. Reilly TP, Lash LH, Dollo MA, et al. (2000) A role for bioactivation and covalent binding within epidermal keratinocytes in sulfonamide-induced cutaneous drug reactions. J Invest Dermatol 114:1164–1173
46. Ring J (1978) Anaphylaktoide Reaktionen nach Infusion natürlicher und künstlicher Kolloide. Springer, Berlin Heidelberg New York
47. Ring J (1986) Exacerbation of eczema by formalin-containing hepatitis B vaccine in a formaldehyde-allergic patient. Lancet 2:522–523
48. Ring J (1987) Diagnostik von Arzneimittel-bedingten Unverträglichkeiten. Hautarzt 38:516–522
49. Schaub N, Bircher AJ (2000) Severe hypersensitivity syndrome to lamotrigine confirmed by lymphocyte stimulation in vitro. Allergy 55: 191–193
50. Schnyder B, Pichler WJ (2000) Skin laboratory tests in amoxicillin- and penicillin-induced morbilliform skin eruption. Clin Exp Allergy 30: 590–595
51. Schulz KH, Kasemir HD (1990) Arzneimittelallergie. In: Fuchs E, Schulz KH (eds) Manuale allergologicum, vol 3. Dustri, München-Deisenhofen, pp 1–71
52. Solensky R, Earl HS, Gruchalla RS (2000) Clinical approach to penicillin-allergic patients: a survey. Ann Allergy Asthma Immunol 84:329–333
53. Stejskal VDM, Olin RG, Forsbeck M (1986) The lymphocyte transformation test for diagnosis of drug-induced occupational allergy. J Allergy Clin Immunol 77:411–426
54. Sullivan TJ (1982) Antigen-specific desensitization of patients allergic to penicillin. J Allergy Clin Immunol 69:500–508
55. Templeton B (1965) Suicide by anaphylaxis attempted with penicillin. JAMA 192:264
56. Van Arsdel PP Jr (1982) Allergy and adverse drug reactions. J Am Acad Derm 6:833–845
57. Velcovsky H-G, Federlin K (1987) Unverträglichkeitsreaktionen gegenüber Insulin, auch Humaninsulin, bei Diabetikern. Allergologie 10:287–296
58. Vervloet D, Durham S (1998) Adverse reactions to drugs. Br Med J 316:1511–1514
59. Vieluf D (2000) Arzneimittelreaktionen. In: Przybilla B, Bergmann K, Ring J (eds) Praktische allergologische Diagnostik. Steinkopff, Darmstadt, pp 224–242
60. Vieluf D, Ring J (2001) Der Allergie-Paß. MMW Fortschr Med 143:608–610
61. Vittorio CC, Muglia JJ (1995) Anticonvulsant hypersensitivity syndrome. Arch Intern Med 155:2285–2290
62. De Weck AL, Bundgaard M (eds) (1984) Allergic reactions to drugs. Handbook of experimental pharmacology, vol 63. Springer, Berlin Heidelberg New York
63. De Weck AL (1997) Zellulärer Allergen-Stimulierungstest (CAST). Allergologie 20:487–502
64. Weiss ME, Adkinson NF (1991) Allergy to protamine. Clin Rev Allergy 9:339–355
65. Zanni MP, von Greyerz S, Schnyder B, et al. (1998) HLA-restricted, processing- and metabolism-independent pathway of drug recognition by human ab T lymphocytes. J Clin Invest 102:1591–1598

5.7.2 Pseudo-allergic Drug Reactions

5.7.2.1 Definition and Elicitors

Adverse reactions mimicking clinically allergic diseases without detectable immunologic sensitization are called "pseudo-allergic" reactions [9, 13, 15, 28]. In principle, pseudo-allergic reactions exist for all types of allergic reactions (see Table 5.85); the most frequent pseudo-allergic reactions, however, are immediate-type reactions resembling anaphylaxis [23].

The most common drugs eliciting pseudo-allergic anaphylactic reactions are radiographic contrast media, local anesthetics, i.v. anesthetics, volume substitutes, acetylsalicylic acid, and other non-steroidal anti-inflammatory drugs (Table 5.86). The case of a severe anaphylactic reaction after infusion of a colloid volume substitute (hydroxyethyl starch HES) is shown in Fig. 5.70.

Asthma and urticaria are the most common clinical manifestations of acetylsalicylic acid

Clinical symptoms	Allergy	Pseudo-allergy
Anaphylactic reaction	IgE, IgG	Direct mediator release Direct complement activation Neuropsychogenic reflexes Embolic-toxic reaction
Cytotoxic reaction	IgG, IgM	G6PDH deficiency
Serum sickness, vasculitis	IgG, IgM	Shwartzman-Sanarelli phenomenon Aggregate-induced reaction Jarisch-Herxheimer reaction Embolia cutis
Eczema, exanthema	T lymphocytes	Phototoxic dermatitis B-cell stimulation (ampicillin), lichen planus (gold)
Granuloma	T lymphocytes + macrophages	Foreign body granuloma
Organopathy or autoallergy	Autoantibodies (drug-induced LE)	Cholestasis

Table 5.85. Mechanisms of different types of drug-induced allergy and pseudo-allergy (examples)

Table 5.86. Drugs eliciting pseudo-allergic anaphylactic reactions (examples)

- Radiographic contrast media
- Colloidal volume substitutes
- Gammaglobulins
- Antibiotics
- Intravenous anesthetics
- Opioids
- Muscle relaxants
- Local anesthetics
- Cyclooxygenase inhibitors
- Drugs increasing microcirculatory flow

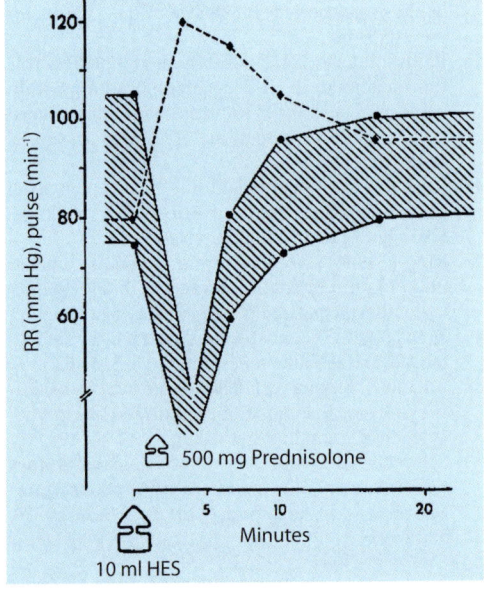

Fig. 5.70. Clinical symptoms of an anaphylactic reaction following the infusion of hydroxyethyl starch (HES)

idiosyncrasy. These patients are often also suffering from nasal polyps and chronic sinusitis (Samter's triad) [30]. Certain forms of drug-induced hepatopathy possibly may be regarded as pseudo-allergic reactions, such as cholestatic (phenothiazine, imipramine) or hepatocellular icterus (amphotericin B, furosemide, isoniazid).

Hemolytic anemias in patients with specific enzyme deficiencies (glucose-6-phosphate dehydrogenase or glutathione reductase) occur after administration of certain drugs, corresponding to "pseudo-allergic" reactions of type II (Table 5.87).

The pathophysiology of pseudo-allergic reactions is variable and not well understood (Table 5.88): Besides direct complement activation, direct mediator liberation as well as enzyme deficiencies, also embolic-toxic reactions, neuropsychogenic mechanism reflex reactions, and Jarisch-Herxheimer reaction may be mentioned here. For only a few drugs are the pathomechanisms established. The situation is complicated by the fact that one and the same drug may elicit both allergic and pseudo-allergic reactions! Table 5.89 gives some rules for

Table 5.87. Drugs and other substances able to induce hemolysis in patients with enzyme deficiency (from [11])

Glucose-6-phosphate dehydrogenase deficiency		Glutathione reductase deficiency	
Drug	Food	Drug	Other substances
Primaquine	Fava beans	Nitrofurantoin	Nitro solvent
Atebrin	Leguminosae	Primaquine	Thallium
Anilin derivatives	Red- and black currants		Resochin
Acetanilide		Azulfidine	
Naphthalene and derivatives		Dapsone (DADPS)	
Phenylhydrazine		Chloramphenicol	
Acetylphenylhydrazine		Phenacetin	
Methylene blue		Pentazolidine	
Phenacetin		Coumarin	
Aminopyrine			
p-Aminosalicylic acid			
Sulfones and Sulfonamides			
Chloramphenicol			
Vitamin K and analogues			
Azulfidine			
Dimercaprol			

Table 5.88. Examples of possible mechanisms of pseudo-allergic reactions

Direct complement activation (Classic)	Gammaglobulin (standard) (aggregated IgG)
	Plasmaprotein solutions (aggregated IgG)
(Bypass activation)	Radiographic contrast media
	Intravenous anesthetics
Direct mediator release	Gelatin
	Radiographic contrast media
	Relaxants
	Intravenous anesthetics
	Antibiotics (polymyxin)
	(Acetylsalicylic acid?)
Enzyme defects	
C1 inactivator	Hereditary angioneurotic edema
Glucose-6-phosphate dehydrogenase	Hemolytic anemia
(cholinesterase)	(Succinylcholine incompatibility)
Neuropsychogenic reflexes	Local anesthetics
Embolic-toxic reaction	Depot-penicillin (intravascular)
Jarisch-Herxheimer reaction	Destruction of cells (e.g., syphilis treatment with penicillin)
Increase of blood flow	Nicotinic acid esters

Table 5.89. Rough criteria for distinction of allergic from pseudo-allergic reactions

Allergy	Pseudo-allergy
Sensitization	No sensitization
Reaction after repeated contact	Reaction at first contact
Rare (<5%)	Frequent (>5%)
Typical clinical symptoms	"Unspecific" symptoms
Low eliciting doses	Dose dependent (speed dependent in infusions)
Family history sometimes positive	Family history negative (exception: enzyme defects)
Moderate psychologic influence	Strong psychologic influence

the differentiation of pseudo-allergic and allergic reactions (cum grano salis).

In the following, some clinically common pseudo-allergic reactions will be discussed.

5.7.2.2 Radiographic Contrast Media

The majority of adverse reactions after radiographic contrast media (RCM) are non-immunologic in origin. Occasional cases of true allergy have been published. In recent years, late or delayed reactions (4–8 h) after RCM infusion have been reported, which may correspond to a true type IV reaction (positive patch tests) [1, 32]. RCM are direct histamine and serotonin liberators [25] as well as complement activators [38]. Interactions with the coagulation and kallikrein-kinin system have been reported [17, 28].

While 20 years ago toxic effects of ionic contrast media as well as high osmolarity were considered pathophysiologically important, we now know that even after non-ionic solutions with physiological osmolarity, severe side reactions (even fatalities) may occur.

There is no reliable method of predicting the risk of an RCM reaction in the individual patient. Iodine allergy is a type IV reaction in the sense of a classic allergic contact dermatitis and is not primarily linked to anaphylactic reactions after iodinated RCM, where iodine is bound within the benzoic acid ring structure! Occasional cases of systemic contact dermatitis may be elicited by iodine since in some RCM solutions minute amounts of free iodine (picogram range) have been detected.

According to our experience, the risk of an RCM reaction is not increased in atopics or patients with other drug reactions. Only in patients with a clear-cut history of severe anaphylactic reactions after RCM infusion is the risk significantly elevated to 30% (normal individuals around 10%) (cited in [24]).

Some patients may react to a prick test with systemic reactions. Therefore, we perform skin tests as a minimum variant of provocation under emergency conditions. The occasional intravenous provocation testing with RCM is a matter of clinical research.

Uncontrolled "test injections" of small volumes may elicit severe anaphylactic reactions.

For prophylaxis, antihistamines and glucocorticosteroids, beta-adrenergics, antidepressives, as well as hypnotic suggestion have been recommended.

In a prospective placebo-controlled study of our own, we were able to show a significant prophylactic effect of a combined H_1 and H_2 antagonist intravenous pretreatment (clemastine + cimetidine 5 min prior to RCM infusion) [26].

5.7.2.3 Plasma Protein Solutions

After intravenous injection of standard gammaglobulin, severe anaphylactic reactions may occur; therefore, these preparations are only applied intramuscularly. Gammaglobulin aggregates present in the solutions activate the complement system via the classic pathway (reverse immune complex reaction). Protein aggregates are also present in other plasma protein solutions and severe systemic reactions have been observed [23]. The liberation of kinins and kinin-activating substances present in some human serum albumin batches is discussed. The common intravenous gammaglobulins are chemically or physically modified on the Fc part, thus preventing aggregate formation and complement activation. Therefore, they are generally well tolerated.

5.7.2.4 Gelatine Volume Substitutes

After infusion of gelatine volume substitutes – especially the urea-linked modification using di-isocyanate (Haemaccel) – a dose- and speed-dependent histamine liberation has been described [8, 19]. Anaphylactic reactions after gelatine infusion were very frequent in the 1980s (up to 30%!), but have been reduced by better production with lower isocyanate concentrations. Pretreatment with histamine H_1 and H_2 antagonists is an effective prophylaxis. Occasional true IgE-mediated reactions to gelatine have been reported [42].

5.7.2.5 Intravenous Anesthetics

Intravenous anesthetics (Table 5.90) have pharmacological effects, giving rise to complica-

Table 5.90. Intravenous anesthetics

Barbiturates	Opiates
• Thiopental	• Morphine
• Methohexital	• Fentanyl
• Hexobarbital	• Alfentanil
• Thiobutabarbital	• Droperidol
Diazepines	**Others**
• Diazepam	• Propanidide
• Medazolam	• Ketamine
	• Etomidate
	• Althesin

tions like hypotension or tachycardia or have central stimulating effects such as ketamine and propanidide, or sedative effects like barbiturates.

Various mechanisms have been discussed to explain anaphylactic reactions. Besides classic IgE-mediated reactions (barbiturates), pseudo-allergic mechanisms with direct complement activation and histamine liberation may play a role (especially opioids) [8, 24]. Recently, IgE-mediated reactions to opiates and relaxants have been reported [19].

A careful history is the mainstay of diagnosis of these adverse reactions. The allergist needs the cooperation of the anesthetist, who should record the exact time sequence of the substances administered! When skin tests are performed, the histamine-liberating properties of certain anesthetics need to be considered.

5.7.2.6 Muscle Relaxants

The most important side effects of muscle relaxants are:

- Prolonged muscle relaxation
- Anaphylactic reaction
- Malignant hyperthermia

Prolonged muscle relaxation mostly is due to a genetic or drug-induced inhibition of cholinesterase (e.g., neostigmine, organophosphates, hexafluronium, quinidine, cyclophosphamide, aprotinin) or a muscular disease (myasthenia gravis).

Muscle relaxants are direct histamine liberators. It is under discussion whether this property is connected with the frequently observed tachycardia and hypotension. However, in severe anaphylactic reactions, true IgE-mediated allergies against muscle relaxants have been observed with cross-reactivity related to the quarternary ammonium group [39].

If a depolarizing relaxant (e.g., succinylcholine) is not tolerated, a non-depolarizing agent (e.g., alcuronium) may be tolerated.

Malignant hyperthermia occurs in patients with myopathy due to increased calcium influx and contractility with rapid increase in body temperature without shivering, tachycardia, tachypnea, muscle rigidity, and cardiac arrhythmia. The disease is familiar. For diagnosis, muscle biopsy with in vitro stimulation and contractility study is available. Molecular genetic tests found a relevant mutation in the ryanodin receptor 1 gene (RYR-1) [38]. Effective therapy uses the hydantoin derivative dantrolen (1 mg/kg body wt. i.v.), oxygen, and slow reduction of body temperature.

5.7.2.7 Local Anesthetics

So-called allergic reactions against local anesthetics are common in the allergist's office; however, true allergies are rare, except for the type IV reactions in classic allergic contact dermatitis [29]. Most anaphylactic reactions are non-immunologic in origin with unspecific symptoms. Intradermal tests cannot be related to clinical manifestation [14]. As pathomechanism, psychoneurogenic reflex mechanisms with vasovagal components have been suggested. In practice, the procedure of "subcutaneous provocation testing" (Table 5.91) is recommended with slowly increasing doses under careful observation in emergency conditions subcutaneously.

The role of preservatives contained in some solutions, especially in larger bottles, has to be

Table 5.91. Local anesthetics: provocation tests, 20-min interval

Prick test if negative:			
	1. I.d.	1:10	0.1 ml
	2. S.c.	1:10	0.1 ml
	3. S.c.	Undiluted	0.1 ml
	4. S.c.	Undiluted	0.5 ml
	5. S.c.	Undiluted	1.0 ml
↓	6. S.c.	Undiluted	2.0 ml

Table 5.92. Local anesthetic (LA) incompatibility: "reverse placebo provocation" (in patients reacting to placebo and psychological influence)

Procedure	Patient information
1. Skin test	Open
2. S.c. provocation with LA 1	"with LA"
3. S.c. provocation with LA 2	"another LA"
4. S.c. provocation with NaCl	"another LA"
5. S.c. provocation with LA 1	"NaCl"
6. S.c. provocation with LA 1	LA 1

Table 5.94. Hypothetical concepts for pathophysiology of ASA idiosyncrasy

- Cyclooxygenase inhibition leads to diminished protective prostaglandins
- Cyclooxygenase inhibition leads to increased formation of lipoxygenase products
- Cyclooxygenase 1-inhibition is decisive
- Direct release of vasoactive mediators
- Activation of complement system
- Activation of coagulation and/or kallikrein-kinin system
- Increased platelet reactivity
- Immune reaction against ASA metabolites or impurities

evaluated by testing preservative-free substances (mostly in ampules).

If there is psychologic influence and patients also react to placebo, we use the procedure of "reverse placebo provocation" (Table 5.92), giving the patient "verum" under the label "placebo." If the local anesthetic then is well tolerated, the patient is completely informed and the same procedure is repeated on the next day openly.

5.7.2.8 Acetylsalicylic Acid and Non-steroidal Anti-inflammatory Drugs (NSAIDs)

Toxic effects of NSAIDs such as gastric irritation and inhibition of platelet aggregation need to be differentiated from pseudo-allergic hypersensitivity reactions with variable manifestation (Table 5.93).

The pathomechanism of acetylsalicylic acid (ASA) idiosyncrasy (15% of asthma patients) has not yet been clearly elucidated. Direct mediator liberation [3, 4, 5, 15, 21, 27, 36, 40, 41] has been discussed as well as direct complement activation, platelet stimulation and a shift in eicosanoid metabolism (Table 5.94). The concomitant administration of NSAIDs and allergen can lead to increased reactions (ASA augmentation [20]) (see Sect. 5.1.4 on "Anaphylaxis").

The most prominent feature of analgesic idiosyncrasy (sometimes also called "intolerance syndrome" [20, 40] is the lack of immunologic cross-reactivity with other chemically related substances. However, there are pharmacologic cross-reactivities with similarly acting substances, e.g., other NSAIDs, but also chemicals such as food colorings (tartrazine) and preservatives (see Sect. 5.1.5 on "Food Allergy").

For diagnosis the provocation test is most important (see Sect. 5.7.1). Caveat: with too high doses of ASA, patients with aspirin-asthma may develop acute severe asthma attacks! We recommend beginning according to the intensity of symptoms in the history with 5–50 mg ASA and increasing doses at 2-h intervals to 100, 200–500 and eventually 500 mg.

Patients with chronic urticaria often react to ASA as well as other additives and colorings (see Sect. 5.1.6 on "Urticaria").

Several in vitro diagnostic techniques have been attempted in ASA idiosyncrasy; however, the observed effects (e.g., histamine release by ASA) have also been observed in patients tolerating ASA [3, 5, 27, 39]. Recently the cellular allergen stimulation test (CAST) has been favored, when after stimulation with C5a, PAF or F-Met-Leu-Phe increased leukotriene secretion is measured in patients with chronic urticaria and a positive ASA provocation test [5, 43]. Direct stimulation with ASA in vitro, however, has yielded controversial results [5, 21, 43].

Table 5.93. Clinical manifestations of NSAID incompatibility

Eye
- Conjunctivitis

Respiratory tract
- Rhinitis
- Sinusitis
- Asthma

Urticaria and angioedema

Anaphylactic reaction

Photodermatosis

For therapy, avoidance is the primary principle: in nasal polyposis polypectomy is indicated; equally infectious sinusitis has to be treated.

By administrations of slowly increasing doses of ASA, in some patients "adaptive deactivation" is possible, leading to ASA tolerance, which makes the daily intake of 500 mg or 650 mg ASA necessary [34, 27, 40]. In some patients a decrease in relapses of nasal polyposis has been observed [34].

Adaptive deactivation with ASA in patients with chronic urticaria or anaphylactic reactions has not been convincingly achieved.

After the introduction of cyclooxygenase (COX) 2 inhibitors [10], many people were hopeful of having safe alternatives for patients with ASA idiosyncrasy [6, 31, 36, 37, 45]. There are, however, patients who react particularly to COX 2 inhibitors [12]. COX 2 inhibitors, therefore, cannot generally be regarded as safe alternatives in ASA idiosyncrasy.

5.7.2.9 Additives

Adverse drug reactions may not only be elicited by the active substance but also by additives in the preparation. Most additives have been added for galenic reasons (preservatives, antioxidants, stabilizers, filling substances, etc.); however, undesired ingredients may also be considered [16, 23, 28]. Some may be legal (such as high molecular residues or small particles < 30 μm in infusion solutions) or illegal such as bacterial contaminants or pyrogens (Table 5.95).

Table 5.95. Additives in drugs as elicitors of anaphylactic reactions (examples)

• Depot mediators	(Penicillin preparations)
• Micell formers	(Cremophor EL)
• Sulfites	(Injection solutions, local anesthetics)
• Protein stabilizers	(Protein solutions)
• Benzylalcohol	(Injection solutions, sterile H_2O or saline)
• Colorings	(In tablets)
• Acetate	(Dialysis)

5.7.2.10 Other Pseudo-allergic Reactions

For the sake of completeness the classical *Jarisch-Herxheimer reaction* should be mentioned in a chapter on pseudo-allergic reactions; by cell destruction (penicillin in syphilis), pyrogenic or vasoactive substances may be released and activate the complement system.

After administration (mostly intramuscular) of depot-penicillins occasional pseudo-allergic reactions have been observed with central nervous disturbances and cardiovascular symptoms, which have been called *"embolic-toxic reactions" (Hoigné syndrome)* [13]. Oily material of the depot emulsion may reach the intravasal lumen after injection and lead to microemboli. Whether a direct pharmacologic effect of procaine – sometimes also contained in these preparations – plays a pathogenic role remains open.

For the mechanisms of ampicillin rash see Sect. 5.7.3.

Generally, contaminants and impurities have to be considered whenever an adverse reaction remains unclear.

5.7.2.11 Therapy and Prophylaxis

The treatment of pseudo-allergic anaphylactic reactions follows the principles of anti-anaphylactic regimens (see Sect. 5.1.4). In unclear cases and with a history of pseudo-allergic reactions the prophylactic administration of histamine H_1- and H_2-antagonists (intravenously 5 min prior to the drug) or orally together with glucocorticosteroids (18 h prior to administration) is recommended.

References

1. Brockow K, Ring J (1996) Mechanisms of pseudo-allergic reactions due to radiographic contrast media. Allergy Clin Immunol Int 8:123–125
2. Brockow K, Vieluf D, Püschel K, Grosch J, Ring J (1999) Increased postmortem serum mast cell tryptase in a fatal anaphylactoid reaction to nonionic radiocontrast medium. J Allergy Clin Immunol 104:237–238
3. Capron A, Ameisen J, Joseph M, Auriault C, Tarnel AB, Caen J (1985) New functions for platelets and their pathological implications. Int Arch Allergy Appl Immunol 77:107–114

4. Conroy MC, de Weck AL (1981) Effect of aspirin and indomethacin on histamine release from leukocytes of patients with suspected intolerance to aspirin. Int Arch Allergy Appl Immunol 66 [Suppl 1]:152–153
5. Czech W, Schöpf E, Kapp A (1995) Release of sulfidoleukotrienes in vitro: Its relevance in the diagnosis of pseudoallergy to acetylsalicylic acid. Inflamm Res 44:291–295
6. Dahlen B, Szczeklik A, Murray JJ (2001) Celecoxib in patients with asthma and aspirin intolerance (letter). N Engl J Med 344:142
7. Denborough MA, Lovell RRH (1960) Anaesthetic deaths in a family. Lancet II:362
8. Doenicke A, Koenig UD (eds) (1983) Immunologie in Anästhesie und Intensivmedizin. Sertürner Workshops Einbek. Springer, Berlin Heidelberg New York
9. Dukor P, Kallos P, Schlumberger HD, West GB (eds) (1980) Pseudo-allergic reactions, 3 vols. Karger, Basel
10. Fitzgerald GA, Patrono C (2001) The coxibs, selective inhibitors of cyclooxygenase-2. N Engl J Med 345:433–442
11. Gaetani GF, Luzatto L (1980) Haemolytic reactions induced by drugs and other agents: the role of red cell enzyme abnormalities and of abnormal haemoglobins. In: Dukor P, Kallos P, Schlumberger HD, West GB (eds) Pseudo-allergic reactions; involvement of drugs and chemicals. vol. 2, Karger, Basel, pp 1–19
12. Grimm V, Rakoski J, Ring J (2004) Selective COX-2 inhibitors also can elicit symptoms in patients with aspirin idiosyncrasy. J Allergy Clin Immunol (in press)
13. Hoigné R (1962) Allergische und pseudo-allergische Reaktionen auf Penicillinpräparate. Acta Allergol 17:521
14. Incaudo G, Schatz M, Patterson R, Rosenberg M, Yamamoto E, Hamburger RN (1978) Administration of local anesthetics to patients with a history of prior adverse reaction. J Allergy Clin Immunol 61:339–345
15. Kallos P, Kallos L (1980) Histamine and some other mediators of pseudo-allergic reactions. In: Pseudo-allergic reactions: involvement of drugs and chemical, vol. 1. Karger, Basel, p 28
16. Kleinhans D, Galinsky T (1982) Zur möglichen Provokation eines Bronchialasthmas und einer Urtikaria durch Natriumdisulfit. Allergologie 4:120–121
17. Lasser EC, Lang JH, Lyon SG, Hamblin AE, Howard MM (1981) Prekallikrein-kallikrein conversion rate as a predictor of contrast media catastrophes. Radiology 140:11–15
18. Lorenz W, Doenicke A (1978) Histamine release in clinical conditions. Mt Sinai J Med N Y 45:357–386
19. Meßmer K, Lorenz W, Sunder-Plassmann L, Klövekorn WP, Hutzel M (1970) Histamine release as cause of hypotension following rapid colloid infusion. Arch Pathol Pharm 267:433–439
20. Paul E, Gall H-M, Mechlin A, Möller R, Müller I (2001) Acetylsalicylic acid (ASA)-augmentation in relation to ASA-intolerance. Allergo J 10:269–272
21. Pierzchalska M, Mastalerz L, Sanak M, et al. (2000) A moderate and unspecific release of cysteinyl leukotrienes by aspirin from peripheral blood leucocytes preludes its value for aspirin sensitivity in asthma. Clin Exp Allergy 30:1785–1791
22. Przybilla B, Ring J (1987) Pseudo-allergische Arzneimittelreaktionen: Pathophysiologie und Diagnostik. Z Hautkr 62:430–443
23. Ring J (1978) Anaphylaktoide Reaktionen nach Infusion natürlicher und künstlicher Kolloide. Springer, Berlin Heidelberg New York
24. Ring J, Brockow K (2004) Pseudo-allergische Arzneimittelreaktionen. In: Schultze-Werninghaus G, et al. (eds) Manuale allergologicum, 2nd edn. Dustri, Munich (in press)
25. Ring J, Arroyave CM, Fritzler MJ, Tan EM (1978) In vitro histamine and serotonin release by radiographic contrast media (RCM). Complement dependent and independent release reaction and changes in ultrastructure of human blood cells. Clin Exp Immunol 32:105–118
26. Ring J, Rothenberger KH, Clauß W (1985) Prevention of anaphylactoid reactions after radiographic contrast media in fusion by combined histamine H_1- and H_2-receptor antagonists: results of a prospective controlled trial. Int Arch Allergy Appl Immunol 78:9–14
27. Ring J, Walz U (1985) Indomethacin enhances in vitro histamine release induced by anti-IgE and Ca-Ionophore but inhibits C5a-induced release reactions from basophils of atopics and normals. Int Arch Allergy Appl Immunol 77:225–227
28. Ring J (1992) Pseudo-allergic reactions. In: Korenblat PE, Wedner HJ (eds) Allergy: theory and practice. Saunders, Philadelphia, pp 243–264
29. Ruzicka T, Gerstmeier M, Przybilla B, Ring J (1987) Allergy to local anesthetics: comparison of patch test with prick and intradermal test results. J Am Acad Dermatol 16:1202–1208
30. Samter M, Beers RF (1968) Intolerance to aspirin. Clinical studies and consideration of its pathogenesis. Ann Intern Med 68:975–983
31. Sánchez-Borges M, Capriles-Hulett A, Caballero-Fonseca F (2001) NSAID hypersensitivity in the COX-2 inhibitor era. ACI Int 13:211–218
32. Schick E, Weber L, Gall H (1996) Delayed hypersensitivity reaction to the non-ionic contrast medium iopromide. Contact Dermatitis 35:312
33. Simon RA (1984) Adverse reactions to drug additives. J Allergy Clin Immunol 74:623
34. Stevenson DD (1984) Diagnosis, prevention, and treatment of adverse reactions to aspirin and nonsteroidal antiinflammatory drugs. J Allergy Clin Immunol 74:617–622

35. Stevenson DD, Simon RA (2001) Lack of cross-reactivity between rofecoxib and aspirin in aspirin-sensitive patients with asthma. J Allergy Clin Immunol 108:47–51
36. Szczeklik A, Sanak M (2000) Genetic mechanisms in aspirin-induced asthma. Am J Resp Crit Care Med 161:S142–146
37. Szczeklik A, Nizankowska E, Sanak M, Swierczynska M (2001) Aspirin-induced rhinitis and asthma. Curr Opin Allergy Clin Immunol 1:27–33
38. Till G, Rother U, Gemsa D, Gerhardt P (1977) Aktivierung des Komplementsystems bei Zwischenfällen nach Kontrastmittelinjektionen. Verh Dtsch Ges Inn Med 83:1589–1591
39. Vervloet DL, Dor P, Arneud A, Senft M, Alazia M, Charpin J (1985) Anaphylactic reactions to succinylcholine. Prevention of mediator release by choline. J Allergy Clin Immunol 75:150
40. Virchow C (ed) (1986) Analgetika, Asthma. Medidact 6. Programmed, Frankfurt
41. Voigtländer V, Walter E, Siess R, Rother U (1981) Acetylsalicylic acid intolerance: a possible role of complement. Int Archs Allergy Appl Immunol 66 [Suppl 1]:154–155
42. Wahl R, Kleinhans D (1989) IgE-mediated allergic reactions to fruit gums and investigation of cross-reactivity between gelatine and modified gelatine-containing products. Clin Exp Allergy 19:77–80
43. Wedi B, Kapp A (2000) Aspirin induced adverse skin reactions: new pathophysiological aspects. Thorax 55 [Suppl 2]:S70–S71
44. Wüthrich B (1983) Allergische und pseudo-allergische Reaktionen der Haut durch Arzneimittel und Lebensmitteladditiva. Schweiz Rdsch Med (Praxis) 72:691–699
45. Yoshida S, Ishizaki Y, Onuma K, Shoji T, Nakagawa H, Amayasu H (2000) Selective cyclo-oxygenase 2 inhibitor in patients with aspirin-induced asthma. J Allergy Clin Immunol 106:1203–1204

5.7.3 Exanthematous Drug Eruptions

5.7.3.1 Prevalence

Adverse drug reactions occur preferably on the skin. Three percent of all drug treatments give rise to adverse drug reactions on the skin [3, 10, 62], not including contact allergic reactions after external application of topicals (see Sect. 5.5.2). Exanthematous drug eruptions occur after systemic administration of a drug, manifesting mostly symmetrically with a predilection of the extensor surfaces of extremities [10, 12, 24, 35, 53, 56, 62]. The morphology of exanthematous drug eruptions is very colorful. Skin reactions mostly are not specific but may be elicited through allergic, toxic, or infectious processes. There are, however, conditions which are elicited more frequently by certain drugs than by others [10, 60, 62]. Knowledge of these facts is crucial in the causal diagnosis [3, 10, 25, 39, 62] (Tables 5.96, 5.97).

On the other hand, an underlying disease of the patient does influence the occurrence of

Table 5.96. Prevalence of drug-induced allergic skin reactions (from [3])

	Prevalence (%)		Prevalence (%)
Cotrimoxazole	5.90	Trimethobenzamide	0.66
Ampicillin	5.20	Phenazopyridine	0.65
Other semisynthetic penicillins	3.60	Methenamine	0.64
Corticotropin	2.80	Cyanocobalamin	0.62
Erythromycin	2.30	Barbiturate	0.47
Salicylazosulfapyridine	2.10	Glutethimide	0.45
Sulfisoxazole	1.70	Indomethacin	0.44
Penicillin G	1.60	Chlordiazepoxide	0.42
Gentamycin	1.60	Metoclopramide	0.40
Practolol	1.60	Diazepam	0.38
Cephalosporin	1.30	Propoxyphene	0.34
Quinidine	1.20	Isoniazid	0.30
Metamizol (dipyrone)	1.10	Nystatin	0.29
Mercury diuretics	0.95	Chlorothiazide	0.28
Nitrofurantoin	0.91	Furosemide	0.26
Heparin	0.77	Insulin	0.13
Chloramphenicol	0.68	Phenytoin	0.11
		Phytonadione	0.09

Table 5.97. Common elicitors of certain cutaneous drug eruptions

Morphology	Elicitor (examples)
Urticarial eruptions	see Sect. 5.1.3 on "Urticaria" and Sect. 5.1.4 on "Anaphylaxis"
Erythematovesicular eruptions	see Sect. 5.5.2 on "Dermatitis"
Purpura/hemorrhagic eruptions	see Sect. 5.2 on "Cytotoxic Reactions" and Sect. 5.3 on "Immune Complex Reactions"
Erythema multiforme	Barbiturates Sulfonamides Hydantoin Hydralazine Carbamazepine Diuretics NSAIDs
Erythema nodosum	Anticonceptives Halogens Sulfonamides
Macular and maculopapular	Penicillin Ampicillin Allopurinol Sulfonamides NSAIDs
Exfoliative dermatitis	Antiepileptics Phenylbutazone Heavy metals (e.g., arsenic)
Fixed drug eruption	Barbiturates Analgesics NSAIDs Tetracyclines Sulfonamides Anticonceptives Hydantoin Laxants Metronidazole
Lichenoid drug eruptions	Thiazides Phenothiazine Captopril Gold Sulfonamides
Acneiform drug eruptions	Steroid hormones Halogens Lithium Isoniazin Vitamins (B) Hydantoin
Lymphocytic infiltration	Analgesics (plus alcohol?)
Psoriasiform eruptions	Beta-blockers Gold salts Lithium

drug eruptions: Increased prevalences of drug eruptions are common in HIV infection and AIDS (sulfonamides, etc.) while in early stages of HIV, IgE-mediated reactions may be diminished [36, 47].

5.7.3.2 Clinical Classification of Exanthematous Drug Eruptions

The prevalences of the most important types of drug eruptions from a Finnish study are shown in Table 5.98.

Urticarial Drug Eruptions. These represent mostly allergic reactions due to IgE-mediated phenomena (urticaria, anaphylaxis) (see Sects. 5.1.3, 5.1.4) or IgG/IgM immune complexes as serum sickness (after 8–14 days!) (see Sect. 5.3.2).

Erythematovesicular Drug Eruptions. These correspond clinically to systemic contact dermatitis whereby the allergens are administered systemically (e.g., sulfonamides, metal ions) (see Sect. 5.5.2).

Hemorrhagic Drug Eruptions. Some exanthematous drug eruptions may become hemorrhagic in nature when they are very intense or

Table 5.98. Prevalence of clinical types of drug eruptions in 446 patients (from Kauppinnen and Stubb [26])

Type	Number of patients
Macular und maculopapular eruptions	189
Fixed eruptions	92 (16 multi-locular)
Urticaria/angioedema	57
Eczema	47
Erythema multiforme	18
Stevens-Johnson syndrome	8
Lyell's syndrome (toxic epidermal necrolysis)	8
Photosensitization	5
Purpura	4
Lupus erythematosus-like lesions	2
Erythema nodosum	1
Fever	5
Total	436

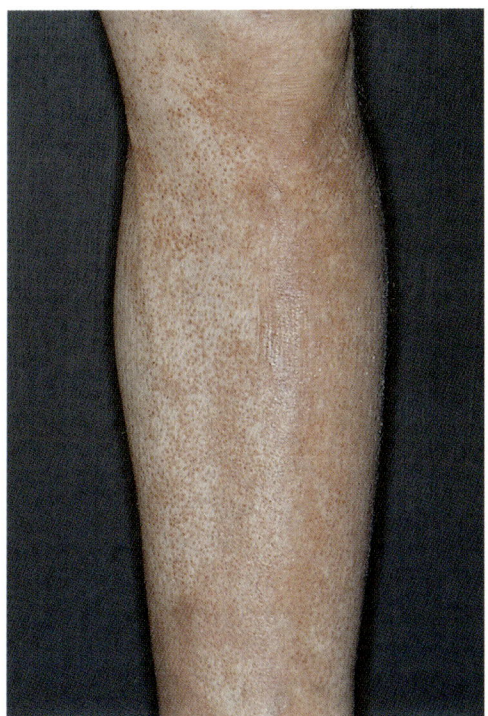

Fig. 5.71. Clinical manifestation of purpura chronica progressiva (Schamberg's disease)

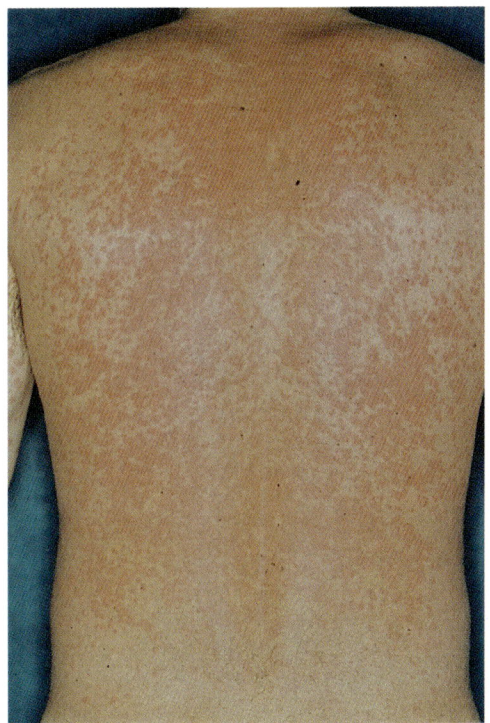

Fig. 5.72. Measles-like drug exanthema following the oral administration of penicillin

due to hydrostatic pressure (legs). There is, however, primary drug-induced purpura corresponding to cytotoxic reactions (allergic thrombocytopenic purpura) (see Sect. 5.2) or as immune complex vasculitis (see Sect. 5.3).

Purpura chronica progressiva (M. Schamberg) is characterized by small petechial bleedings with a reddish-brownish (Cayenne pepper) skin lesion and is elicited by drugs (bromide carbamide) or additives (Fig. 5.71).

Histologically, lymphocytic infiltration around the vessels is seen; sometimes patch tests are positive. Some authors regard progressive pigmentary purpura as the vascular type IV reaction (" dermatitis of the vessels") [35].

Macular and Maculopapular Drug Eruptions. These are the most common exanthematous drug eruptions with histologically perivascular lymphocytic infiltrates. The skin lesions manifest 8–12 days after the first treatment (Fig. 5.72), in repeated treatment much faster. Pathogenetically, a type IVc reaction is probable (CD8 cells), which can be demonstrated as delayed-type reactions in the intradermal or patch test [14, 35, 42, 54]. Infectious diseases (measles, rubeola) are a differential diagnosis.

A special problem is ampicillin exanthema, which occurs in 10% of ampicillin-treated patients and is probably due to unspecific B-cell stimulation as it occurs with certain viral infections (e.g., Epstein-Barr virus). Infection and drug effect may potentiate in the example of infectious mononucleosis where 90–100% of ampicillin-treated patients develop ampicillin rash (almost pathognomonic).

Exfoliative Dermatitis. Some drugs elicit generalized exfoliative dermatitis (Fig. 5.73) ranging up to erythroderma (e.g., sulfonamides, antimalarials, penicillin, mercury-containing diuretics, barbiturates). The pathomechanism is not clear; in the differential diagnosis, toxic shock syndrome should be considered [15, 23, 58].

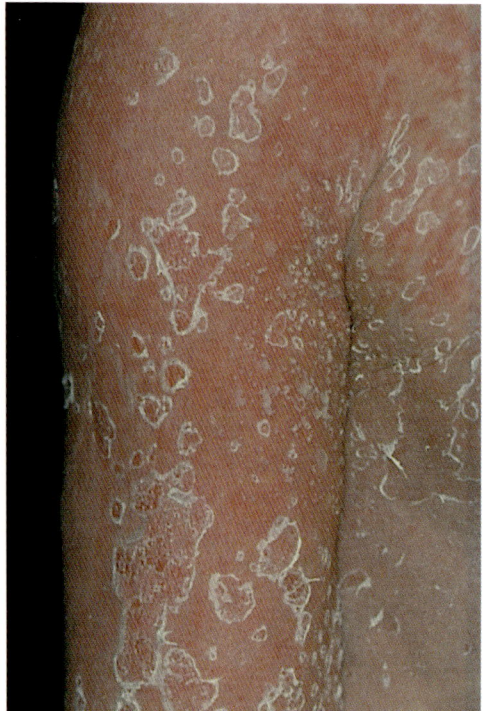

Fig. 5.73. Drug exanthema: exfoliative dermatitis

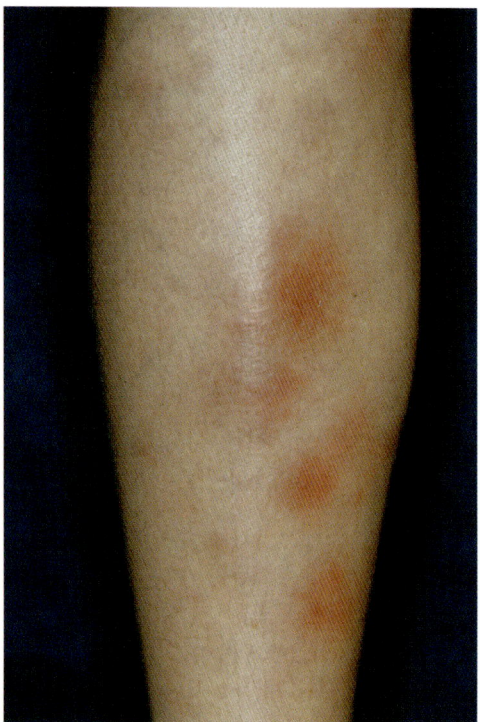

Fig. 5.74. Drug-induced erythema with nodosum-like skin lesions

Drug-Induced Erythema Nodosum. Erythema-nodosum-like skin lesions may be drug induced (anticonceptives, sulfonamides, phenylbutazone) (Fig. 5.74). In the pathogenesis, immune complexes but also cellular reactions have been discussed.

Lymphohistiocytic Reaction. This is a localized reaction mostly in the face with livid-red infiltrates (Fig. 5.75), sometimes occurring 12–24 h after intake of analgesics together with alcohol. Histologically, perivascular infiltrates of lymphocytes and histiocytes together with edema of the dermis are characteristic.

Bullous Drug Eruptions

Fixed Drug Eruptions. These are sharply marginated dark red to livid macules, which can be blistering with predominant acral localization (hands, feet, glans penis) 24–48 h after drug intake (Figs. 5.76, 5.77). The characteristic feature is the occurrence on exactly the same skin

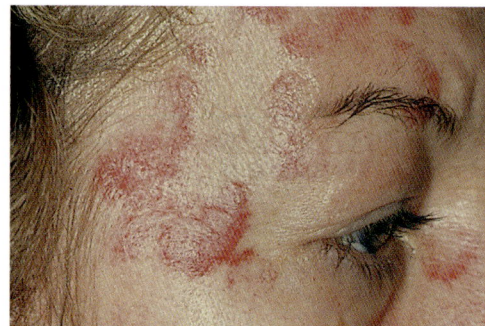

Fig. 5.75. Lymphohistiocytic reaction

area after repeated administration. With increasing number of relapses, skin lesions may be more brownish. Specifically sensitized lymphocytes may stay over longer periods of time in the area. Patch tests only will be positive in loco during remission (Fig. 5.78). New investigations describe an early vascular phase with CD4 infiltrates followed by an epidermal phase with CD8 cells and HLA-DR-expressing, partly destroyed keratinocytes [41].

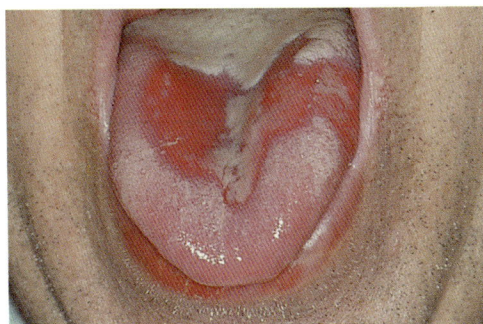

Fig. 5.76. Fixed drug-induced exanthema of the oral mucosa

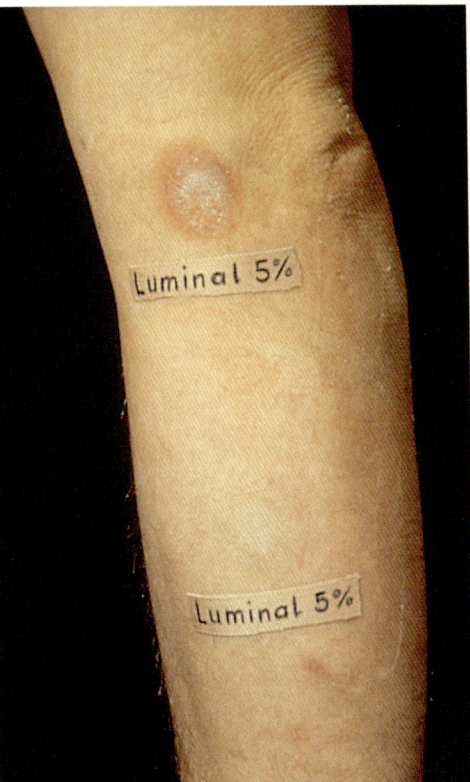

Fig. 5.78. Positive epidermal reaction to patch test in loco during remission (K.H. Schulz)

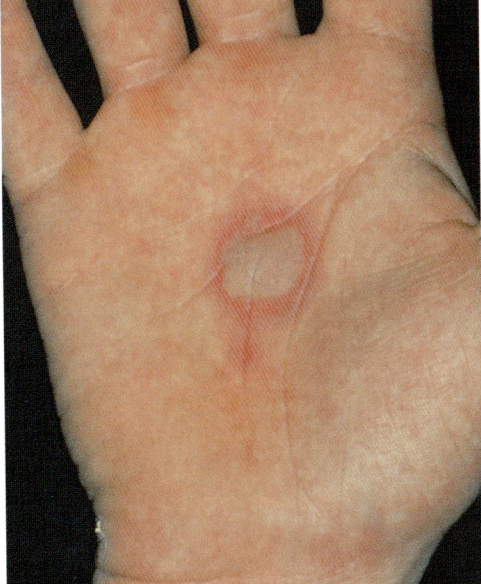

Fig. 5.77. Fixed drug-induced exanthema following the oral administration of phenylbutazone

Erythema Multiforme. Erythema multiforme-like skin lesions with typical target formations (Fig. 5.79) may be triggered by viral, bacterial infection or drugs. Sulfonamides and barbiturates are common, also tetracyclines. Pathogenetically, type IV reactions but also immune complex mechanisms are suspected [27]. In the histology, subepidermal blistering is characteristic.

A serious complication of erythema multiforme is mucosal involvement (conjunctival, oral, genital) (Figs. 5.80, 5.81) such as in Stevens-Johnson syndrome. In rare cases, there is

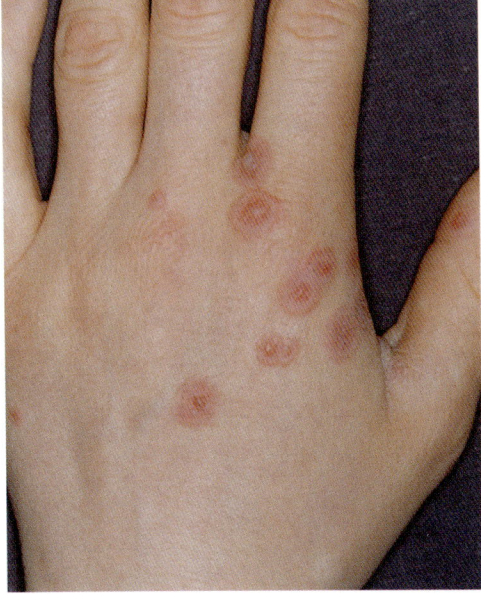

Fig. 5.79. Exudative erythema multiforme

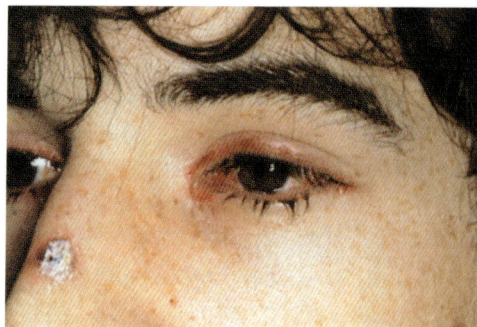

Fig. 5.80. Exudative erythema multiforme with mucosal involvement

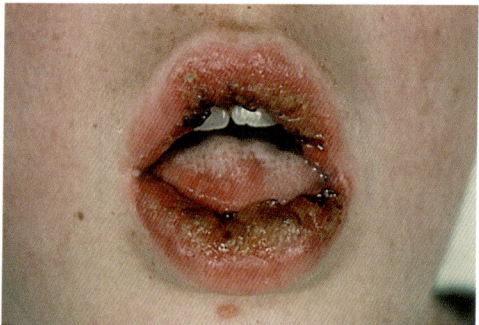

Fig. 5.81. Erosive reaction of the oral mucosa (Stevens-Johnson syndrome)

transition possible into drug-induced Lyell's syndrome (toxic epidermal necrolysis) (see below). Clinical and dermatopathological characteristics (Table 5.99), however, argue for the individual entity of the different diseases [39, 51].

Toxic Epidermal Necrolysis (Drug-Induced Lyell's Syndrome). Drug-induced Lyell's syndrome ("toxic epidermal necrolysis" or "syndrome of burnt skin") represents the maximal variant of bullous drug eruptions.

In 1956, Allen Lyell coined the term "toxic epidermal necrolysis" (TEN) for diseases which had been published earlier under different names (Table 5.100). In a retrospective study of 1967, Lyell postulated four subgroups of TEN [34]: drug-induced, staphylococcal-induced, miscellanea (sepsis, viral infections, vaccination, GVH, or malignancy) as well as idiopathic TEN.

Today two forms of Lyell's syndrome can be well differentiated clinically and pathophysiologically (Table 5.101): staphylococcal Lyell's syndrome, also staphylococcal scalded skin syndrome (SSSS) [10, 12, 39], whereas TEN in the actual definition comprises diseases where

Table 5.99. Clinical characteristics of various bullous drug eruptions (according to [39]). *SJS*, Stevens-Johnson syndrome; *TEN*, toxic epidermal necrolysis

	Extent (% body surface)	Target lesions	Macules	Large erythemas	Mucosal involvement
Erythema multiforme	<10%	++	–	–	–
SJS	<10%	– (atypical)	+	–	++
SJS/TEN (mixed)	10–30%	– (flat)	++	–	++
TEN with macules	>30%	– (flat)	+++	+	++
TEN	>10%	–	–	+++	++

Exfoliative dermatitis	Rittershain 1878	**Table 5.100.** History and terminology of Lyell's syndrome (from [45])
Erythrodermie avec epidermolyses	Debré 1939	
Toxicoderma bullosum	Guszman 1940	
Pemphigus aigu febrile	Griveaud and Mitarb 1946	
Toxic epidermal necrolysis	Lyell 1956	
Universelle epidermolysis acuta toxica	Korting and Holzmann 1960	
Syndrome de Lyell	Dugois and Mitarb 1961	
Syndrom der verbrühten Haut	Braun-Falco and Geissler 1962	
Lyell's syndrome	Jung and Mitarb 1964	
Staphylococcal scalded skin syndrome	Melish and Glasgow 1970	
Acute disseminated epidermal necrolysis (type III)	Ruiz-Maldonado 1985	

Table 5.101. Differences between staphylococcal and drug-induced Lyell's syndrome (from [28])

	Staphylococcal	Drug-induced
History	Mostly first episode	Sometimes previous incompatibility
Family history	*S. aureus* in family	∅
Drugs	Variable	Obligatory
Age	Newborn babies	Elderly
Skin pain	+++	±
Mucosal involvement	++	++
Conjunctival involvement	+	++
Blister formation	Subcorneal	Junctional

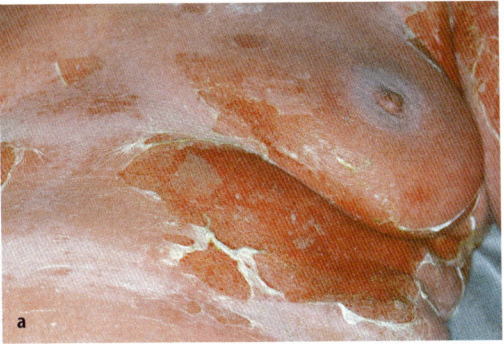
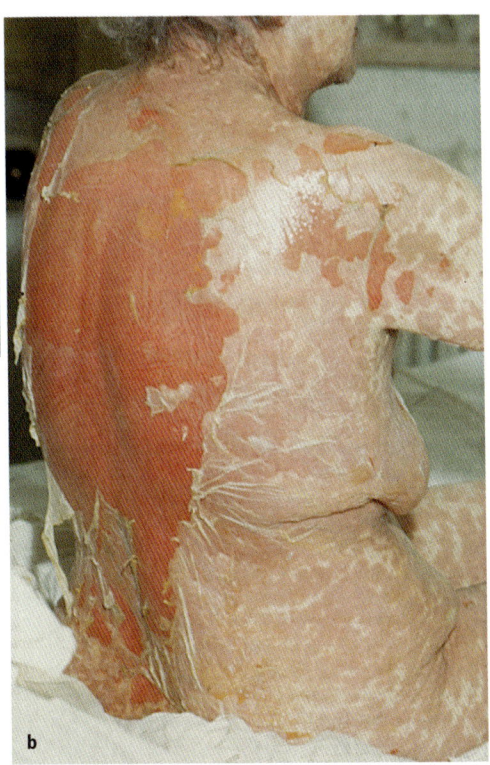

Fig. 5.82a,b. Detachment of large areas of the epidermis in a patient with a drug-induced Lyell's syndrome

the whole epidermis is filled with necrotic keratinocytes in the blister roof [39].

Clinical Symptoms and Dermatopathology. The clinical symptoms of Lyell's syndrome are dramatic in nature. After a prodromal phase with fever and unspecific complaints of the upper respiratory tract, often misinterpreted as a viral infection, macular eruptions occur, sometimes confluent and leading to large areas of epidermolysis (Fig. 5.82a,b). Nikolski I and II signs are positive. The patient is "swimming in his own skin." Mucous membranes are involved, and sometimes hair loss occurs.

After successful therapy, skin will heal within 2–4 weeks with large scaling of epidermal components. Finger- and toenails may be lost. Postinflammatory hyperpigmentation is common. Mucosal changes heal more slowly, especially in the eye, giving rise to synechia (Fig. 5.83). Generally, there is a severe disease (high fever!). Through the fluid loss, hypovolemia occurs, leading to shock. Superinfection may compromise other organs (pneumonia). Mucosal involvement gives rise to intestinal

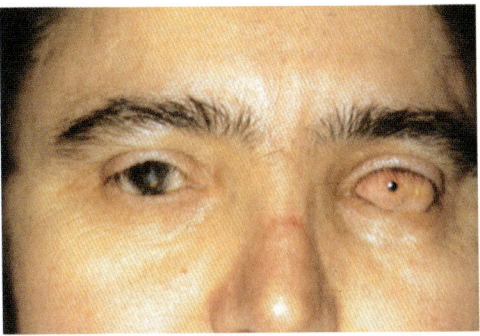

Fig. 5.83. Status post-Lyell's syndrome with scarified conjunctival lesions

bleeding. Toxic changes of the liver (dystrophy, toxic fattening) and the kidneys (tubular necrosis, interstitial nephritis) have been described as well as endocarditis, myocarditis, or central nervous involvement (cerebral edema, encephalomalacia) [11].

In dermatopathology, there is necrosis of the whole epidermis with only minimal inflammatory changes in the dermis ("empty corium"). Monoclonal antibodies may detect an increase in monocytoid cells in the epidermis [20, 51], which is in the blister roof (Fig. 5.84), in contrast to staphylococcal scalded skin syndrome with subcorneal blistering (Fig. 5.85, Table 5.102). The blister formation is junctional with the destruction of basal cells (Fig. 5.86).

Higher age groups are more often affected with female sex predilection (2:1). Rarely, there is a history of allergy. In France, a linkage to the HLA haplotypes A2, B12, and DR4 has been found [49].

Prognostic infaust factors include advanced age, late hospitalization, extent of blister formation, early leukopenia, initial renal insufficiency, as well as increased glucosemia. Lethality is around 30% in spite of the availability of most modern therapeutic modalities (15–50% in the literature) [45].

According to Schöpf, the risk of drug-induced Lyell's syndrome in the total population is 0.7 per 1 million inhabitants [53].

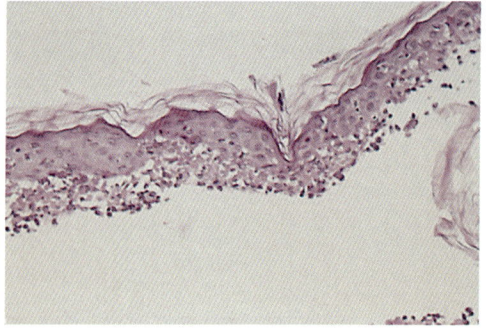

Fig. 5.84. Histological picture of a drug-induced Lyell's syndrome. The entire epidermis with necrotic keratinocytes is in the blister roof

Table 5.102. Comparison between staphylococcal scalded skin syndrome (SSSS), toxic shock syndrome (TSS), and toxic epidermal necrolysis (TEN)

	SSSS	TSS	TEN
Etiology	S. aureus (II)	S. aureus (I)	Drug (?)
Toxin	Exfoliatin	TSST-1	?
Blister formation	Subcorneal	Subgranular	Junctional
Mucosal involvement	±	++	++
Organ involvement		++	++

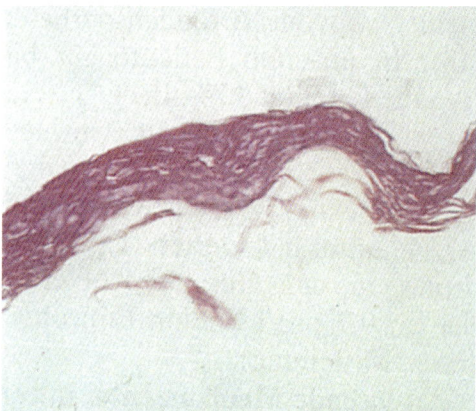

Fig. 5.85. Histological picture of a staphylogenic Lyell's syndrome: subcorneal blistering

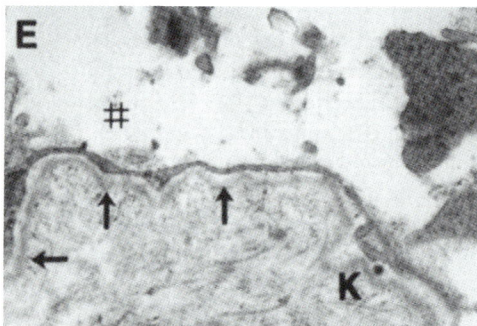

Fig. 5.86. Drug-induced Lyell's syndrome. The basement membrane (*arrow*) remains intact at the base of the continuity boundary. Above the lamina lucida there are cytoplasmic residues of necrotic keratinocytes (electron microscope magnification: 25,000:1). *E*, epidermis; *K*, corium; ↑ basement membrane; #, cytoplasmic residue of a necrotic keratinocyte (reprinted with the consent of Prof. Dr. C. Luderschmidt)

Eliciting Drugs. Many textbooks contain "hit lists" based on the literature, naming sulfonamides, analgesics, CNS-active drugs such as barbiturates and phenytoin besides many other drugs. The causal relation is difficult and sometimes arbitrary. Often, drugs are administered simultaneously (especially in elderly patients with 15 and more different drugs). The danger of "tautology" following reports from the literature is evident, leading to increased mentions of certain substances which have been mentioned before.

In a study of our own evaluating 306 cases, in only 67 patients, clear-cut evidence for a suspected drug was found (criterion: single or only recently introduced drug or proved by reexposure). However, we have seen a patient who reacted to carbamazepine, which he had been taking over 4 years as a single drug prior to TEN [45].

In a critical evaluation, there is no totally safe drug. We observed a case elicited by a herbal tea (devil's claw) as well as cases elicited by eyedrops (Borelli, personal communication), isoproterenol powder or tonic water [11, 18, 45].

In Germany, the documentation center for severe cutaneous reactions has been recording for 10 years all bullous drug eruptions occurring in Germany. Evaluation and classification is done through an expert committee leading to a list of eliciting drugs (Table 5.103).

Diagnostic Procedures in TEN. Besides the clinical and dermatopathological diagnosis (Table 5.104), allergy tests may be helpful in single cases. Positive skin tests or in vitro lymphocyte transformation tests have revealed sensitizations [54]. We observed positive skin tests in two out of four tested persons with severe TEN [32, 45]. Looking through the literature, there is no evidence that a careful skin test (prick or patch test) may induce generalized TEN symptoms.

Rarely oral provocation has been tried [28] successfully. Many authors, however, do not recommend it. If there is an indication, one should use an extremely low starting dose (1/1,000 of a single dose and lower) and apply only one substance per day under inpatient conditions.

Therapy of TEN. Therapy consists of general, local, and systemic procedures (Table 5.105), as well as the observation of certain items to avoid (Fig. 5.87). Local therapy includes early ophthalmologic counseling for prevention of synechia with hourly application of eyedrops!

Table 5.103. Suspected drugs as elicitors of TEN

Sulfonamides
Aminopenicillins
Quinolones
Chlormezanone
Carbamazepine
Phenobarbital
Phenytoin
Valproic acid
NSAIDs
Allopurinol

Table 5.104. Diagnosis of Lyell's syndrome

- Dermatological examination
- Blister cryosection
- Biopsy (immunochemistry)
- Asservation of serum (for later investigation)
- Bacteriological swabs (skin, mucosa, specific foci)
  - Phage typing and toxin detection
  - Blood culture
- In vitro diagnosis (e.g., lymphocyte transformation, controls!)
- Skin test (after 2–3 months)
  - Patch test
  - Prick, intradermal (dilution! one substance/day)

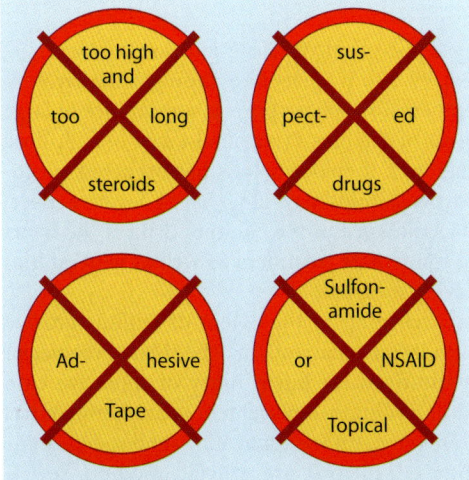

Fig. 5.87. Four important "Don'ts" when treating Lyell's syndrome

Table 5.105. Drug-induced Lyell's syndrome therapy

General measures
Hospitalization in single room, intensive care or burn center
Warmth
Special bedding
Fluid, electrolytes, colloid replacement[a]
Nutrition through gastric tube
Withdrawal of suspected drugs
Plasmapheresis?

Local therapy
Balneotherapy (antiseptics)
Metallic foil
Debridement of necrotic epidermis
Antiseptics ($AgNO_3$, crystal violet, 0.1%, chlorhexidine)
Antibiotic gaze (furantoin, povidone iodine)
Covering (polyurethane)
Mucosal care (oral mucosa, genitals)
Eye prophylaxis (scleral lenses, artificial tears, hourly)
Avoid suspected topicals!
No adhesive tape!!

Systemic drug therapy
In the acute phase (prior to necrolysis) glucocorticosteroids
(e.g., days 1–4: 1,000, 250, 100, 20 mg prednisolone)
Caveat: high-dose long-term treatment!
Antibiotics
If sepsis is suspected or leukopenia (prophylactic?)
Choice of not suspected agents (e.g., cephalosporins, imipenem)
Heparin (thrombosis prophylaxis)
Central analgesics (selection according to history)

[a] Not only according to the "rule of 9" but controlled according to excretion, body weight, urine, and serum electrolytes, etc.

Systemic glucocorticosteroids are controversial [30, 49, 50]. We give steroids only in the early exanthematous phase prior to appearance of large areas of necrolysis (maximal 4 days of high-dose therapy). If epidermolysis has occurred, glucocorticosteroids may rather have a negative effect.

Avoidance of the eliciting drug is the focus of immediate treatment as well as general life-saving measures.

According to the extent of bullous erosive skin lesions, patients may be treated in special institutions for burn injury or intensive care units. Volume replacement, parenteral nutrition, temperature application, and special bedding (Clinitron) are crucial. Medium-severe cases have been treated successfully isolated under hygienic conditions in a single room.

In order to influence the immune reaction, the following drugs have been tried:

- Cyclophosphamide
- Cyclosporin A
- Thalidomide as TNF inhibitor
- Intravenous immunoglobulin G
- Protease inhibitors (ulinastatin)
- Plasmapheresis

But only case reports or small numbers have been published [13, 17, 25, 30, 45, 49, 56, 59].

The immediate and adequate general therapy is the performance of life-saving measures. Due to pathophysiologic considerations and possible involvement of microbial toxins as well as the avoidance of sepsis, prophylactic antibiotics with unsuspicious agents are recommended by some authors.

5.7.3.3 Pathophysiology of Cutaneous Drug Eruptions

While urticarial reactions may often be due to IgE-mediated or pseudo-allergic reactions, thrombocytopenic purpura represents a cytotoxic reaction, hemorrhagic vasculitic phenomena an immune complex reaction. The mechanisms of the colorful spectrum of exanthematous drug eruptions, however, are not well established (Table 5.106).

In dermatopathology, superficial perivascular mononuclear cell infiltrate is seen sometimes with eosinophils. Often a so-called interface dermatitis with lymphocytes at the dermoepidermal junction is seen [61].

Immunohistochemistry shows a predominant T-cell (CD3+) infiltrate with both CD4 and CD8 cells. CD1a+ dendritic cells and CD68 macrophages are also increased as well as CD56+ natural killer cells. Major basis protein from eosinophils can be detected.

Activated T cells are also CLA positive and may maintain inflammatory reactions through cytokines (IL-5, IL-6, TNFα) or chemokines (eotaxin, RANTES) [19, 36, 43].

Furthermore, cytotoxic T cells may directly destroy keratinocytes either via Fas/Fas ligand (rather unlikely) or more probably via a cytotoxic mechanism through perforin and granzyme B.

Table 5.106. Pathophysiology of various forms of drug eruptions

Clinical manifestations	Suspected pathomechanism	Differential diagnosis
Urticarial eruption	IgE, serum sickness	Focus (infection, tumor)
Erythematovesicular	Systemic contact	Toxic dermatitis, eczema atopic eczema
Purpura		
– Thrombopenic	Type II	Coagulation defect
– Vasculitic	Type III	Infection, tumor
– Purpura chronica progressiva	?	
– Purpura senilis	Cortisone effect	Atrophy, vitamin deficiency
Macular and maculopapular (special case: ampicillin rash)	Type IV? (B-cell stimulation?)	Viral exanthema
Exfoliative dermatitis, scarlatiniform eruption	Type IV?	Scarlet fever (toxic shock syndrome)
Bullous drug eruption (erythema exsudativum multiforme, EEM)	Type III/type IVc	Postherpetic EEM
Erythema nodosum	Type III?	Sarcoidosis, infection
Fixed drug eruption	Type IVc	
Toxic epidermal necrolysis	Type IVc	Staphylococcals, scalded
Skin syndrome		
Lichenoid eruption	?	Lichen planus
Acneiform eruption	?	Acne vulgaris
Psoriasiform eruption	?	Psoriasis vulgaris
Lymphohistocytic reaction	Type IV	Pseudolymphoma

The role of proinflammatory cytokines is supported by the common coincidence of concomitant infections in the eliciting phase. It may be that different cell populations (CD4 or CD8 cells) with different activation mechanisms induce different clinical symptoms. The metabolism of the drug via different routes (acetylation, glutathione transferase, cytochrome P450, etc.) is important [22, 37].

Table 5.107 lists some possible immunologic and non-immunologic reactions which play a role in the pathogenesis of TEN (hypothetical). Animal experiments have shown similarities between GVH and TEN [38].

The differential diagnosis between TEN and toxic shock syndrome (TSS) may be difficult [23, 58]. TSS is defined by: fever, exanthema (diffuse, sometimes with erythroderma or vesiculation), mucous membrane involvement, hypotension, multiorgan affection, as well as exclusion of other infectious diseases [15].

TEN and TSS have some things in common: prodromi, certain laboratory findings (liver enzymes), mucosal involvement, multiorgan affection. However, in the majority of TSS patients, no large epidermolysis occurs, but rather desquamative exfoliative dermatitis (especially palmoplantar) after 8–10 days (similar to scarlet fever).

Table 5.107. Toxic epidermal necrolysis: pathophysiological concepts

Immunologic reactions
Allergy (type II): antibodies or cytotoxic T cells against keratinocytes?
Allergy (type III): immunoglobulin and complement deposits
Allergy (type IV): positive patch tests and lymphocyte transformation
Graft versus host reaction: altered self?
Monocyte-mediated cytotoxicity?
Combination of infection and drug
Photosensitization
Non-immunologic reaction
Pharmacotoxicity in enzyme deficiency
Enzyme activation
Activated oxygen species
Combination: virus/drug?
Combination: UV/drug?
Microbial toxins (prodromi through toxin, interleukin-1)?

The staphylococcal toxin of TSS (TSST-1) induces necrosis in the stadium granulosum in animal experiments with keratinocyte necrosis in contrast to the exfoliatin of staphylococcal Lyell's syndrome with subcorneal blisters. Dermatologically, TEN can be clearly differentiated from other bullous drug eruptions (Table 5.108).

Table 5.108. Dermatopathological patterns of bullous drug eruptions

Fixed drug eruption
Vacuolar degeneration of basal keratinocytes
Single cell keratinization
Single cell necrosis
Superficial and deep perivascular infiltrate (lymphohistiocytic and neutrophils)
Erythrocyte extravasate
Pigment incontinence

Erythema multiforme
Vacuolar degeneration of basal keratinocytes
Single cell keratinization
Single cell necrosis
Interface dermatitis
Superficial perivascular infiltrate (lymphohistiocytic)
Erythrocyte extravasate

Drug-induced Lyell's syndrome (toxic epidermal necrolysis)
Complete necrosis of epidermis
Junctional blister formation
Little inflammatory infiltrates ("empty corium")
Possibly thrombi in dermal vessels

Table 5.110. Genuine skin diseases provoked by drugs

Acanthosis nigricans	Gestagens
Acne vulgaris	Androgens, gestagens
Bullous pemphigoid	Furosemide, salazosulfapyridine
Dermatitis herpetiformis	Halogens, progesterone
Lichen planus	Gold, arsenic, quinine, sulfonamides
Lupus erythematosus	Hydralazine, isoniazid, procainamide, phenytoin, phenylbutazone
Pemphigus vulgaris	D-Penicillamine
Porphyria cutanea tarda	Alcohol, analgesics, androgens, barbiturates, contraceptives, sulfonamides

5.7.3.4 Special Forms of Drug-Induced Skin Diseases

After intake of some drugs, specific dermatologic symptoms may be induced (Table 5.109).

Some genuine dermatoses may be provoked by drugs such as lichen planus by gold and sulfonamides, lupus erythematosus by hydralazine and procainamide, or psoriasiform drug eruptions by beta-blockers (Table 5.110).

Many cases are characterized by mucosal membrane involvement only ("stomatitis medicamentosa") [2]. These conditions need to be distinguished from contact-allergic reactions (against dental prostheses) as well as the toxic effects of some drugs as cytostatics. Drugs inducing stomatitis medicamentosa include

Table 5.109. Skin changes due to drugs (selection)

Morphology	Example
Exanthematous drug eruptions	(see Table 5.98)
Pruritus	Opioids, belladonna, laxatives
Sebostasis	Retinoids
Pigmentary changes	Metals (silver, gold, bismuth, mercury), antimalarials (gray-yellow), clofazimine (red), gestagens, estrogens (melasma)
Atrophy/striae	Glucocorticosteroids
Keratoses, tumors	Arsenic, cytostatics, levodopa (melanoma?)
Nail changes	Cytostatics, photosensitization, beta-blockers
Alopecia	Cytostatics, steroids, anticoagulants, retinoids
Skin color changes	Chloroquine, mephenesin, bleomycin
Hypertrichosis	Diazoxide, minoxidil, cyclosporin
Iododerma/bromoderma	Halogens
Palmoplantar pustulosis	Lithium
Pseudolymphoma	Phenytoin, analgesics, menthol
Photosensitization	See Sect. 5.6
Granuloma	See Sect. 5.8
Embolia cutis	Antirheumatics, steroids
Necroses	Coumarin, barbiturates, ergotaminine, see vasculitis allergica (Sect. 5.3)
Mucosal changes	See Sect. 5.5

heavy metals (mercury, gold), antibiotics (sulfonamides, chloramphenicol, streptomycin), local anesthetics, hypnotics (barbiturates, hydantoin), and analgesics (phenylbutazone, aminopyrine) [2].

References

1. Aberer W, Stingl G, Wolff K (1982) Stevens-Johnson-Syndrom und toxische epidermale Nekrolyse nach Sulfonamideinnahme. Hautarzt 33:484–490
2. Archard HO (1979) Stomatologic disorders of an internal and integumental nature. In: Fitzpatrick TB, Eisen AZ, Wolff K, Freedberg IM, Austen KF (eds) Dermatology in general medicine. McGraw Hill, New York, p 834
3. Arndt KA, Jick H (1976) Rate of cutaneous reactions to drugs. J Am Med Assoc 235:918
4. Bachot N, Roujeau J-C (2001) Physiopathology and treatment of severe drug eruptions. Curr Opin Allergy Clin Immunol 1:293–298
5. Barreiro P, Soriano V, Casas E, et al. (2000) Prevention of nevirapine-associated exanthema using slow dose escalation and/or corticosteroids. AIDS 14:2153–2157
6. Behrendt H, Gollnick H, Bonnekoh B (2000) Upregulated perforin expression of CD8+ blood lymphocytes in generalized non-anaphylactic drug eruptions and exacerbated psioriasis. Eur J Dermatol 10:365–369
7. Bergner T, Przybilla B, Ring J (1989) Anaphylactoid reaction to the coloring agent Erythrosine in an antiallergic drug. Allergy Clin Immunol News 1:177–179
8. Bigby M, Stern R (1985) Cutaneous reactions to nonsteroidal anti-inflammatory drugs. J Am Acad Dermatol 12:866–876
9. Billingham RE, Streilein JW (1968) Toxic epidermal necrolysis and homologous disease in hamsters. Arch Dermatol 98:528
10. Bork K (1985) Kutane Arzneimittelnebenwirkungen. Unerwünschte Wirkungen systemisch verabreichter Medikamente an Haut und hautnahen Schleimhäuten bei Erwachsenen und Kindern. Schattauer, Stuttgart
11. Braun-Falco O, Bandmann HJ (eds) (1970) Das Lyell-Syndrom. Das Syndrom der verbrühten Haut. Huber, Bern
12. Braun-Falco O, Plewig G, Wolff HH (1998) Dermatologie und Venerologie, 4th edn. Springer, Berlin Heidelberg New York
13. Craven NM (2000) Management of toxic epidermal necrolysis. Hosp Med 61:778–781
14. Crowson AN, Magro CM (1999) Recent advances in the pathology of cutaneous drug eruptions. Dermatol Clin 17:537–560
15. Davis JP, Chesney PJ, Wand PJ, LaVenture M (1980) Toxic-shock syndrome: Epidemiologic features, recurrence, risk factors and prevention. N Engl J Med 303:1429–1435
16. Fellner MJ, Prutkin L (1970) Morbilliform eruptions caused by penicillin. A study by electron microscopy and immunologic tests. J Invest Dermatol 55:390–395
17. French LE, Tschopp J (2000) Fas-mediated cell death in toxic epidermal necrolysis and graft-versus-host disease; potential for therapeutic inhibition. Schweiz Med Wochenschr 130:1656–1661
18. Goerz G, Ruzicka T (1978) Lyell-Syndrom. Grosse, Berlin
19. Gutierrez-Ramos JC, Lloyd C, Gonzalo JA (1999) Eotaxin from an eosinophilic chemokine to a major regulator of allergic reactions. Immunol Today 20:500–504
20. Hari Y, Frutig-Schnyder K, Hurni M, Yawalkar N, Zanni MP, Schnyder B, Kappeler A, von Greyerz S, Braathen LR, Pichler WJ (2001) T cell involvement in cutaneous drug eruptions. Clin Exp Allergy 31:1398–1408
21. Hofmann C, Burg G, Jung C (1986) Kutane Nebenwirkungen der Goldtherapie. Klinische und histologische Ergebnisse. Z Rheum 45:100–106
22. Hertl M, Jugert F, Merk HF (1995) CD8+ dermal T cells from a sulphamethoxazole-induced bullous exanthem proliferate in response to drug-modified liver microsomes. Br J Dermatol 132: 215–220
23. Hurwitz M, Rivera HP, Gooch MH, Slama TG, Handt A, Weiss J (1982) Toxic shock syndrome or toxic epidermal necrolysis? J Am Acad Dermatol 7:246–254
24. Kaplan AP (1984) Drug induced skin disease. J Allergy Clin Immunol 74:573–579
25. Kasemir H, Kerp L (1980) Arzneimittel-Allergene und Arzneimittel-Allergien. In: Filipp G (ed) Allergologie, vol 1. Ätiopathogenese. Werk-Verlag, Gräfelfing, p 144
26. Kauppinen K, Stubb S (1984) Drug eruptions: Causative agents and clinical types. A series of inpatients during a 10-year period. Acta Derm Venereol (Stockh) 64:320–324
27. Kazmierowski JA, Wuepper KD (1981) Erythema multiforme: Clinical spectrum and immunopathogenesis. Springer Semin Immunopathol 4:45
28. Kleinhans D, Fuchs T (1984) Orale Provokation bei einem durch Barbitursäure verursachten Lyell-Syndrom. Akt Derm 10:122–124
29. Knowles SR, Uetrecht J, Shear NH (2000) Idiosyncratic drug reactions: the reactive metabolite syndromes. Lancet 356:1587–1591
30. Konstantinow A, Mühlbauer W, Balda BR, Ring J (2001) Toxische epidermale Nekrolysen (Arzneimittel-induziertes Lyell-Syndrom). Dtsch Med Wochenschr 126:141–144, 177–179
31. Le Cleach L, Delaire S, Boumsell L, et al (2000) Blister fluid T lymphocytes during toxic epidermal necrolysis are functional cytotoxic cells

which express human natural killer (NK) inhibitory receptors. Clin Exp Immunol 119:225–230
32. Luderschmidt C, Linderkamp O, Ring J (1985) Drug-induced toxic epidermal necrolysis (Lyell's syndrome) in a 4-year-old girl. Eur J Pediatr 14:91–93
33. Lyell A (1956) Toxic epidermal necrolysis: an eruption resembling scalding of the skin. Br J Dermatol 68:355–361
34. Lyell A (1967) A review of toxic epidermal necrolysis in Britain. Br J Derm 79:662–671
35. Marghescu S (1978) Allergische Arznei-Exantheme. Pathomechanismus – Klinik – Testung – Therapie. Perimed, Erlangen
36. Merk H, Gerecke D (1986) Arzneimittelnebenwirkungen bei Patienten mit LAV/HTLV-III-Infektion. AIDS-Bericht 2. Grosse, Berlin, pp 139–142
37. Merk HF, Hertl M (1996) Immunologic mechanisms of cutaneous drug reactions. Semin Cutan Med Surg 15:228–235
38. Merot Y, Saurat JH (1985) Clues to pathogenesis of toxic epidermal necrolysis. Int J Dermatol 24:165–168
39. Mockenhaupt M, Norgauer J (2001) Schwere arzneimittelinduzierte Hautreaktionen. Allergologie 24:419–432
40. Mougdil A, Porat S, Brunnel P, Jordan SC (1995) Treatment of Stevens-Johnson syndrome with pooled human intravenous immune globulin. Clin Pediatrics 34:47–51
41. Murphy GF, Guillén FJ, Flynn TC (1985) Cytotoxic T lymphocytes and phenotypically abnormal epidermal dendritic cells in fixed cutaneous eruptions. Hum Pathol 16:1264–1271
42. Pichler WJ, Yawalkar N (2000) Allergic reactions to drugs: involvement of T cells. Thorax 55 [Suppl 2]:S61–S65
43. Pichler WJ, Zanni M, von Greyerz S, et al. (1997) High IL-5 production by human drug-specific T cell clones. Int Arch Allergy Immunol 113:177–180
44. Ring J (1987) Diagnostik von Arzneimittel-bedingten Unverträglichkeitsreaktionen. Hautarzt 38:16–22
45. Ring J (1989) Drug-induced Leyell's syndrome (toxic epidermal necrolysis). In: Pichler WJ, et al. (eds) Progress in allergy and clinical immunology. Hogrefe & Huber, Toronto, pp 455–461
46. Ring J, Przybilla B, Gollhausen R (1989) Progressive pigmentary purpura provoked by a phytotherapeutic drug containing Echinacea extract. Allergy Clin Immunol News 114:108–109
47. Ring J, Kraus K, Fröschl M, Brunner R, Przybilla B, Burg G, Braun-Falco O (1987) AIDS, HIV-Infektion und allergische Reaktionen. AIDS Forschung 2:643–646
48. Roujeau JC, Kelly JP, Naldi L, et al. (1995) Medication use and the risk of Stevens-Johnson syndrome or toxic epidermal necrolysis. N Engl J Med 333:1600–1607
49. Roujeau J-C, Stern RS (1994) Severe cutaneous adverse reactions to drugs. N Engl J Med 331:1272–1285
50. Ruiz-Maldonado R (1985) Acute disseminated epidermal necrosis types 1, 2, and 3: Study of sixty cases. J Am Acad Dermatol 13:623–635
51. Rzany B, Hering O, Mockenhaupt M, et al. (1996) Histopathological and epidemiological characteristics of patients with erythema exudativum multiforme major, Stevens-Johnson syndrome and toxic epidermal necrolysis. Br J Dermatol 135:6–11
52. Sachs B, Merk H (2001) Demonstration and characterization of drug-specific lymphocyte reactivity in drug allergies. Allergy Clin Immunol Int 13:91–98
53. Schöpf E, Stühmer A, Rzany B, Victor N, Zentgraf R, Kapp JF (1991) Toxic epidermal necrolysis and Stevens-Johnson syndrome. An epidemiologic study from West Germany. Arch Dermatol 127:839–842
54. Schulz KH (1966) Stellenwert und Aussagekraft von Testmethoden bei allergischen Arznei-Exanthemen. In: Braun-Falco O, Wolff HH (1979) Fortschritte der praktischen Dermatologie und Venerologie, vol 9. Springer, Berlin Heidelberg New York, p 71
55. Steigleder GK (1966) Haut. In: Heintz R (ed) Erkrankungen durch Arzneimittel. Diagnostik, Klinik, Pathogenese und Therapie. Thieme, Stuttgart, pp 103–130
56. Schulz JT, Sheridan RL, Ryan CM, et al. (2000) A 10-year experience with toxic epidermal necrolysis. J Burn Care Rehabil 21:199–204
57. Smith CL, Brown I, Torraca BM (1997) Acetylator status and tolerance of high-dose trimethoprim-sulfamethoxazole therapy among patients infected with human immunodeficiency virus. Clin Infect Dis 25:1477–1478
58. Todd J, Fishaut M, Kapral F, Welch T (1978) Toxic-shock syndrome associated with phage-group-I staphylococci. Lancet II:1116–1118
59. Viard I, Wehrli P, Bullani R, et al. (1998) Inhibition of toxic epidermal necrolysis by blockade of CD95 with human intravenous immunoglobulin. Science 282:490–493
60. Stern RS, Wintroub BU (1999) Cutaneous reactions to drugs. In: Freedberg IM, Eisen AZ, Wolff K, et al. (eds) Fitzpatrick's dermatology in general medicine, 5th edn. McGraw Hill, New York, pp 1633–1642
61. Wolff HH, Winzer M (1986) Histopathological patterns of drug eruptions. In: Ring J, Burg G (eds) New trends in allergy II. Springer, Berlin Heidelberg New York, pp 240–253
62. Zürcher K, Krebs A (1992) Cutaneous drug reactions. Karger, Basel

5.8 Granulomatous Reactions

In some textbooks, type IV reactions include both allergic contact dermatitis and tuberculin reactions under the common pathophysiology of sensitized T-lymphocyte reaction with a difference of route of administration (epidermal versus intradermal). The kinetics of tuberculin correspond to a maximum between 48 and 72 h after intradermal administration of allergen to those with epidermal patch test reactions.

Quite different kinetics (3–5 weeks) are characteristic of the lepromin reaction as well as some other granulomatous infectious diseases characterized by typical histopathology with epithelioid cell granulomas [6, 11, 26]. The clear-cut differences in clinical symptomatology, dermatohistopathology, and kinetics [3, 29, 30] justify a separate classification of granulomatous hypersensitivity reactions as type V (see Chap. 1).

Granulomatous reactions are inflammatory changes occurring with slow development over 3–5 weeks and long-lasting persistence; histologically, they are characterized by typical epithelioid cell granuloma formation in the upper and mid dermis. In the skin brownish-red or livid nodules are characteristic, sometimes showing a "lupoid" infiltrate under the diascope [6].

5.8.1 Clinical Examples

Common clinical examples of allergic reactions of the granulomatous type V are the zirconium granuloma after application of zirconium-containing deodorants with histologically typical epithelioid cell granulomas without necrosis together with lymphocytic infiltrates with foreign bodies in polarization microscopy [30].

Rare subcutaneous granuloma formations after allergen-specific subcutaneous immunotherapy can equally be classified as type V, especially after application of aluminum hydroxide adsorbed allergen extracts [2]. In some cases, these granulomas may change into subcutaneous pseudolymphomas [15].

After repeated intradermal administration of procaine polyvinylpyrrolidone (PVP) for back pain, one of our patients developed multi-

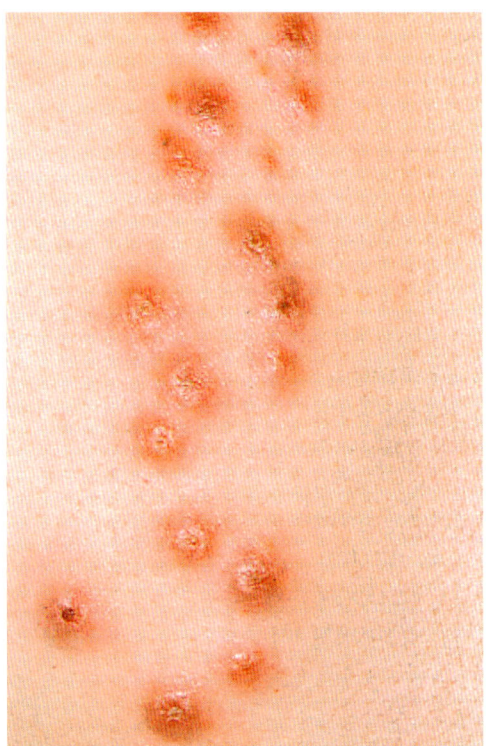

Fig. 5.88. Multiple circumscribed brownish-red nodules at the injection site following the repeated intradermal administration of procaine polyvinylpyrrolidone (PVP) to alleviate back pain (from [3])

ple brownish-red sharply margined nodules at the injection sites, histologically resembling sarcoid granuloma without clinical evidence for sarcoidosis (Figs. 5.88, 5.89). Earlier administrations had been tolerated without adverse reaction. In the intradermal test, a positive granulomatous reaction was observed [3]. Similar granulomas have been described after administration of other PVP-containing substances [4], whereby often clear storage processes were evident in contrast to the hypersensitivity reaction to minute amounts as observed in our patient.

In dermatological practice, granulomatous reactions have gained relevance against soluble bovine collagen used for the correction of scars and wrinkles [7, 8, 12, 16–20, 27, 29]. Therefore, prior to such treatment, a test injection needs to be performed, which can lead to clinically visible nodule formation in 0.3% of the

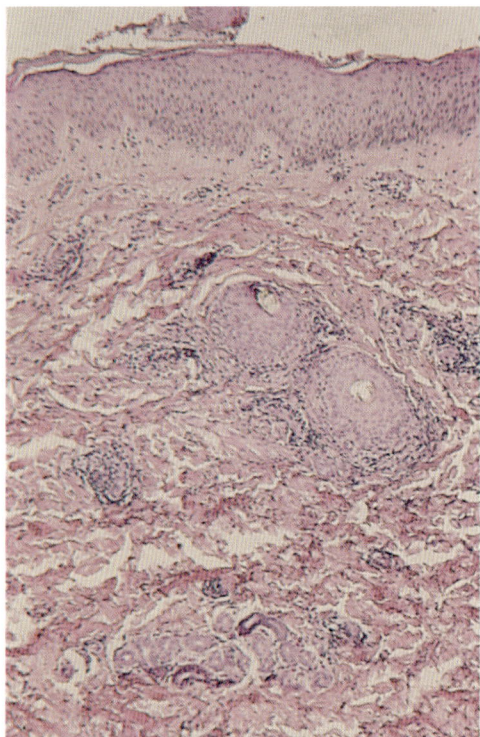

Fig. 5.89. Histological examination of the lesions shown in Fig. 5.88 yields the picture of sarcoid granuloma even though there is no clinical evidence of sarcoidosis (from [3])

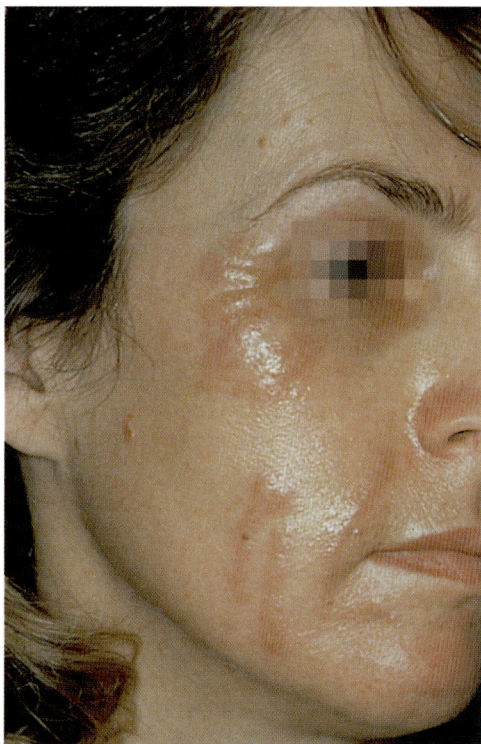

Fig. 5.90. Protruding hard inflammatory lesions following the injection of soluble bovine collagen in a patient with type V allergy (from [29])

patients [7]. Without this test injection or when sensitization occurs during the first treatment, long-lasting persistent granulomatous inflammatory skin reactions may develop at the injection site (Figs. 5.90, 5.91) [29].

5.8.2 Pathophysiology

Activation of T cells and macrophages for elimination of infectious agents plays a major role in immune defense (especially against intracellular microorganisms). When antigen cannot be eliminated totally, this can lead to continuous T-cell activation and macrophage reactions with accumulation of epithelioid cells and formation of giant cells. Macrophages which have taken up bacterial antigens and present those may be destroyed by cytotoxic T cells, as well as by natural killer cells in an unspecific manner. Therefore, in granulomatous reactions, immunophenotyping often shows T cells, NK cells, and macrophages together with activated fibroblasts.

The mechanism of activation of NK cells – especially the recently discovered NKT-cell subpopulation – is not well understood [22]. It seems that NKT cells appear early in the reaction while classic NK cells may stay for a longer time at the inflammatory site [23] and mediate or elicit functions of innate immunity. Among the various cytokines, especially a member of the lymphotoxin family, namely LTα3, plays a major role in the recruitment of lymphocytes and macrophages and, thus, the persistence of granuloma formation [24].

In the complex interaction between sensitized lymphocytes producing certain cytokines [22] and macrophages, possibly also immune complex phenomena (high antibody titers of the IgG class) may be involved. In the above-described case of bovine collagen hypersensitivi-

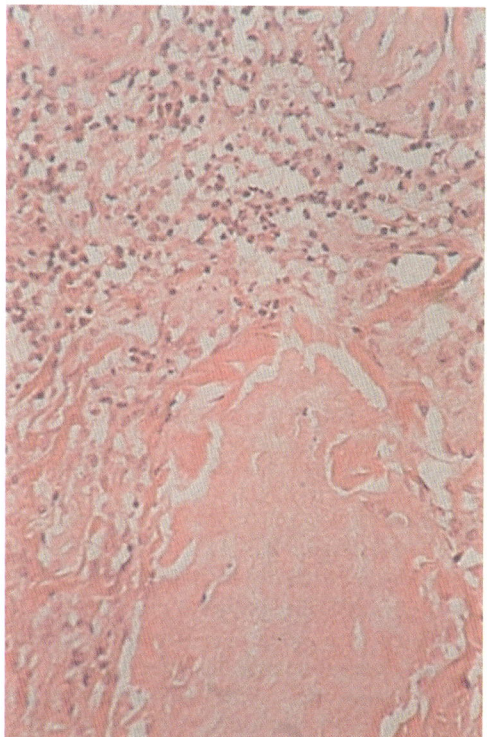

Fig. 5.91. Granulomatous infiltrate surrounding streaky eosinophilic material (injected collagen) seen in the histological preparation (from [29])

ty, a high IgG antibody antititer against bovine collagen was found [29].

A concomitant or subsequent following of immune complex reaction and granulomatous inflammation also is characteristic for the chronic stage of extrinsic allergic alveolitis (hypersensitivity pneumonitis). On the basis of these considerations, a hypothetical concept may be suggested: Persistent antigen induces after an initial type III reaction with vasculitis a strong activation of macrophages, leading finally to granulomatous inflammation. In hypersensitivity pneumonitis in the early phase changes similar to leukocytoclastic vasculitis can be seen together with high titers of precipitating antibodies, while in the chronic course the histologic pattern of granulomatous inflammation develops (see Sect. 5.4 on "Hypersensitivity Pneumonitis").

It is tempting to speculate about the pathophysiology of some other granulomatous inflammatory skin diseases such as granuloma anulare, sarcoidosis, Melkersson-Rosenthal syndrome, M. Crohn, Wegener's granulomatosis, or Churg-Strauss granulomatosis. Some common features of these diseases might be explained by a deposit of a persisting yet unknown antigen.

In granuloma anulare in the early phase, signs of vasculitis with positive immunofluorescence [9, 14] can be found. It is a well-known clinical experience that granuloma anulare sometimes develops after insect stings or minimal trauma and can heal spontaneously after skin biopsy (removal of persistent antigen?). Development of granuloma anulare after injection of soluble collagen has been described [22]. We observed an exacerbation of scar sarcoidosis under immunotherapy with interferon which had been silent for decades [10].

5.8.3 Therapy

Treatment uses glucocorticosteroids (according to the organ manifestation). In granulomatous reactions of the skin, intralesional steroids or occlusion treatment should be tried [3, 6, 29]; also cytostatic therapy, tuberculostatic drugs as well as UVA-1 irradiation have been used.

References

1. Apostolou I, Takahama Y, Belmant C, Kawanos T, Huerre M, Marchal G, Cui J, Taniguchi M, Nakauchi H, Fournié J-J, Kourilsky P, Gachelin G (1999) Murine natural killer cells contribute to the granulomatous reaction caused by mycobacterial cell walls. Proc Natl Acad Sci USA 96:5141–5146
2. Baumgarten C (1978) Häufigste Nebenwirkungen bei der spezifischen Hyposensibilisierung. Allergologie 1:223–228
3. Bode U, Ring J, Schmoeckel Chr (1984) Granulombildung nach intrakutaner Applikation von Procain-Polyvinylpyrrolidon (PVP). Hautarzt 35:474–477
4. Bork K, Hoede N (1982) Vortäuschung maligner Tumoren durch nicht deklariertes PVP in Arzneimitteln. Hautarzt 33:373–377
5. Boros DL (1981) The role of lymphokines in granulomatous inflammations. Lymphokines 3:257–281
6. Braun-Falco O, Plewig G, Wolff HH (1998) Derma-

tologie und Venerologie, 4th edn. Springer, Berlin Heidelberg New York
7. Castrow FF II, Krull E (1983) An injectable collagen implant – update. J Am Acad Dermatol 9: 889–893
28. Cooperman LS, Mackinnon V, Bechler G, Pharriss BB (1983) Injectable collagen: A six-year clinical investigation. Aesth Plast Surg 9:145–151
9. Dahl M, Ullmann S, Goetz RW (1977) Vasculitis in granuloma anulare. Arch Dermatol 113:463–467
10. Eberlein-König B, Hein R, Abeck D, Engst R, Ring J (1999) Cutaneous sarcoid foreign body granulomas developing in sites of previous skin injury after systemic interferon-alpha treatment for chronic hepatitis C. Br J Dermatol 140:370–372
11. Eder M, Gedigk P (1986) Lehrbuch der allgemeinen Pathologie und pathologischen Anatomie. Springer, Berlin Heidelberg New York
12. Ellingsworth LR, DeLustro F, Brennan JE, Sawamura S, McPherson J (1986) The human immune response to reconstituted bovine collagen. J Immunol 36:877–882
13. Harms M, Masouyé I, Saurat JH (1990) Silica granuloma mimicking granulomatous cheilitis. Dermatologica 181:246–247
14. Kleinhans D, Knoth W (1977) Immunhistochemischer Fibrin-Nachweis beim Granuloma anulare. Arch Dermatol Res 258:231–234
15. Klepzig K, Ring J, Burg G (1987) Pseudolymphom nach Hyposensibilisierung. Allergologie 10:432
16. Kligman AM, Armstrong RC (1986) Histologic response to intradermal zyderm und zyplast (glutaraldehyde crosslinked) collagen in humans. J Dermatol Surg Oncol 12:351–357
17. Konz B (1983) Injizierbares Kollagen. In: Braun-Falco O, Burg G (eds) Fortschritte der praktischen Dermatologie und Venerologie, vol. 10, pp 193–198. Springer, Berlin Heidelberg New York
18. Kuhn K, Timpl R (1984) Collagens. Molecular and antigenic structure. In: Myelofibrosis and the biology of connective tissue, p. 45. Liss, New York
19. Lombardi T, Kuffer R, Dubrez B (2001) Polishing-paste-induced silica granuloma of the gingiva. Dermatology 203:177–179
20. McCoy JP, Schade WJ, Siegle RJ, Vanderveen EE, Zachary CB, Waldinger TP, Swanson NY (1987) Immune responses to bovine collagen implants. J Am Acad Dermatol 16:955–960
22. Rapaport M (1984) Granuloma annulare caused by injectable collagen. Arch Dermatol 120:837
23. Raupach B, Kaufman S (2001) Immune responses to intracellular bacteria. Curr Opin Immunol 13:417–428
24. Roach DR, Briscoe H, Saunders B, France MP, Riminton S, Britton WJ (2001) Secreted lymphotoxin-alpha is essential for the control of an intracellular bacterial infection. J Exp Med 193:239–246
25. Roitt I, Delves P (2001) Essential immunology, 10th edn. Blackwell, Oxford
26. Sandritter W, Beneke G (1984) Allgemeine Pathologie. Schattauer, Stuttgart
27. Sellem PH, Caranzan FR, Bene MC, Faure GC (1987) Immunogenicity of injectable collagen implants. J Dermatol Surg Oncol 13:1199–1202
28. Shelley WB, Hurley HJ (1960) The pathogenesis of silica granulomas in man: A nonallergic colloidal phenomenon. J Invest Dermatol 34:107–123
29. Schurig V, Konz B, Ring J, Dorn M (1986) Granulombildung an Test- und Behandlungsstellen durch intrakutan verabreichtes, injizierbares Kollagen. Hautarzt 37:42–45
30. Shelley WB, Hurrley HJ (1958) The allergic origin of zirconium deodorant granulomas. Br J Dermatol 70:75–82

5.9 Type VI Reactions (Stimulating/Neutralizing Hypersensitivity)

While the pathology of allergic diseases types I–V is mainly due to activation of humoral or cellular inflammatory systems, the pathologic response of type VI reactions occurs through direct interaction of an antibody molecule with a receptor mediating a signal without inflammation (comparable to a hormone) leading to the untoward reaction.

5.9.1 Clinical Examples of Autoimmune Diseases

The best-known examples of type VI reactions are classical autoimmune disease [2, 6, 8, 9, 11].

Autoimmune Thyreoiditis. The autoantibody acts like a hormone. Thyroid-stimulating activity (long-acting thyroid-stimulating factor, LATS) was found decades ago in patients with Hashimoto's thyreoiditis. These autoantibodies stimulate specifically the TSH receptor and may elicit a thyreotoxic crisis. As IgG antibodies they pass through the placenta and may induce reversible thyreotoxicosis in neonates.

Myasthenia Gravis. Autoantibodies in myasthenia gravis do not stimulate but have a blocking effect, directed against the acetylcholine receptor on the motoric endplate of the muscle [1, 9, 14].

Table 5.111. Direct pathogenic effects of autoantibodies

Disease	Specificity	Clinical symptoms
Thyreotoxicosis	TSH receptor	Stimulation, hormone formation
Myasthenia gravis	Acetylcholine receptor	Blockade, muscle weakness
Antiphospholipid syndrome	Cardiolipin/β_2-glycoprotein	Thromboembolic complications
Pernicious anemia[a]	ATPase, gastrin receptor	Decreased acid production, decreased B_{12} resorption
Male infertility	Spermatozoa	Agglutination and immobilization of spermatozoa
Wegener's granulomatosis	Proteinase III (neutrophil granulocytes)	Endothelial damage
Acanthosis nigricans (type B)	Insulin receptor	Receptor blockade, proliferation
Pemphigus vulgaris	Desmoglein 3	Bulla formation (acantholysis)

[a] Hematological cytopenias (anemia, thrombocytopenia); see Sect. 5.2

Other Autoimmune Diseases. Similar mechanisms can be found in a variety of other autoimmune diseases although the actual pathogenic role of autoantibodies has not been proven for each disease entity (Table 5.111) [4, 6, 7, 8, 15].

5.9.2 Stimulating Hypersensitivity in Bacterial Infection

Some authors regard the severe acute disease of "multiorgan failure" occurring in certain bacterial infections as hypersensitivity of components of innate immunity, e.g., as overstimulation of macrophages and endothelial cells by endotoxin (lipopolysaccharide S = LPS) or unspecific T-cell activation by superantigens of Gram-positive organisms.

5.9.3 Stimulating/Neutralizing Reactions in Classic Allergic Diseases

In a variety of classic allergic diseases with well-known antibody formation against exogenous allergens, recently autoantibodies of different classes against cells or surface receptors autologous with possible pathogenic importance have been found (Table 5.112). These include:

Table 5.112. IgE and autoimmune reactions

Autoantibody	Specificity	Disease
IgG	IgE	Immunotherapy
IgG	FcεRI	Chronic urticaria
IgE	Hom s 1–5 (epidermal proteins)	Severe atopic eczema

- IgG antibodies against platelet factor 4 in heparin-associated thrombocytopenia (see Sect. 5.2)
- Anti-IgE antibodies in patients with high total serum IgE or in the course of allergen-specific immunotherapy [10]
- Antibodies against the high-affinity IgE receptor (FcεR I) in some patients with chronic urticaria and positive skin reaction to autologous serum [5]
- IgE autoantibodies against epidermal proteins (Hom s 1–5) in patients with very severe atopic eczema and high serum IgE levels [12]
- In severe asthma, antibodies against the β-adrenergic receptor have been described [13]

In clinical experimental models, it has been known for a long time that IgG antibodies against IgE or IgE receptors may elicit in vitro and in vivo similar reactions as allergen (e.g., in vitro histamine release from peripheral basophil leukocytes with anti-IgE as positive control).

The positive wheal and flare reaction after injection of anti-IgE in the passive cutaneous anaphylaxis (PCA) has been known as "reverse anaphylaxis" for a long time [7].

The better we understand the molecular mechanisms of these reactions, the more it is to be expected that overlaps between type VI and other allergic reaction types (e.g., type II) will be detected.

5.9.4 Therapy

The existence of a stimulating/neutralizing hypersensitivity is not an esoterical-philosophical idea but has important practical and therapeutic implications: In patients with autoantibodies against the IgE receptor, chronic urticaria does not respond to antihistamines and should be treated with cortisone or immunosuppressives.

The skin lesions of patients with atopic eczema and high IgE autoantibodies against epidermal proteins will not improve by allergen avoidance. Active anti-inflammatory or immunosuppressive treatment is indicated.

In certain antibody-mediated autoimmune diseases, the intravenous administration of immunoglobulin G in high doses has proven beneficial [4, 7, 8] (see Sect. 5.2).

References

1. Almon RR, Andrew CG, Appel SH (1974) Serum globulin in myasthenia gravis: inhibition of alpha-bungarotoxin binding to acetylcholine receptors. Science 186:55–57
2. Atkinson MA, Maclaren NK (1994) The pathogenesis of insulin-dependent diabetes mellitus. N Engl J Med 331:1428–1436
3. Beck K, Hertel J, Rasmussen NG, et al. (1991) Effect of maternal thyroid antibodies and postpartum thyroiditis on the fetus and neonate. Acta Endocrinol 125:146:149
4. Chapel H, Haeney M (1993) Essentials of clinical immunology, 3rd edn. Blackwell, Oxford
5. Hide M, Francis DM, Grattan CE, Hakimi J, Kochan JP, Greaves MW (1993) Autoantibodies against high-affinity IgE receptor as a cause of histamine release in chronic urticaria. N Engl J Med 328:1599–1604
6. King C, Sarvetnick N (1997) Organ-specific autoimmunity. Curr Opin Immunol 9:863–871
7. Peter HH, Pichler WJ (1996) Klinische Immunologie, 2nd edn. Urban & Schwarzenberg, Munich
8. Roitt IM (1996) Essential immunology, 8th edn. Blackwell, Oxford
9. Shoenfeld Y, Isenberg D (eds) (1993) Natural autoantibodies. CRC Press, Boca Raton, Florida
10. Stadler BM, Miescher S, Horn M, et al. (2001) Allergic manifestations as the results of a conditional autoimmune response. Int Arch Allergy Immunol 124:411–413
11. Tan EM (1982) Autoantibodies to nuclear antigens (ANA): their immunobiology and medicine. Adv Immunol 33:167–240
12. Valenta R, Seiberler S, Natter S, et al. (2000) Autoallergy: a pathogenetic factor in atopic dermatitis? J Allergy Clin Immunol 105:432–437
13. Venter JC, Fraser CM (1981) The development of monoclonal antibodies to beta-adrenergic receptors and their use in receptor purification and characterization. In: Eisenbarth G, Fellows R (eds) Monoclonal antibodies in endocrine research. Raven Press, New York, pp 119–134
14. Vincent A, Mewsom-Davis J (1982) Acetylcholine receptor antibody characteristics in myasthenia gravis. I. Patients with generalized myasthenia or disease restricted to ocular muscles. Clin Exp Immunol 49:257–265
15. Wegmann DR (1996) The immune response to islets in experimental diabetes and insulin-dependent diabetes mellitus. Curr Opin Immunol 8:860–864

5.10 "Eco-syndrome" ("Multiple Chemical Sensitivity," MCS)

5.10.1 Classification

An increasing number of patients visit the doctor because of supposed incompatibility reactions against environmental pollutants with quite variable complaints, often involving several organ symptoms which are difficult to reproduce objectively. The patients have often undergone an odyssey of visits to various specialists, so-called special clinics, or "gurus" without having found help. The problem is well

Table 5.113. "Eco-syndrome": identical or related syndromes

- "Multiple chemical sensitivity" (MCS)
- "Multiorgan dysesthesia"
- "Idiopathic environmental intolerance"
- "Environmental illness"
- "Allergy to the 20th century"
- "Total allergy syndrome"
- "Chronic fatigue syndrome"
- "Candidiasis hypersensitivity syndrome" ("yeast connection")
- "Wood furnishing syndrome"
- "Living room poison"
- "Toxicopia"

Table 5.114. Eco-syndrome: common complaints (selection)

Neurologic symptoms	Skin and mucous membranes	General complaints
Fatigue, malaise, headache, vertigo, concentration disturbance, sleep disturbance, psychologic symptoms (confusion, anxiety, memory loss, irritability, depression)	Itch, burning of the skin, eye irritation, dry larynx and nose, rhinorrhea, dyspnea, hair loss	*Gastrointestinal:* nausea, diarrhea, obstipation, flatulence, gastric pain
		Cardiovascular: cardiac pain, anxiety, tachycardia
		Flu-like symptoms: mild fever, arthralgia

covered in the media and has received attention under different names (Table 5.113).

The mostly subjective complaints may be classified roughly into skin and mucous membrane symptoms, neurologic and general symptoms (Table 5.114) [2, 8, 13, 15, 24, 31, 34]. Many patients have fear of the "environment" and apply excessive avoidance behavior with chemicals, foods, drugs, fragrances, etc. The most common name for this condition today is "multiple chemical sensitivity" (MCS); it has to be remarked that in most of these patients, this sensitivity is not objectively measurable. The term "supposed multiple chemical sensitivity" would be better, but it seems to contradict the opinions of the patients, who are convinced of their hypersensitivity. On the other hand, there are patients who objectively suffer from multiple hypersensitivity against various chemicals, namely patients with multiple drug allergies. This, however, is a totally different group with objective signs and symptoms.

When in the early 1980s we saw the first patients with these conditions we suggested the term "eco-syndrome" as a working diagnosis for "patients suffering from mostly subjective symptoms affecting different organ systems who are convinced that the disease is due to environmental noxes."

The definition of MCS (according to Cullen) [8] is:

- Elicitation of symptoms by a variety of factors in low dose exposure
- Various symptoms manifesting in more than one organ system and improving after avoidance of exposure
- The complaints cannot be explained by classical examination
- There is a tendency to chronification
- There is immense suffering
- Exclusion of other well-defined diseases

From this list it is clear that the diagnosis "MCS" can never be made in a clear-cut fashion since certain criteria are not defined exactly (what are "classical examinations" or "other well-defined diseases"?).

Since the factors suspected are not only chemicals, but also physical factors (e.g., electromagnetic radiation, radioactive radiation), an expert committee of the WHO has proposed the term "idiopathic environmental intolerances" (IEI) [16].

5.10.2 Differential Diagnoses

The "eco-syndrome" partly has similarities with some differently defined but also environment-associated conditions:

- Chronic fatigue syndrome (virus infections like EBV, HHV 6, etc., are discussed) [1].
- Fibromyalgia syndrome with muscle pain in the center and disturbed pain regulation with possible disturbance in serotonin metabolism.
- Candida syndrome with mainly irritable bowel symptoms and candida phobia and immune weakness.

Complaints related to indoor exposure comprise the sick building syndrome (SBS) and building-related illnesses (BRI) (Table 5.115) [18, 19, 33].

BRI are well-known and objective diseases, and include infectious diseases and allergies.

SBS is due to a complex interaction between physical, chemical, and biological exposure as well as psychological factors with occurrence of subjective complaints in a large number of people employed in one building.

Table 5.115. Differential diagnosis between building-related illness (BRI), sick building syndrome (SBS), and eco-syndrome

	Building-related illness	Sick building syndrome	Eco-syndrome (MCS)
Occurrence	Clearly building-associated, individual or several persons	At least 10–20% of persons employed in a building are affected	Individual complaints
Symptoms	Objective (e.g., infection, allergy)	Mucous membrane and skin irritations, neurologic complaints	Many organ systems involved, diffuse psychologic and physical complaints
Pathophysiology	Monocausal: • Infectious • Irritative-toxic • Allergic	Multifactorial (physical, chemical, psychological)	Unknown (only hypotheses)
Risk factors	Atopy, higher age, immunosuppression	Atopy, air conditioning, occupation in low social grade	Atopy
Female:male	1:1	Predominantly female	Predominantly female
Psyche	Not prominent	Psychosomatic-psychiatric factors, not causal	Strong psychosomatic involvement

5.10.3 Pathophysiological Concepts

Toxicological Concept. Intoxication by environmental noxious agents is regarded as causal especially by followers of the so-called "clinical ecology" in the United States. Large toxicologic measurements including biomonitoring of affected individuals, however, have not yet given evidence for intoxications by environmental noxes [34]. Enzyme defects have been discussed [12, 14].

Immunological Concept. Another theory describes damage of the immune system by chemicals leading to disturbance of cellular and humoral immunity. However, no deviations of immune response were measurable in objective trials [30].

Allergological Concept. Many patients believe strongly that they are allergic against minute amounts of environmental poisons. In our own intensive investigations in approximately 100 patients, we found objective hypersensitivity phenomena (both allergic and pseudo-allergic in nature) in approximately one-third of our patients; this could explain some of the complaints; however, rarely were they directed against the originally suspected environmental noxes [13, 23, 24, 25]. The majority of patients have an atopic diathesis and are familiar with the experience of becoming sick from the environment. So it is tempting to look at the environment for elicitors of unexplained disturbances.

Neurological Concept. Many environmental noxes have an impact on the nervous system leading to psychiatric phenomena, concentration disturbance, or fatigue. The low reproducibility and subjectivity of the complaints may be the reason that this theory has not yet been proven [1, 2, 3, 7, 28, 31].

Olfactoric Concept. Many patients suffer from increased olfactory sensitivity and believe they can detect (smell) very low concentrations of environmental chemicals as unpleasant odors (kakosmia). According to this hypothesis, an olfactoric-hypothalamic-limbic stimulus transfer may induce symptoms in the sense of conditioned learning and amplification to olfactory stimulation [4, 22]. In clinical practice using olfactometry, this hypothesis has not been proven.

Psychiatric Concept. Many physicians believe that patients with "eco-syndrome" suffer from psychiatric disease. Indeed, some cases of true endogenous psychoses (schizophrenia, manic-depressive reactions, etc.) were present among our patients. One of my first patients, a 35-year-old female, believed herself to be allergic against

"Radio Free Europe"; this highly intelligent woman had previously been totally psychologically normal and healthy and only then was diagnosed as having schizophrenia. In intensive investigations comprising allergy and consultations together with exposure challenges, it was not possible to elicit the observed symptoms by the respective electromagnetic waves. In the course of our diagnostic activities, finally the diagnosis of schizophrenia was ascertained. The majority of patients, however, do not suffer from psychiatric disease [10, 13, 16, 26, 27, 31, 32].

Psychosomatic Concept. The symptoms of eco-syndrome are very similar to a condition very common in the 19th century and called "neurasthenia" [1]. Anxiety reactions, disproportional conflict coping, as well as "somatization disturbance" in hidden depression are factors [5, 6, 15, 17, 21, 25, 27, 31, 36]. It is important for the patient to gain a socially acceptable diagnosis such as "nerval disturbance" in the 19th century and "allergy" today, which are easier to bear than psychiatrization.

Similar to neurasthenia, "eco-syndrome" affects mainly females (2.5:1 female-male ratio). Some of our patients reported after careful exploration a history of sexual abuse in early childhood [23, 29].

In interdisciplinary expert committees, mostly no one feels responsible: the toxicologist sees psychological phenomena, the psychiatrist thinks of allergies, and the allergist discusses toxicological effects.

Although the definition and etiopathophysiology of "eco-syndrome" are controversial and ill understood, something needs to be done for the affected patients, who suffer considerably.

It cannot be excluded that environmental noxes in low concentrations have true effects which are not yet measurable at this time or are not yet understood. Exposure of patients with atopic eczema in stable remission to low concentrations of formaldehyde in indoor air led to objectively measurable changes of transepidermal water loss, e.g., a disturbance of barrier function of the skin without subjective complaints of the patients [10].

5.10.4 Management of Patients with "Eco-syndrome"

Therapy of the condition follows the results of the investigations, which should be performed

Table 5.116. Recommendations for the management of patients with "eco-syndrome"

- Since many patients suffer from being neglected or primarily regarded as "psychologic," a physician-patient relationship based on mutual confidence is most important. This needs time, patience, and talking.
- The problem has to be taken seriously; at the same time, irrational expectations have to be calmed down.
- The examination requires a general understanding of the whole human being and includes the psychosocial aspects as well as possible environmental influences.
- Through cooperation with other disciplines, diseases sometimes disguised under the term "eco-syndrome" have to be excluded, such as:
  - Infectious diseases (sinusitis, mononucleosis, respiratory infection)
  - Allergies (rhinoconjunctivitis, atopic eczema, allergic contact eczema, urticaria)
  - Metabolic toxic diseases (diabetes mellitus, drug abuse, hypo- or hyperthyreoidism)
  - Malignant neoplasias
  - Psychiatric disease
- Polypragmatic diagnostics and therapy have to be avoided:
  - Only recommend measurements when results can be interpreted!
  - Only recommend acceptable procedures (avoid prophylactic measures in houses and apartments connected with high financial and personal input).
  - Do not treat laboratory results but individual disease conditions.
  - Avoid "depoisoning" techniques which may be risky.
  - Avoid social and human isolation.
- The evaluation of environmental parameters should be done on a strictly scientific basis, e.g.
  - Objective environmental toxicological dose-response relationships and epidemiological evidence
  - Allergologic-immunological examinations for detection of allergy or pseudo-allergy
  - Besides rational recommendations for therapy based on diagnosis of eliciting causes, a supportive attitude is crucial including if needed psychologic-psychiatric consultations and therapies.

with interdisciplinary cooperation. The avoidance of relevant elicitor factors is crucial, be it in the treatment of underlying diseases (e.g., chronic cholecystitis, ostemyelitis), the avoidance of allergens, the administration of specific diets (e.g., pseudo-allergic reactions to food additives), change of living conditions or psychosomatic or psychiatric counseling (Table 5.116). There is considerable need for research. The major advice I give my co-workers in dealing with these patients is: "Take the patient seriously!"

There is no need for pessimism: In a long-term follow-up over 2–5 years we found that two-thirds of our patients had remarkably improved or were almost symptom free.

References

1. Abbey SE, Garfinkel PE (1991) Neurasthenia and chronic fatigue syndrome: The role of culture in making of a diagnosis. Am J Psychiatry 148: 1638–11646
2. Altenkirch H (1995) Multiple chemical sensitivity (MCS)-Syndrom. Gesundheitswesen 57:661–666
3. Bartenstein PF, Grundwald F, Herholz K, Kuwert T, Tatsch K, Sabri O, Weiller C (1999) Rolle der Positronen-Emissions-Tomographie (PET) und Single-Photon-Emissions-Tomographie (SPECT) bei der sogenannten "Multiple Chemical Sensitivity" (MCS). Nuklearmedizin 38:297–301
4. Bell IR, Miller CS, Schwarz GE, et al. (1996) Neuropsychiatric and somatic characteristics of young adults with and without self-reported chemical odor intolerance and chemical sensitivity. Arch Environ Health 51:9–21
5. Binkley K, King N, Poonai N, Seeman P, Ulpian C, Kennedy J (2001) Idiopathic environmental intolerance: Increased prevalence of panic disorder-associated cholecystokinin B receptor allele 7. J Allergy Clin Immunol 107:887–890
6. Bornschein S, Hausteiner C, Zilker Th, Bickel H, Förstl H (2000) Psychiatrische und somatische Morbidität bei Patienten mit vermuteter Multiple Chemical Sensitivity (MCS). Nervenarzt 71: 737–744
7. Bullinger M (1989) Psychological effects of air pollution on healthy residents – a time-series approach. J Environ Psychol 9:103–118
8. Cullen MR (1987) The worker with multiple chemical sensitivities: An overview. State Art Rev Occup Med 2:655–661
9. Derbolowsky J (1999) Die Glaubwürdigkeit wieder herstellen. Zeitschr Umweltmed 7:2–4
10. Eberlein-König B, Przybilla B, Kühnl P, Pechak J, Gebefügi I, Kleinschmidt J, Ring J (1998) Influence of airborne nitrogen dioxide or formaldehyde on parameters of skin function and cellular activation in patients with atopic eczema and control subjects. J Allergy Clin Immunol 101: 141–143
11. Eikmann T, Herr C (2001) Ein Paradigmenwechsel in der Umweltmedizin? Umwelt Forschung Prax 6:179–180
12. Fabig K-R (1999) Glutathion-S-Transferase T_1 und Multiple Chemikaliensensitivität (MCS). Umwelt Medizin Gesellschaft 12:226–232
13. Gieler U, et al. (1998) Therapeutische Aspekte des MCS-Syndroms. Umweltmed Forschung Praxis 3:3–10
14. Grimm V, Ruhdorfer S, Eberlein-König B, Scherer G, Engst R, Ring J (1999) Defizit der Glutathiontransferase bei Patienten mit Öko-Syndrom? Allergo J 8 [Suppl 1]:32
15. Hüppe M, Bullinger M (1997) Verfahren zur MCS-Diagnostik. Zusammenfassung und Bewertung einer Umfrage. Umweltmed Forschung Prax 2:291–294
16. IPCS (International Programme on Chemical Safety) (1996) Report of Multiple Chemical Sensitivities (MCS) Workshop. Berlin, Inst Arch Occup Environ Health 69:224–226
17. Kofler W (1993) Umweltängste, Toxikopie-Mechanismus, komplexes evolutionäres Coping-Modell und die Notwendigkeit neuartiger Auflagen für genehmigungspflichtige Anlagen. In: Aurand K, Hazard BP, Tretter F (eds) Umweltbelastungen und Ängste. Westdeutscher Verlag, Wiesbaden, pp 225–226
18. Kröling P (1989) Zur Problematik des "Sick building"-Syndroms. Allergologie 3:118–129
19. Molina C, Caillaud D, Molina N (1993) Sick building syndrome and atopy. Indoor Air 1:369–373
20. Neuhann HF, Wiesmüller GA (1994) Diagnostische Strategien bei gebäudebezogenen Gesundheitsstörungen. In: Luftverunreinigung in Innenräumen. VDI Berichte 1122
21. Nixon PGF (1982) "Total allergy syndrome" or fluctuating hypercarbia? Lancet I:516
22. Österberg OP, Akesson B, Bergendorf U, Karlson B, Seger L (1998) Suprathreshold intensity and annoyance reactions in experimental challenge to toluene and n-butyl acetate among subjects with long-term solvent exposure. Scand J Work Environ Health 24:432–438
23. Ring J, Gabriel G, Vieluf D, Przybilla B (1991) "Das klinische Ökologie-Syndrom" ("Öko-Syndrom"): Polysomatische Beschwerden bei vermuteter Allergie gegen Umweltschadstoffe. Münch Med Wochenschr 133:50–55
24. Ring J, Eberlein-König B, Behrendt H (1999) "Eco-Syndrome" ("multiple chemical sensitivity" – MCS). Zbl Hyg Umweltmed 202:207–218
25. Ring J, Triendl C, Behrendt H, Borelli S (2000) Das Öko-Syndrom (multiple chemical sensitivi-

ty) und verwandte Syndrome. In: Przybilla B, Bergmann KCh, Ring J (eds) Praktische allergologische Diagnostik. Steinkopff, Darmstadt, pp 351–371
26. Röttgers HR (2000) Psychisch Kranke in der Umweltmedizin. Deutsches Ärzteblatt 97:A835–A840
27. Selner JC, Staudemayer H (1992) Neuropsychophysiologic observation in patients presenting with environmental illness. Toxicol Indust Health 8:145–155
28. Staudenmayer H, Selner J, Buhr M (1993) Double-blind provocation chamber challenges in 20 patients presenting with "multiple chemical sensitivity". Regul Toxicol Pharmacol 18:44–53
29. Staudenmayer H, Selner M, Selner J (1993) Adult sequelae of childhood abuse presenting as environmental illness. Ann Allergy 71:538–546
30. Terr A (1993) Immunological issues in "multiple chemical sensitivities". Regul Toxicol Pharmacol 18:54–60
31. Tretter F (1996) Umweltbezogene funktionelle Syndrome. Int Praxis 37:669–686
32. Triendl C, Borelli S, Rakoski J, Herschbach P, Behrendt H, Ring J (1999) Das "Öko-Syndrom" (multiple chemical sensitivity"): Allergologisch-umweltmedizinisches Management. Allergologie 22:744–760
33. Voack C, Borelli S, Ring J (1997) Der umweltmedizinische 4-Stufenplan. Münch Med Wochenschr 139:69–72
34. Wiesmüller GA, Hornberg D (2001) Multiple Chemikalienüberempfindlichkeiten (MCS). Eine Herausforderung moderner Diagnostik und Therapie. Allergologie 24:507–514
35. Zilker M (1991) Pathophysiological mechanisms of fibromyalgia. Clin J Pain 7 [Suppl 1]:8–15
36. Wüthrich B (2001) Allergien: Umweltkrankheiten Nummer 1. Der Allergie-Patient im Spannungsfeld zwischen Schul- und Alternativmedizin. Dermatol Beruf Umwelt/Occup Environ Dermatol 49:136 141
37. Walkowiak J, Wiener J-A, Fastabend A, Heinzow B, Krämer U, Schmidt E, Steingrüber H-J, Wundram S, Winneke G (2001) Environmental exposure to polychlorinated biphenyls and quality of the home environment: effect on psychodevelopment in early childhood. Lancet 358:1602–1607

6 Allergy Prevention and Therapy

6.1 General Concept of Allergy Treatment

The most efficient causal method of allergy treatment is the avoidance of the eliciting allergen (Fig. 6.1). This underlines the immediate importance of careful allergy diagnosis. There are few disciplines in medicine in which diagnosis and therapy are as closely connected as in allergology. Note: "Not every cold in summer is hay fever, not every cold in winter is a viral infection!"

Allergen avoidance comprises not only the avoidance of pets, sanitizing measures in the apartment, anti-housedust mite strategies, but also the elimination of unspecific irritants, as well as dietetic regimens in food allergy; finally changes in occupation as well as rehabilitation treatments in an allergen-poor climate (North Sea, high altitude as in Davos, Switzerland) have to be considered.

The next causal therapeutic option is allergen-specific immunotherapy (hyposensitization), where it is possible to change the abnormal pathologic immune reaction into normal immunity.

The final aim of any treatment is that the patient will be free of symptoms. The single steps in the general concept of allergy treatment do not exclude each other! Also during allergen-specific immunotherapy, symptomatic treatment has to be given. Table 6.1 shows the most important steps of a treatment strategy ranging from allergen avoidance to psychosomatic counseling or psychotherapy.

After prophylactic treatment with mast cell stabilizers (e.g., cromones), anti-inflammatory strategies are the most important symptomatic treatment. Here glucocorticosteroids are in first place, and these have gained much in efficacy and safety by the development of

Table 6.1. General concept of allergy treatment

Level of action	Procedure
Allergen exposure	Avoidance (e.g., apartment, mite protection, rehabilitation in occupational allergy, climatic therapy, diet)
Pathogenic immune reaction	Allergen-specific immunotherapy (hyposensitization), immunosuppression, immunomodulation
Inhibition of mediator release	Mast cell stabilizers
Inhibition of inflammation	Glucocorticosteroids
Receptor antagonists	
Histamine	Antihistamines (sedating, non-sedating)
Leukotrienes	Leukotriene antagonists, lipoxygenase inhibitors
Specific therapy at organ level	Bronchodilation, secretolysis, physical therapy, skin care, restoration of disturbed barrier
Psyche	Antidepressives, psychotherapy, psychosomatic counseling

6.1 General Concept of Allergy Treatment

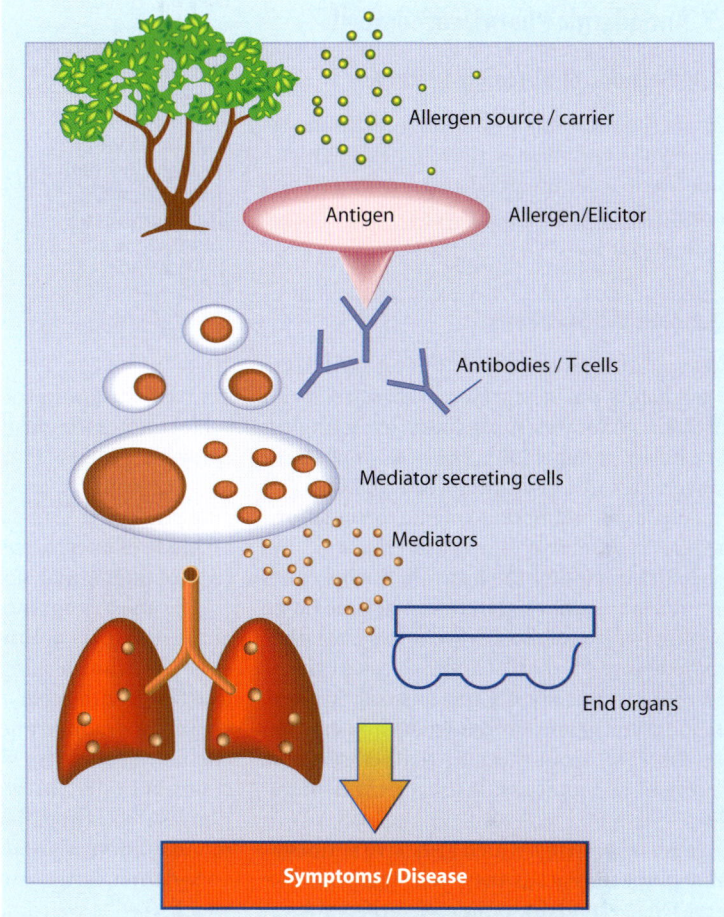

Fig. 6.1. General concept of allergy treatment (points of intervention)

topical products for mucous membranes and skin.

Antagonists of proinflammatory mediators are the most commonly used antiallergic drugs. Apart from antihistamines, also antagonists of leukotrienes or inhibitors of lipoxygenase should be mentioned.

Finally, the specific therapy at the diseased organ – in asthma bronchodilation, secretolysis, physical therapy, in eczema skin care, antimicrobial treatment, and restoration of impaired barrier function – is crucial.

Allergic reactions show a well-known interaction with psychologic factors; therefore, psychosomatic counseling may be important.

Phytopharmacological preparations are used in allergy treatment and "unconventional" or "complementary" therapeutic procedures have gained a high degree of popularity in many countries, but rarely show evidence-based efficacy. Depending on the definition of "complementary," some procedures (e.g., autogenic training, Kneipp's hydrotherapy) can be supplementary in some conditions (see Sect. 6.4).

The novel experimental therapeutic concepts which are undergoing clinical trials may be the therapeutic options of the future and should not be called "complementary."

6.2 Antiallergic Pharmacotherapy

6.2.1 Inhibition of Histamine Synthesis

Previously, substances inhibiting histidine decarboxylase and thereby the synthesis of histamine were recommended (e.g., tritoqualine). Flavonoids may have a similar action. Studies are in progress.

6.2.2 Mast Cell Stabilizers

These substances are able to inhibit the release of mediators on the surface of mast cells and basophil leukocytes most likely by acting on the calcium channel [30]. The best known substance is disodium cromoglycate (DSCG) [3], which is used in different galenic formulations for the conjunctiva, the nasal mucosa, the bronchial tract, and the gastrointestinal tract. Cromones are also used in veterinary medicine (obstructive bronchitis in racehorses). Another cromone is nedocromil. Cromoglycates can only be used topically on the mucosal surface. They do not penetrate the epidermis and are not absorbed from the gut. Neither systemic treatment nor topical skin treatment is possible.

Some other drugs which also have antihistamine properties act as mast cell stabilizers like ketotifen [29] and oxatomide. Ketotifen not only is effective against allergen-induced but also against bronchoconstriction due to platelet-activating factor and is able to influence bronchial hyperreactivity over longer periods of time.

6.2.3 Antihistamines

Since the first antihistamine (Bovet and Staub [10]), a multitude of H_1 antagonists (in Germany more than 50 preparations are on the market) have been developed (Table 6.2); they compete with histamine on the H_1 receptor and can be further distinguished in different pharmacological groups (Fig. 6.2). The sidechains R1 and R2 contain aromatic or heteroaromatic ring structures. Furthermore, mention should be made of tricyclic systems, which are derivatives of phenothiazine.

The most commonly used so-called classic antihistamines are not totally specific and apart from antihistamine also show antagonistic effects with other receptors such as acetylcholine, serotonin, and dopamine. Due to anticholinergic effects, some antihistamines are contraindicated in glaucoma, urinary retention, as well as in patients under treatment with monoaminooxidase (MAO) inhibitors.

Sedation is the most common side effect, which may be welcome under some conditions (against itch during the night). There are, however, paradoxical reactions especially in children, who show signs of hyperactivity after antihistamines.

Sedation is especially undesired in patients who have to be well oriented in their occupation [8, 9]. Therefore, the development of the new non-sedating H_1 antagonists (Table 6.2) is one of the major advances of allergy therapy [37, 39, 42]. Most of the substances are also available for children in liquid form.

Table 6.2. Histamine H_1 receptor antagonists

Classic antihistamines	New less sedating antihistamines
Alimemazine	Azelastine
Bamipine	Cetirizine
Clemastine	Desloratadine
Cyproheptadine	Ebastine
Dexchlorpheniramine	Fexofenadine
Dimetinden	Levocabastine
Diphenhydramin	Levocetirizine
Doxylamine	Loratadin
Hydroxyzine	Mizolastine
Meclozine	Terfenadine
Mequitazine	

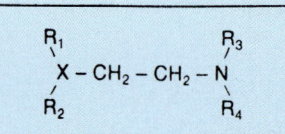

– Ethylendiamine-Type: X = N-Atom
– Colamine-Type: X = O-Atom
– Propylamine-Type: X = C-Atom

Fig. 6.2. Classification of the H_1 antagonists

In severe cases of chronic urticaria or for prophylaxis of anaphylactoid reactions, the combined administration of H_1 and H_2 antagonists (see Sect. 5.1.4 on "Anaphylaxis") has been recommended.

The topical use of antihistamines as antipruritics (e.g., after insect stings) is controversial. The possible beneficial effect of some antihistamine gels is most likely due to the alcoholic vehicle more than the drug.

6.2.4 Leukotriene Inhibitors

Leukotrienes are among the most active proinflammatory mediators and have principally two quite different effects: LTB4 is chemotactic for neutrophil and eosinophil granulocytes, and the sulfidoleukotrienes LTC4, LTD4, and LTE4 have a long-acting bronchoconstrictory effect (previously called "slow-reacting substance of anaphylaxis SRS-A").

6.2.4.1 Lipoxygenase Inhibitors

By inhibiting 5-lipoxygenase (5-LO), reduction of both LTB4 and sulfidoleukotriene is possible. Specific 5-LO inhibitors (e.g., zileuton, genleuton) may be distinguished from inhibitors of an interaction between 5-LO- and the "5-lipoxygenase-activating protein FLAP" (e.g., MK886, BAYx1005) [35].

Zileuton is used against asthma in the United States; it has to be given 3–4 times per day and can induce disturbance of liver function. It affects allergen-induced bronchoconstriction and decreases the use of cortisone in asthmatics.

6.2.4.2 Leukotriene Antagonists

Sulfidoleukotriene Antagonists
Several companies have developed specific antagonists of sulfidoleukotrienes such as:

- Zafirlukast (Astra-Zeneca)
- Montelukast (MSD)
- Pranlukast (in preparation, ONO)

These substances inhibit allergen-induced bronchoconstriction [6, 20, 28]. In the allergist's office, however, while they can reduce cortisone use in severe asthma, they are no miracle drugs. The history of leukotriene antagonists is a good example of the advances made in practical medicine: From the characterization of the substance in 1979 by Samuelson until the first practically available antagonist for the patient, there was a time lag of almost 20 years in spite of very intensive research being carried out.

LTB4 Antagonists
The search for LTB4 antagonists was not as successful although a variety of substances have been tried in experimental and clinical trials (e.g., LY293111, Lilly, CGS25019C, Novartis, BI-IL284BS, Boehringer-Ingelheim). These substances have an effect in in vitro and in experimental models, but have produced controversial results in clinical trials.

6.2.5 Glucocorticosteroids

Glucocorticosteroids (GC) play a central role in antiallergic treatment since almost all inflammatory phenomena elicited during an allergic reaction may be inhibited. GC act after passive penetration through the cell membrane and binding to a GC receptor in the cytoplasm, which is normally protected by heat-shock proteins from dimerization. The novel complex then enters into the nucleus and binds to the promoter region of certain genes (GC-responsive elements) inducing the well-known catabolic effects by increased transcription. At the same time, GC bind to intracellular regulator proteins (transcription factors NF-κB or activator protein 1AP1) and inhibit mRNA formation. This is the basis of anti-inflammatory and in allergy therapy desired effects [5, 21, 22, 33] (Table 6.3).

In practice, the distinction between systemic and topical GC therapy is essential. The most important and unpleasant side effects of cortisone occur after long-term systemic treatment, which is necessary for severe asthma, autoimmune disease, or rare cases of chronic urticaria. Side effects of topical GC on the skin are covered in Sect. 5.5.4.

Side effects of inhalatory GC comprise hoarseness, oropharyngeal candidosis, and dysphonia (the "smoky" voice of a pop singer).

Table 6.3. Glucocorticosteroid effects on transcription of various genes (according to Barnes [5])

Increased transcription
α_2-Adrenoceptors
Lipocortin
IL-1 receptor II
IL-1 receptor antagonist

Inhibition of transcription
Cytokines (IL-1 - -6, IL-11, IL-13, TNFα, SCF, GM-CSF)
Chemokines (IL-8, RANTES, eotaxin, MIP-1α, MCP-1, MCP-3)
COX1 and COX2
Phospholipase A2
Adhesion molecules
Neurokinin receptors
Endothelin1

Table 6.4. Glucocorticosteroids for inhalation

Beclometasone dipropionate
Budesonide
Dexamethasone-21-isonicotinate
Fluocortinbutyl
Flunisolide
Fluticasone-17-propionate
Triamcinolonacetonide
Mometasonfuroate

Combination:
Fluticasone-17-propionate
and salmeterol

It is surprising that the respiratory mucosa obviously is more resistant to atrophy-inducing GC effects than the skin.

Table 6.4 lists the available inhalative GC, which can also be combined successfully with other drugs such as β_2-adrenergics. Further improvement can be seen through the development of substances with fewer side effects (e.g., fluocortinbutyl, which is rapidly inactivated by unspecific esterases, loteprednoletabonate or cyclesonide). After long-term administration of inhalative GC in childhood, reversible growth retardation may occur.

6.2.6 Sympathicomimetics

6.2.6.1 α-Adrenergics

The previously very common α-sympathicomimetics adrenaline und ephedrine and their derivatives are only available in combination prep-

Table 6.5. α-Sympathicomimetics

Topical decongestants	Systemic preparations
Indanazoline	Phenylpropanolamine
Naphazoline	Pseudoephedrine
Oxymetazoline	
Tetryzoline	
Tramazoline	
Xylometazoline	

arations. Adrenaline (epinephrine) has its main indication in anaphylactic shock (see Sect. 5.1.4). Today for treatment of mucosal swelling, synthetic drugs, mostly imidazole derivatives, are used (Table 6.5). All these substances should only be given over a short time period since the mucosal epithelium may be damaged through the vasoconstriction ("privinism").

Apart from solutions and sprays, some patients with very sensitive nasal mucosa prefer the application of an ointment or gel (e.g., oxymetazoline or tramazoline). For mucosal care, vehicle preparations, some of them containing vitamins in emollients, are used.

6.2.6.2 β_2-Adrenergics

β_2-Adrenergics act especially in the bronchial tract as dilatory substances (Table 6.6) with reduced cardiac side effects. They also show mast-cell-blocking activity, inhibit edema formation, enhance mucociliary transport, and decrease the risk of infection. Most substances are available for inhalation as well as systemic treatment. The advantage of inhalatory therapy can be seen in the lower dosage, fewer systemic side effects, and rapid onset of action. Disadvantages are sometimes wrong use by the patient and the tendency to overdose. For children, β_2-adrenergics are available in liquid form.

Table 6.6. Selective β_2-adrenoceptor agonists

Systemic	Inhalation, short-acting
Bambuterol	Fenoterol
Clenbuterol	Salbutamol
Reproterol	Terbutaline
Salbutamol	Pirbuterol
Terbutaline	Prosaterol
Tolbuterol	Bitolterol
	Inhalation, long-acting
	Formoterol fumarate
	Salmeterol xinafoate

Newer developments comprise the long-acting β_2-agonists salmeterol and formoterol as well as mixed β_2 + dopamine receptor antagonists (Viozan, in development).

6.2.7 Anticholinergics

Cholinergic hyperreactivity is the major characteristic of patients with bronchial asthma. Clinically useful anticholinergics are the muscarine receptor antagonists atropine sulfate, atropine methylnitrate, as well as the more recent substances ipratropium bromide, oxitropium bromide, and tiotropium. One hundred years ago, "asthma cigarettes" containing atropine were used for the treatment of asthma (stramonium cigarette according to Trousseau).

Anticholinergics have a place, especially for intrinsic (cryptogenic) asthma as well as nonallergic vasomotor rhinitis. Side effects are dryness of the mucous membranes, which needs special care.

6.2.8 Phosphodiesterase Inhibitors

Since the 1920s, xanthine derivatives – especially theophylline – have been used as bronchodilators. The non-selective inhibition of phosphodiesterase is responsible for the poor compatibility. The poor solubility in water requires the addition of complex-forming agents such as ethylenediamine or glycine. Certain solutions also contain sulfites, which may elicit severe asthma attacks in hypersensitive patients (see Sect. 5.1.5 on "Food Allergy"). Some solutions contain carbamoylphenoxyacetic acid (= salicylamide-o-acetate sodium), which does not seem to show cross-reactivity to acetylsalicylic acid in patients with ASA idiosyncrasy.

Side effects of xanthine derivatives are nausea, headache, anxiety, and sleeplessness; an adequate dosage is mandatory requiring efficient monitoring of blood levels between 10 and 20 µg/ml. Certain factors influence theophylline metabolism (e.g., in small children and infants, as well as after certain other medications like phenytoin or barbiturates, or in smokers); with concomitant use of erythromycin or other antibiotics, metabolism is slower.

Circadian rhythm should be considered [27, 34]. Many preparations are in slow release form. Also combination preparations of theophylline, diprophylline, and proxyphylline are available. Newer developments can be seen in selective PDE-IV inhibitors, which are undergoing clinical trials.

6.2.9 Secretolytics

These substances are able to split the very large molecules (>1 million kDa) of mucus in the bronchial mucosa by cutting disulfide bridges and increasing water retention, which also induces expectoration [16]. In animal experiments, blockade of in vitro allergen tachyphylaxis after pretreatment with acetylcysteine [14] may lead to an increase in asthmatic reactions; however, this has not been investigated so far in humans.

Most important in secretolysis is adequate fluid intake (see Sect. 5.1.2 on "Asthma"), which also humidifies the inspiratory air.

6.2.10 Preparations with Doubtful Efficiency

Apart from therapeutic modalities which are evidence based, many procedures are commonly used in the treatment of allergy diseases where the efficacy has not really been proven. The immunomodulating substance inosiplex may have mast-cell-stabilizing activity [37]. The peptide *N*-acetyl-aspartyl-glutamic acid (Rhinaaxia) has antagonistic effects against some lipoxygenase metabolites. Pharmacologically, calcium preparations are ineffective; however, they are widely used by general practitioners and patients [16, 26]. Phytotherapeutic substances comprise *Echinacea* extracts, extracts from *Ginkgo biloba,* benzyl mustard oil, as well as homeopathic therapy using *Cardiospermum, Chelidonium, Galphimia glauca,* etc. (see Sect. 6.4).

6.2.11 New Developments

New developments in pharmacotherapy of allergic diseases comprise calcium antagonists, flavonoids, indolbenzodiazepines, possible inhibitors of synthesis of mediators or antagonists of vasoactive mediators (e.g., AHR 5333, C11949, ICI 204 219, Sch 37 224, neurotropin) [20] as well as antiallergic substances from onion extracts [13] or fish oil (see Sect. 6.3 for immunotherapy).

6.2.12 Antipruritic Treatment

6.2.12.1 General Introduction

Itch is an untoward sensation inducing the urge to scratch (Fig. 6.3). There is no better modern definition. Itch is the most common and most crucial – impairing quality of life – symptom of allergic skin diseases [7, 12]. Similar to pain, itch is a sensation with strong subjective components and individual variants. Itch is mediated via a subpopulation of demyelinated C-fibers and differs qualitatively also in peripheral and central nervous conduction from pain. Small children and infants often cannot clearly describe itch; infants only learn to scratch between the 3rd and 6th months of life.

The basis of each antipruritic treatment is the avoidance of specific and non-specific provocation factors (see other chapters of this book). There are various qualities of itch which differ considerably as can be seen on the scratch reaction:

- "Wheal" itch in urticaria (never excoriated until bleeding, but only rubbed)
- "Eczema" itch in atopic and contact dermatitis (superficial excoriations)
- "Prurigo" itch (extremely itchy nodules, which are dug out while scratching)

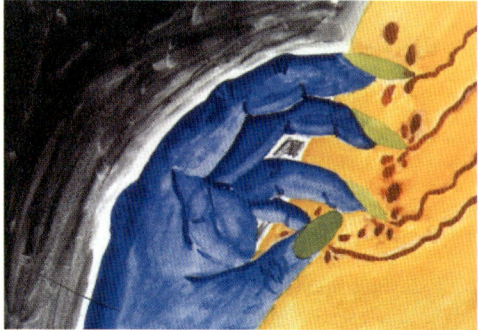

Fig. 6.3. Representation of itching in a drawing by a teenage allergy patient

Table 6.7. Antipruritic therapy

Central nervous action
Patient education (itch-scratch cycle)
Systemic: H_1 antagonists (sedating), sometimes combined with H_2 antagonists, cholestyramine, opiate antagonists, acetylsalicylic acid (polycythemia vera), tricyclic antidepressants
Acupuncture, TENS
Stress reduction

Action on the skin
Patient education (skin care)
Elimination of provocation factors (allergens, infestation)
Unspecific topical therapy (capsaicin, polidocanol, doxepine)
Physical treatment (UVB, PUVA, cooling)
Steroids only when indicated for underlying disease

Recently, it has been possible to visualize the itch sensation by positron emission tomography (PET) [11] (see Sect. 5.5.3).

In the treatment of itch, one distinguishes between central and peripheral mechanisms of action (Table 6.7). Each antipruritic treatment modality has to be integrated into a general concept of treatment of the underlying disease.

6.2.12.2 External Treatment of Itch

In the treatment of acutely itching dermatoses, the application of cold (stimulation of Aδ fibers) is effective, e.g., using wet wraps ("wet pyjamas"), lotio alba, or menthol. Antihistamines do not have an effect when used externally. Possibly the tricyclic antidepressant doxepin with combined H_1 and H_2 antagonistic action may also be used topically [4, 15]. The long-known topical local anesthetic Thesit can be used as a lotion or in a cream. Itch on the basis of disturbed nerval functions (e.g., in zoster neuralgia) can be treated with capsaicin leading to depletion of sensory nerve endings. In prurigo itch due to internal diseases (liver, kidney), UV treatment (UVB) has proven helpful.

6.2.12.3 Systemic Antipruritic Treatment

The most commonly used systemic antipruritics are antihistamines, which are especially effective in urticaria. In eczema, antihistamines show a limited effect, and classic antihista-

Table 6.8. Systemically acting antipruritics

Substance	Dose/day	Remarks
Antihistamines		Sedative preparations
– Dimetinden maleate	3 × 1–2 mg	
– Alimemazine	3 × 5 mg	Max. 50–100 mg/day
ASS	3 × 500 mg	In polycythemia vera
Cholestyramine	8–16 g	In renalem and hepatic pruritus
Cyclosporin A	5 mg/kg	In atopic eczema (caveat: nephrotoxicity!)
Doxepine	3 × 10–25 mg	Tricyclic antidepressant
Mycophenolatmofetil	1–2 g	In atopic eczema, immunosuppressive
Ondansetron	2–3 × 8 mg	Serotonin antagonist
Opiate antagonists		
– Naloxone	0.8 mg s.c.	In primary biliary cirrhosis
– Naltrexone	25–50 mg	
– Nalmefen	2 × 5 mg	Caveat: opiate withdrawal
Propofol	10-mg bolus	Experimentally used in cholestasis
Rifampicin	1–2 × 300 mg	In cholestasis; caveat: toxicity

mines with sedative properties may be helpful especially when given intravenously as infusion in acute itch crisis (e.g., dimetinden) (Table 6.8).

Antipruritic therapy has to be supported by other measures such as adequate cutting of fingernails, soft gloves, as well as covering itching skin areas with fatty-moist bandages (e.g., Tubifast). Chronic itch can be treated using behavioral therapy (itch diary, "scratch device") [1, 2, 35].

In urticarial itch, antihistamines are effective. In eczema, antihistamines with sedating components like doxylamine succinate, dimetinden maleate, clemastine, and hydroxyzine are preferred [2, 35, 39]. In 10–15% of children, after antihistamines paradoxical reactions leading to hyperactivity may occur. Then another antihistamine may be used; possible overdosage should be considered. Antihistamines should only be given during acute phases of exacerbation, especially at night and in adequate dosing. In acute itch crises dimetinden maleate should be given intravenously!

In a double-blind study using the combined H_1 antagonist promethazine and the H_2 antagonist cimetidine in 21 young adults with atopic eczema, there was no additional effect of cimetidine [17].

6.2.13 Antiallergic Pharmacotherapy and Pregnancy

There is little information regarding the risks of antiallergic drugs during pregnancy. Most producers therefore recommend using the utmost care. From long-lasting experience and wide international use, β_2-adrenergic aerosols as well as topical glucocorticosteroids are considered fairly safe [23]. Fenoterol has been used after the 16th week as a tocolytic. Systemic glucocorticosteroids over a short period are well tolerated.

Due to forensic considerations, antihistamines should be used only in selected cases. Drugs which have been in worldwide use for decades against hyperemesis gravidarum also have antihistamine action.

References

1. Abeck D, Ring J (1998) Etablierte medizinische Therapieansätze. In: Ring J (ed) Neurodermitis. Expertise zur gesundheitlichen Versorgung und Vorsorge bei Kindern mit atopischem Ekzem. Ecomed, Landsberg, pp 93–105
2. Abeck D, Werfel S, Brockow K, Ring J (1997) Die Behandlung des atopischen Ekzems im Kindesalter. Hautarzt 48:379–383
3. Altounyan REC (1967) Inhibition of experimental asthma by a new compound disodium cromoglycate – "Intal". Acta Allerg (Kbh) 22:487–489
4. Anonymous (2000) Doxepin cream for eczema? Drug Ther Bull 38:31–32

5. Barnes PJ (1996) Molecular mechanism of steroid action in asthma. J Allergy Clin Immunol 97: 159–168
6. Barnes W, Piper P, Castello J (1987) The effect of an oral LT antagonist L-649923 on histamine and leukotriene D_4-induced bronchoconstriction in normal man. J Allergy Clin Immunol 79:816–821
7. Bernhard JD (1994) Itch. McGraw-Hill, Philadelphia
8. Betts T, Markman D, Debenham S, Mortiboy D, McKevitt T (1984) Effects of two antihistamine drugs on actual driving performance. Br Med J 288:281–282
9. Bieber T, Ring J (1987) Terfenadin und Kraftfahrzeug-Führung: Eine Placebo-kontrollierte Doppelblind-Studie zum Einfluß verschiedener Antihistaminika auf das Fahrverhalten. Med Klin 82:683–686
10. Bovet D, Staub AM (1937) Action protectrice des éthers-phénoliques au cours de l'intoxication histaminique. CR Soc Biol (Paris) 124:547–549
11. Darsow U, Scharein E, Simon D, Walter G, Bromm B, Ring J (2001) New aspects of itch pathophysiology: component analysis of atopic itch using the 'Eppendorf Itch Questionnaire'. Int Arch Allergy Immunol 124:326–331
12. Darsow U, Mautner V, Scharein E, Bromm B, Ring J (1997) Der Eppendorfer Juckreizfragebogen. Hautarzt 48:730–733
13. Dorsch W, Ring J (1984) Suppression of immediate and late anti-IgE-induced skin reactions by topically applied alcohol/onion extract. Allergy 39:43–49
14. Dorsch W, Auch E, Powerlowicz P (1987) Adverse effects of acetyl cysteine on human and guinea pig bronchial asthma in vivo and on human fibroblasts and leukocytes in vitro. Int Arch Allergy Appl Immunol 82:33–39
15. Drake MD, Millikan LE (1995) The antipruritic effect of 5% doxepin cream in patients with eczematous dermatitis. Arch Dermatol 131:1403–1408
16. Forth H, Henschler D, Rummel W (1987) Allgemeine und spezielle Pharmakologie und Toxikologie, 5th edn. Wissenschaftsverlag, Mannheim
17. Foulds IS, McKie RM (1981) A double-blind trial of the H_2-receptor antagonist cimetidine and the H_1-receptor antagonist promethazine hydrochloride in the treatment of atopic dermatitis. Clin Allergy 11:319
18. Hanifin JM (1991) Atopic dermatitis: New therapeutic considerations. J Am Acad Dermatol 24:1097–1101
19. Fjellner B, Hägermark Ö (1979) Pruritus in polycythemia vera: treatment with aspirin and possibility of platelet involvement. Acta Derm Venereol 59:505–512
20. Hansel TT, Barnes PJ (eds) (2001) New drug for asthma, allergy and COPI. Progr Resp Res 31. Karger, Basel
21. Hatz HJ (1998) Glucocorticoide. Immunologische Grundlagen, Pharmakologie und Therapierichtlinien. Wiss. Verlagsges., Stuttgart
22. Hirata F, Schiffmann E, Venkatasubramanian K, Salomon D, Axelrod J (1980) A phospholipase A_2 inhibitory protein in rabbit neutrophils induced by glucocorticoids. Proc Natl Acad Sci U S A 77:2533–2536
23. Hoffman C, Schatz M, Harden K, Forsythe A, Chillingar L, Porreco R, Benenson A, Sperling W, Kagnoff M, Saunders B, Zeiger R (1986) The safety of inhaled bronchodilators (IB) during pregnancy. J Allergy Clin Immunol 77:249
24. Kaiser H (1977) Cortisonderivate in Klinik und Praxis. Thieme, Stuttgart
25. Klein PA, Clark RAF (1999) An evidence-based review of the efficacy of antihistamines in relieving pruritus in atopic dermatitis. Arch Dermatol 135:1522–15625
26. König W, Baron M, Ehring F (1984) Effect of calcium mineral solutions on the histamine release from human peripheral leukocytes. Arzneimittelforschung 34:52–54
27. Kunkel G, Schupp J, Borner K, Lasius D, Meysel U (1983) Untersuchungen zur Theophyllinwirkung unter besonderer Berücksichtigung der Tagesrhythmik. Therapiewoche 33:1113–1123
28. Manning PJ, Watson RM, Margolskee DJ, Williams VC, Schwartz JI, O'Byrne PM (1990) Inhibition of exercise-induced bronchoconstriction by MK-571, a potent leukotriene D_4 antagonist. N Engl J Med 323:1736–1739
29. Martin U, Römer D (1977) Ketotifen: A histamine release inhibitor. Monogr Allergy 12:145–149
30. Mazurek N, Berger G, Pecht I (1980) Binding site on mast cells and basophils for the anti-allergic drug cromolyn. Nature 286:722–724
31. Melin L, Frederikson T, Noren P, Swebilius BG (1986) Behavioural treatment of scratching in patients with atopic dermatitis. Br J Dermatol 115: 467–474
32. Middleton ER Jr (1985) New drugs in management: calcium antagonists. Chest 87:79
33. Newton R (2001) Molecular mechanisms of glucocorticoid action. What is important? Thorax 55:603–613
34. Nolte D, Krejci G (1983) Methylxanthine beich. Apotheker-Verlag, Stuttgart
35. Ring J, Brockow K, Abeck D (1996) The therapeutic concept of "patient management" in atopic eczema. Allergy 51:206–215
36. Ring J, Fröhlich HH (1985) Wirkstoffe in der dermatologischen Therapie, 2nd edn. Springer, Berlin Heidelberg New York
37. Schmutzler W (1981) Möglichkeiten der Arzneitherapie allergischer Erkrankungen. Pharmakotherapie 4:155–162
38. Schmutzler W, Delmich K, Eichelberg D, Glück S, Greven T, Jürgensen H, Riesener KP, Risse G, Pult P (1985) The human adenoidal mast cell suscepti-

bility to different secretagogues and secretion inhibitors. Int Arch Allergy Appl Immunol 77: 177–178
39. Simons KI, Simons FER (1996) H1-receptor antagonists: Pharmacokinetics and clinical pharmacology. In: Simons FER (ed) Histamine and H1-receptor antagonists in allergic disease. Dekker, New York, 175–213
40. Wassilew SW (2000) Serotoninantagonisten bei Pruritis. In: Plewig G, Degitz K (eds) Fortschritte der praktischen Dermatologie und Venerologie. Springer, Berlin Heidelberg New York, pp 437–440
41. Weinberger MM, Bronsky EA (1974) Evaluation of oral bronchodilator therapy in asthmatic children. J Pediatr 84:421
42. Woodward JK, Munro NL (1982) Terfenadine, the first non-sedating antihistamine. Arzneimittelforschung/Drug Res 32:1154–1159

6.3 Immunotherapy

6.3.1 Allergen-Specific Immunotherapy (Specific Hyposensitization)

6.3.1.1 Definition and History

The classic causal treatment option in allergology is specific hyposensitization (previously "desensitization"), also called allergen-specific immunotherapy, where the relevant allergen is administered repeatedly in increasing doses until reaching a so-called maintenance dose or remission of symptoms.

This maintenance dose is either the dose leading to complete remission or marked improvement or the dose which is tolerated by the patient over a longer period of time without side effects. This procedure has some similarity to active immunization (= vaccination), but differs in principle (vaccination = protective induction of immunity against infectious disease). Some authors use the broader term "immunotherapy." However, immunotherapy also includes many other therapeutic options like the use of antibodies (= immunoglobulins), immunosuppression, as well as the increasingly used immunomodulating therapy with biologicals (cytokine antagonists, receptor antagonists, anti-IgE, etc.). The term "allergen-specific immunotherapy" (specific hyposensitization) characterizes a well-described therapeutic procedure in certain indications.

Hyposensitization has been used for almost 100 years in clinical allergology (Table 6.9) since Noon and Freeman, who continued Noon's work after his death, with so-called "prophylactic inoculations" of pollen were able to cure hay fever [23, 50, 65].

Early precursor treatments of hyposensitization can be found in antiquity when King Mithradates tried to protect himself against poisoning by eating very low amounts of increasing doses of toxic substances (he died by the sword). In modern times, homeopathy as

Table 6.9. History of allergen-specific immunotherapy (specific hyposensitization) (literature cited in [51] and [65])

Immunization against hay fever	Curtis	1900
Passive immunization ("pollantin") against pollen toxin	Dunbar	1903
Decrease of local reactions after increased administration of xenogeneic serum	v. Pirquet	1906
Antianaphylaxis ("Desensibilization")	Besredka	1907
Intranasal immunization	Scheppegrell	1909
Horse serum treatment of conjunctivitis	Stancueanu and Nita	1909
"Prophylactic inoculation"	Noon and Freeman	1911
"Hyposensitization"	Cooke	1922
Blocking antibodies (blood transfusion)	Cooke	1935
Specificity of blocking antibodies	Loveless	1940
First controlled trial	Bruun	1949
Allergoid (formaldehyde)	Marsh and Lichtenstein	1970
Allergoid (glutaraldehyde)	Johansson et al.	1974
T-cell peptides	Norman	1965
Recombinant PLA2 in insect venom allergy	Müller et al.	1998
Role of IL-10 and IgG4	Akdis and Blaser	2000

well as vaccination can be seen as precursors of hyposensitization. The early authors using hyposensitization in hay fever were convinced that the clinical symptoms were due to a pollen toxin.

In 1935 Cooke described blocking antibodies in the serum of hyposensitized patients, who were able to suppress immediate allergic skin reactions (cited in [51]). Only in the 1970s was the long-known principle in vaccination of using toxoids as better compatible preparations also used in allergology in the development of "allergoids," i.e., modified allergens producing a strong immunogenic action with fewer side effects. Currently, glutaraldehyde- or formaldehyde-treated allergens are used as allergoids [51, 76].

6.3.1.2 Mechanism of Action of Hyposensitization

In spite of its practical use over a long period, the exact mechanisms of action of this therapeutic option are only known as hypothetical concepts (Table 6.10).

IgG-Blocking Antibodies

There is no doubt that during subcutaneous hyposensitization, IgG antibodies are formed in increasing concentrations which can be characterized in vivo and in vitro by their blocking activity of certain IgE-mediated reactions (Fig. 6.4).

In the first weeks of allergen-specific immunotherapy, both IgE and IgG antibodies increase; while IgE decreases within the next few months, IgG stays high. However, in the individual case, the antibody pattern does not always follow this schedule [57] as has been shown in insect venom allergy [30, 57, 72]. Maybe locally produced blocking antibodies in

Table 6.10. Possible mechanisms of action of allergen-specific immunotherapy

IgG antibodies (subclass IgG4?)
- Blocking antigen-specific
- IgE synthesis-inhibitory
- IgE receptor-inhibitory

Secretory antibodies (IgA, possibly IgG)
Hapten inhibition
Induction of B-cell tolerance
Induction of suppressor cells
- Soluble factors
- Ag-/isotype-specific
Anti-idiotypic antibodies
Tachyphylaxis
Decrease of releasability
Switch of TH2 to TH1 reactivity
Induction of T-cell tolerance (anergy)
Increase of IL-10

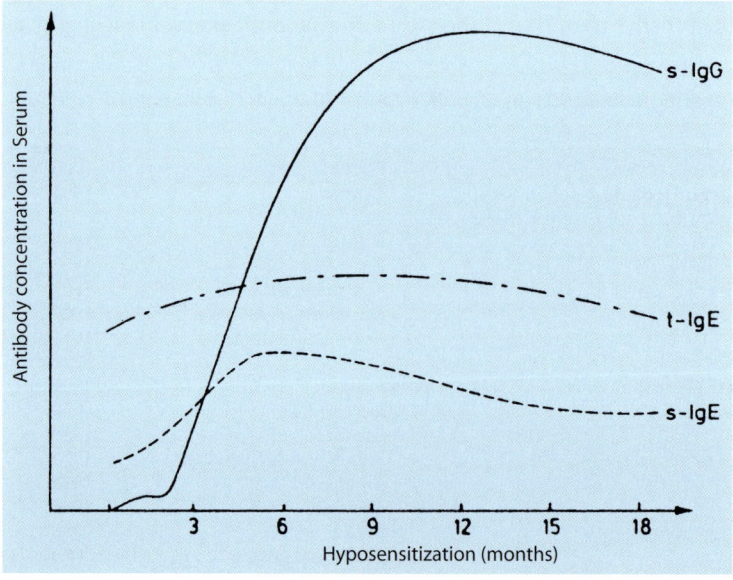

Fig. 6.4. Typical course of the IgE and IgG antibody concentrations during a hyposensitization therapy. *s-IgG*, specific IgG; *t-IgE*, total IgE

the mucous membrane are crucial. Especially the IgG4 subclass seems to be relevant [9]. Apart from a direct blocking effect, IgG antibodies may also inhibit IgE synthesis, possibly via a Fcγ receptor. Gammaglobulin therapy has been used in certain allergies [60]. By administration of specific hyperimmunoglobulin G, allergic reactions can be inhibited as in bee venom allergy [39, 56].

Anti-idiotypic Antibodies

The antigen-binding site of the antibody molecule is the hypervariable region, the personal identity card (individual specificity) of an antibody molecule. Against this idiotypic structure, antibodies may be produced as anti-idiotypic antibodies. Possibly, this idiotype-antiidiotype network (according to N. Jerne) has physiologic importance in the regulation of immune response and also in hyposensitization.

Decrease of Releasability of Mediator-Secreting Cells

The releasability of mediator-secreting cells also decreases during hyposensitization [51, 61]: The same amount of allergen leads to a "marked" diminished release of histamine from basophil leukocytes in patients after allergen-specific immunotherapy.

Tachyphylaxis

The decrease of a reaction after repeated application of the eliciting stimulus is a well-known pharmacologic phenomenon and may also play a role in the early phase of hyposensitization, especially in rush hyposensitization programs.

Suppressor T Cells

Another possible option is the induction of immunological tolerance through suppressor T cells [48, 67], a concept which seems to be a bit out of fashion. However, recently, the regulatory T cells (Tr or also T3 cells) seem to take over the role of the earlier suppressor cells, acting via interleukin (IL)-10 formation.

TH_2-Th_1 Balance

The most important effect of allergen-specific immunotherapy seems to be the successful correction of the deviated immune response from TH_2 to "normal" TH_1 [9, 20, 21, 35, 36, 48], which can be measured as cytokine secretion or isotype antibody pattern. Allergen dose and immunologic milieu (microenvironment) seem to be crucial. Low doses preferably induce IL-4 and TH_2 reactivity with IgE formation, while high doses such as during specific hyposensitization lead to IgG4 antibodies and a TH_1 secretion pattern [3, 9]. Specific hyposensitization follows the rules of the "mass-effect law" as does the process of allergy development (according to K. Blaser).

At the beginning of hyposensitization, T-cell anergy develops: neither TH_1 nor TH_2 cytokines are formed after allergen stimulation, while B-cells produce IgG4 antibodies. This anergy is probably due to IL-10 and reversible [3]. In the TH_1 milieu, interferon-γ induces further IgG4 formation. In a TH_2 milieu together with high concentrations of IL-4, TH_2 reactivity is strengthened. This explains the much better success rates of immunotherapy in patients observing allergen avoidance.

6.3.1.3 Efficacy of Allergen-Specific Immunotherapy

Specific hyposensitization is a causal therapy of allergic disease. Since the first trials were performed some 50 years ago, many randomized placebo-controlled clinical studies have been published clearly showing the efficacy of this therapy [2, 17, 25, 28, 30, 41, 45, 51, 61, 69, 84, 85–87]. The best results have been obtained with insect venoms, pollen, and housedust mites. Positive results have also been reported from animal epithelia and molds. From controlled studies, we know there is a high placebo effect (30–50%!). This, however, may not only derive from the doctor; patients in controlled trials are usually generally better treated than the average patient.

Hyposensitization is especially effective in young patients when the allergic disease has not yet been present for decades.

In various studies, it has been shown that specific hyposensitization is cost-effective and reduces the costs of drugs and hospitalization [13, 44]. Allergen-specific immunotherapy also improves the quality of life and the general health of the patient. In a large study ("Preventive Allergy Treatment," PAT), it was shown that the incidence of bronchial asthma in children with hay fever undergoing specific immunotherapy was 60% lower after a 5 years' observation interval than in controls [31]. Allergen-specific immunotherapy may also be regarded as an option for secondary prevention.

6.3.1.4 Allergen Extracts

For preparation of allergen extracts, specifically collected bulk materials (e.g., pollen grains) are extracted with different solvents to a so-called bulk solution (e.g., carbonate-buffered saline with or without glycerol and 0.4% phenol according to Coca (cited in [65]) (NaCl 5.0 g, NaHCO$_3$ 2.75 g, phenol 4.0, aqua dest. ad 1,000.0). This bulk solution is then diluted further. A major problem of allergen-specific immunotherapy is the standardization of allergen extracts [12, 24, 43, 51, 84].

The commonly used units for allergen extract standardization are shown in Table 6.11 (see also Sect. 3.4 on "Allergens"). Using modern immunological techniques such as radioallergosorbent test (RAST) inhibition, crossed radioimmunoelectrophoresis (CRIE) and other methods together with bioassays in specifically sensitized cell populations or defined volunteers with atopic diseases, a better comparability and standardization of allergen extracts is achieved.

When extracts are used as aqueous solutions, they have to be applied with a relatively high number of injections (2-3 times per week) up to the maintenance dose [25, 28, 51]. Therefore, the addition of depot substances is an attempt to prolong the liberation of the applied allergen. The most commonly method used is the extraction with pyridine and adsorption to aluminum hydroxide (according to Fuchs and Strauss) [24]. A further depot action can be achieved by adsorption to the amino acid L-tyrosine, which as a natural product is normally metabolized without leaving foreign body residues [34]. Newer adjuvants comprise monophosphoryl lipid (MPL) [18, 69] as well as bacterial oligonucleotides in clinical trials (e.g., CpG sequences) [38].

Allergoids are allergen derivatives with reduced allergenic activity (e.g., skin test in sensitized patients) and concomitantly increased immunogenic action (induction of specific IgG antibodies). A large body of experience is available for formaldehyde- and glutaraldehyde-fixed allergoids [34, 51].

Table 6.11. Units for standardization of allergen extracts

Noon unit	Extract of 1 µg allergen source (= 1 NU)
Weight/volume unit	Amount of allergenic bulk material/volume of extraction fluid (e.g., 1:1,000)
Protein nitrogen unit (PNU)	1 µg protein nitrogen = 1 PNU
Histamine equivalent prick (HEP)	Extract concentration provoking in atopic controls the same reaction in prick test as histamine (1 mg/ml)
Biological unit (BU) or bioequivalent allergy unit (BAU)	1 HEP = 1,000 BU/ml
Skin activity reference allergen-histamine (SARAH)	Corresponds to approx. 10 HEP
Activity units by RAST (AUR)	
International reference (IR)	100 IR induces 30 mm^2 wheal
International unit (IU)	WHO reference extracts contain 100,000 IU/ml
Therapeutic units (TU)	Allergen-specific in relation to ODC (optimal diagnostic concentration) in prick test

6.3.1.5 Practical Aspects of Allergen-Specific Immunotherapy

Indication

A specific hyposensitization is indicated when:

- The disease is severe
- Allergen avoidance is difficult or impossible
- IgE-mediated relevant sensitization has been proven

Possibly, the preventive aspect (prevention of increased disease intensity or enlarged allergen spectrum) is of major importance in the future [31].

Contraindications are:

- Acute and chronic infection
- Autoimmune disease
- Secondary damage of the manifestation organ
- Conditions where epinephrine is contraindicated (severe cardiac disease, β-blocker therapy)
- Malignancy (not surgically removed)
- Lack of compliance

The previous contraindications of "cerebral cramps" and "pregnancy" are only of limited value today [6, 47]. In a prospective study with allergic children and epilepsy, no EEG changes were observed after allergen injections [6].

Pregnancy per se also is not a absolute contraindication. We do not start specific hyposensitization during pregnancy, but continue a well-tolerated immunotherapy with a maintenance dose – especially for life-threatening insect venom anaphylaxis.

Careful analysis of 121 pregnancies of 90 atopic mothers undergoing allergen-specific immunotherapy during pregnancy did not yield any evidence or increased prevalence of eclampsia, abortions, premature birth, teratogenicity, increased mortality of newborns, or other complications [47]. On the other hand, the possibility of general active atopy prevention may be considered since an increase in specific IgG antibodies in maternal blood and a protective role with regard to atopy development in the newborn have been discussed [14].

The indication for allergen-specific immunotherapy in patients with atopic eczema needs to be discussed separately. While some patients experience a deterioration of eczematous skin lesions during dose increases, other authors have reported dramatic improvements also of eczematous skin lesions under immunotherapy [27, 62, 63, 81]. Therefore, there is no general contraindication. The literature in this regard shows a state of the art similar to that of allergen-specific immunotherapy for hay fever in 1950. There are few placebo-controlled trials, most of them showing some efficacy. We do not know enough about the vehicle, the dose, the route of administration, or the relevant allergens. There is a need for further studies.

Selection of Allergens (Formulation of Allergen Extract)

The selection of allergens for the individual extract is crucial for the success of specific hyposensitization, which is based on the individual results of careful allergy diagnosis [25, 28, 51, 61, 79, 84, 85–87]. It is here where the most common mistakes take place [25]. The general rule is: fewer rather than too many allergens in one extract!

In this regard, one should remember that the term "allergen" is reserved for the protein molecule while structures like pollen or housedust mites are allergen carriers or allergen sources. This is sometimes not correctly taken into account in the common allergist's nomenclature. Especially suitable allergen sources for allergen-specific immunotherapy are pollen, housedust mite, and insect venom; immunotherapy with animal epithelia, molds, or occupational dusts is more difficult.

Practical Implementation

Specific hyposensitization can be administered in various ways (Table 6.12). The classic and most commonly used method is subcutaneous injection of the allergen extract. Extravasal localization should be checked (several aspirations!) (Fig. 6.5).

In classic hyposensitization with aqueous allergen extracts, the interval between two in-

Table 6.12. Methods of hyposensitization

Method	Interval
Subcutaneous	
Aqueous extracts (classic)	3–5 days
Aqueous extracts (rush hyposensitization)	Hours
Semidepot extracts	7–14 days
Allergoids	7–14 days
Oral/sublingual	
Aqueous extracts	Daily intake
Capsules	Experimental
Nasal	Experimental

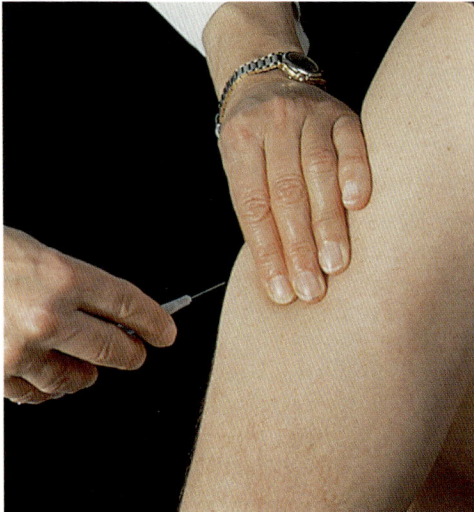

Fig. 6.5. Subdermal injection of allergen extract during hyposensitization treatment

jections is 3–5 days. Hyposensitization with semidepot extracts requires a lower number of injections and with injection intervals between 7 and 14 days. With the introduction of allergoids and new adjuvants, an even further reduced number of injections is possible [18, 36].

Allergen mixtures in solution contain preservatives (e.g., 0.4% phenol) or are lyophilized, which is important for storage (note the date and ensure the correct storage at 4 °C in order to avoid a loss of biological activity).

Most allergen extract producers provide the extract in several bottles of increasing concentrations, which are labeled with different colors, letters, or numbers (e.g., strength 1–3).

Usually, the injections are started with aqueous or semidepot extracts with 0.1 ml at strength 1 and increased up to a maintenance dose of 1 ml at strength 3. The allergen concentrations in the various bottles differ from allergen to allergen and from company to company.

In very sensitive patients with a history of side effects or anaphylaxis, it is recommended to start with an even lower concentration (bottle "0") and a slower increase in concentration than in the routine schedule.

The general rule is: Do not increase the dose schematically but individually, but try to reach remission of symptoms or tolerance of the highest dose [28]. Before each injection, a short history regarding the compatibility of the last injection as well as the general condition of the patient (underlying disease, infection, exercise, stress, allergen exposure) and concomitant medication (β-blocker!) is performed.

The injection interval, which differs according to the type of immunotherapy (aqueous, semidepot, etc.), needs to be watched strictly. If it is prolonged, the dose should be reduced.

After hyperergic local reactions (>15 cm in diameter), it is recommended repeating the last dose; after systemic reactions, the dose is reduced by at least two steps.

Immediately prior to injection and 24 h afterwards, violent physical exercise should be avoided. After the injection, the patient is asked to remain for 30 min in the office and possible side effects are recorded. Severe side reactions usually occur within 30 min and can be treated by the experienced allergist successfully. If a patient who does not stick to this rule notices nausea or unconsciousness on the way home, this may turn out to be fatal! Indeed, most of the severe side effects of allergen-specific immunotherapy can be seen in connection with a disregard for these rules [11, 28, 41].

After infectious disease or vaccinations, the immunotherapy interval is prolonged and the next injection is given 2 weeks later with a reduced dose in two steps.

Seasonal allergies usually are treated preseasonally (in hay fever usually during winter time). During the season, one can either stop the therapy (allergen exposure is difficult to control) or it can be continued over the year with significantly reduced doses (e.g., 1/10).

Oral/sublingual immunotherapy is controversial, although significant effects have been shown in placebo-controlled trials [4, 10, 15, 16, 29, 37, 54, 55, 59, 75]. The efficacy of sublingual/oral immunotherapy is weaker than that of subcutaneous treatment [10, 42].

In an experimental setting, trials for local nasal immunotherapy [26, 68] as well as passive hyposensitization with hyperimmunoglobulin or gammaglobulin [19, 29, 34] have been tried. A possible method of improving efficacy and compatibility can be seen in the simultaneous administration of specific hyperimmunoglobulin prior to allergen-specific immunotherapy [29].

There is no consensus regarding the duration of allergen-specific immunotherapy. Principally, the success rates increase with increasing duration of treatment. Generally, at least a 3-year term of treatment is recommended, in some cases longer.

In order to find evidence for successful immunotherapy, the clinical symptoms as well as the results of specific provocation tests or possibly in vitro tests with IgG/IgG antibodies can be performed.

6.3.1.6 Side Effects of Allergen-Specific Immunotherapy

Possible side effects of specific hyposensitization are listed in Table 6.13. There is no realistic danger of toxic effects of allergen extracts (Table 6.14). The incidence of systemic side reactions of allergen-specific immunotherapy ranges between 1% and 15% per patient or 0.1–1% per injection for aeroallergens. There

Table 6.13. Side effects of allergen-specific immunotherapy

Local reaction
- Erythema, edema, pain, itch
- Infection
- Granuloma
- Pseudolymphoma

Anaphylaxis
Exacerbation of atopic disease
Serum sickness
Unspecific symptoms (headache, vertigo, nervousness)

Table 6.14. Toxicity of allergen extracts (no or negligible risks due to)

- Direct toxicity of allergens
- Teratogenicity
- Cancerogenicity
- Mycotoxins
- Endotoxins
- Aluminum effects
- Metabolic influence

may be higher prevalence rates for insect venom allergy. Fatalities have been reported; often the rules of practical performance of allergen-specific immunotherapy have not been respected [11, 25, 32, 25, 40, 51, 61, 64, 74, 79]. Frankland estimates an incidence of 1 fatality among 750,000 injections [22]. The benefit of a prophylactic antihistamine treatment is discussed [32].

The most dangerous systemic complications are anaphylactic reactions (see chapter on "Anaphylaxis").

Rarely, type III reactions occur during hyposensitization [71, 79] sometimes in relation to inflammatory vascular disease (allergic vasculitis) [8, 55]. Side effects such as serum sickness occurring with arthralgia, fever, urticaria, and sometimes nephritis and lymphadenopathy indicate that the maintenance dose is too high and there is an excess of IgG antibodies leading to circular immune complexes. In the differential diagnosis, the manifestation of a latent autoimmune disease has to be considered.

Occasionally, persisting granulomas at the injection site can occur, most commonly after aluminum-absorbed extracts [7]; rarely they can change into pseudolymphomas (see Sect. 5.8).

Allergen-specific immunotherapy differs from the injection of defined chemical drugs both in its theoretical principles and in its practical performance. It should only be done by physicians with allergological expertise. New developments in allergy research, especially in the explanation of the mechanism of action and the production of better purified and standardized extracts, will greatly improve the efficiency and safety of this well-accepted therapeutic modality.

References

1. Aas K (1975) Clinical and experimental aspects of purification and standardization of allergen extracts. Int Arch Allergy Appl Immunol 49:44
2. Abramsom MJ, Puy RM, Weiner JM (1995) Is allergen immunotherapy effective in asthma? A meta-analysis of randomized controlled trials. Am J Respir Crit Care Med 151:969–974
3. Akdis CA, Blaser K (2000) Mechanisms of allergen-specific immunotherapy. Allergy 55:522–530
4. André C, Vatrinet C, Galvain S, Carat F, Sicard H (2000) Safety of sublingual-swallow immunotherapy in children and adults. Int Arch Allergy Immunol 121:229–234
5. Asero R (2000) Fennel, cucumber, and melon allergy successfully treated with pollen-specific injection immunotherapy. Ann Allergy Asthma Immunol 84:460–462
6. Bauer CP, Czettritz G v, Weinmann HM (1984) Zerebrales Anfallsleiden – eine Kontra-Indikation für die Hyposensibilisierung? Allergologie 7:161–162
7. Baumgarten C (1978) Häufigste Nebenwirkungen bei der spezifischen Hyposensibilisierung. Allergologie I:223–228
8. Berbis Ph, Carena MC, Auffranc JC, Privat Y (1986) Vascularite necrotisante cutaneo-systemique survenue en cours de desensibilisation. Ann Derm Venereol 113:805–809
9. Blaser K (2001) Immunologische Grundlagen der spezifischen Hyposensibilisierung. In: Ring J, Darsow U (eds) Allergie 2000. Dustri, Munich, pp 269–274
10. Bousquet J, Scheinmann P, Guinnepain MT, Perrin-Fayolle M, Sauvaget J, Tonnel AB, Pauli G, Caillaud D, Dubost R, Leynadier F, Vervloet D, Herman D, Galvain S, André C (1999) Sublingual-swallow immunotherapy (SLIT) in patients with asthma due to house-dust mites: a double-blind, placebo-controlled study. Allergy 54:249–260
11. Braun W (1980) Hyposensibilisierung: Bericht über einen Todesfall in der Praxis. Therapiewoche 30:2215–2216
12. Brede HD, Aas K (eds) (1979) Allergen-Extrakte. Fischer, Stuttgart
13. Büchner K, Siepe M (1995) Nutzen der Hyposensibilisierung unter wirtschaftlichen Aspekten. Allergo J 4:156–163
14. Casimir G, Gossart B, Vis HL, Duchateau J (1985) Antibody against beta-lactoglobulin (IgG) and cow's milk allergy, J Allergy Clin Immunol 75:207
15. Clavel R, Bousquet J, André C (1989) Clinical efficacy of sublingual-swallow immunotherapy: a double-blind, placebo-controlled trial of a standardized five-grass-pollen extract in rhinitis. Allergy 53:493–498
16. Creticos PS, Naclerio RM, Adkinson NF, Norman PS (1990) Efficacy, safety and kinetics of oral ragweed immunotherapy in the treatment of allergic seasonal rhinitis (Abstract). J Allergy Clin Immunol 85:165
17. Debelic M (1978) Behandlungserfolge mit Halb-Depot-Extrakten. In: Gronemeyer W, Fuchs E (eds) Allergosen der Atemwege. Dustri, Munich, 78 ff
18. Drachenberg KJ, Wheeler AW, Stuebner P, Horak F (2001) A well-tolerated grass pollen-specific allergy vaccine containing a novel adjuvant, monophosphoryl lipid A, reduces allergic symptoms after only four preseasonal injections. Allergy 56:498–505
19. Düngemann H (1978) Karenz-Expositionsprophylaxe. Atemwegs- u Lungenkr 4:7
20. Durham SR, Walker SM, Varga EM, et al. (1999) Long-term clinical efficacy of grass-pollen immunotherapy. N Engl J Med 341:468–475
21. Ebner C (1999) Immunological mechanisms operative in allergen-specific immunotherapy. Int Arch Allergy Immunol 119:1–5
22. Frankland AW (1980) Anaphylactic reaction to desensitization. Br Med J 281:1429
23. Freeman EJ (1914) Vaccination against hay fever. Lancet 1:1178
24. Fuchs AM, Strauss MB (1959) The clinical evaluation and preparation and standardization of a new water-insoluble whole ragweed pollen complex. J Allergy 30:66
25. Fuchs E (1972) Praktische Durchführung einer spezifischen Hyposensibilisierung. Med Klin 67:988
26. Georgitis JW, Nickelsen JA, Wypych JI, Barde SH, Clayton WF, Reisman RE (1986) Local intranasal immunotherapy with high-dose polymerizid ragweed extract. Int Arch Allergy Appl Immunol 81:170–173
27. Grewe M (2000) Hyposensibilisierung bei atopischem Ekzem. Allergo J 9:351–53
28. Gronemeyer W, Fuchs E (eds) (1983) Karenz und Hyposensibilisierung bei Inhalations- und Insektengift-Allergie, 2nd edn. Dustri, Munich
29. Horak F, Stubner P, Berger UE, Marks B, Toth J, Jäger S (1998) Immunotherapy with sublingual birch pollen extract. A short-term double-blind placebo study. J Invest Allergol Clin Immunol 8:165–171
30. Hunt KJ, Valentine MD, Sobotka AK, Benton AW, Amodio FJ, Lichtenstein LM (1978) A controlled trial of immunotherapy in insect hypersensitivity. N Engl J Med 299:157
31. Jacobsen L, Dreborg S, Moller C, Valovirta E, Wahn U, Niggemann B, Koller D, Urbanek R, Halken S, Host A, Lowenstein H (1996) Immunotherapy as a preventive allergy treatment (abstract). J Allergy Clin Immunol 97:232
32. Jarisch R, Götz Aberer W (1988) Side effects of specific immunotherapy, reduction by pretreatment with antihistamines. J Allergy Clin Immunol 83:262
33. Jarisch R, Wöhrl S, Focke M, Hemmer W (2001)

Anaphylaktische Reaktion bei spezifischer Immuntherapie durch Diaminoxidasehemmung nach Azetylzystein-Therapie. Allergologie 24: 112–115
34. Johansson SGO, Miller ACML, Overell BG, Wheeler AW (1974) Grass pollen-tyrosine adsorbate. Clin Allergy 4:57
35. Jung CM, Funk A, Rakoski J, Ring J (1997) Immunohistochemical analysis of late local skin reactions during rush venom immunotherapy. Allergy 52:717–726
36. Kasai M, Kurasawa K, Nakajima H, Iwamoto I (2001) T cell vaccination eliminates antigen-specific T cells and prevents antigen-induced eosinophil recruitment into the tissue. Int Arch Allergy Immunol 125 [Suppl 1]:59–66
37. Kleinhans D, Zöller I (2000) Therapiestudien zur sublingualen Immuntherapie mit Allergenen. Eine aktuelle Bestandsaufnahme. Allergologie 23:349–353
38. Krieg AM, Hartmann G, Yi AK (2000) Mechanism of action of CpG DNA (review). Curr Top Microbiol Immunol 247:1–21
39. Lessof M, Sobotka AK, Lichtenstein LM (1976) Protection against anaphylaxis in hymenoptera sensitive patients by passive immunization. J Allergy Clin Immunol 57:246
40. Lockey RF, Benedict LM, Turkeltaub PC, Bukantz SC (1987) Fatalities from immunotherapy (IT) and skin testing (ST). J Allergy Clin Immunol 79:660–677
41. Lockey RF, Bukantz SC (eds) (1999) Allergens and allergen immunotherapy, 2nd edn. Marcel Dekker, New York
42. Lowell F, Frankling W (1965) A double-blind study of the effectiveness and specificity of injection therapy in ragweed hay fever. N Engl J Med 273:675–679
43. Løwenstein H (1986) Standardization of allergen extracts. In: Ring J, Burg G (eds) New trends in allergy II. Springer, Berlin Heidelberg New York, pp 266 292
44. Märtens P, Lobermeyer K (2001) Krankheitskosten-Studie und Kosten-Nutzen-Analyse der spezifischen Immuntherapy bei Asthma. Allergo J 10:341–347
45. Malling H-J (2001) Allergen-specific immunotherapy in allergic rhinitis. Curr Opin Allergy Clin Immunol 1:43–46
46. Marsh DG, Lichtenstein LM, Campbell DH (1970) Studies on allergoids prepared from naturally occurring allergens. I. Assay of allergenicity and antigenicity of formalinized rye group component. Immunology 18:705–722
47. Metzger WJ, Turner E, Patterson R (1978) The safety of immunotherapy during pregnancy. J Allergy Clin Immunol 61:268–272
48. Mueller DL, Jenkins MK (199) Molecular mechanisms underlying functional T cell unresponsiveness. Curr Opinion Immunol 7:375–381
49. Nelson HS, Iklé D, Buchmeier A (1996) Studies of allergen extract stability: The effects of dilution and mixing. Mosby Year Book, St. Louis, p 382
50. Noon L (1911) Prophylactic inoculation against hay-fever. Lancet 1572
51. Norman PS (1980) An overview of immunotherapy. J Allergy Clin Immunol 65:87
52. Norman PS, et al. (1996) Treatment of cat allergy with T-cell reactive peptides. Am J Respir Crit Care Med 154:1623–1628
53. Oppenheimer J, Areson JG, Nelson HS (1994) Safety and efficacy of oral immunotherapy with standardized cat extract. J Allergy Clin Immunol 93:61–67
54. Passalacqua G, Albano M, Fragonese L, et al. (1998) Randomised controlled trial of local allergoid immunotherapy on allergic inflammation in mite-induced rhinoconjunctivitis. Lancet 351: 629–632
55. Phanuphak P, Kohler PF (1980) Onset of polyarteritis nodosa during allergic hyposensitization treatment. Am J Med 68:479–485
56. Przybilla B, Ring J, Galosi A, Geursen RG, Stickl HA (1986) Bee-venom immunoglobulin for prophylaxis of anaphylactic reactions during bee venom immunotherapy (rush hyposensitization). Immunol Allergy Practice 8:107–111
57. Przybilla B, Ring J, Grießhammer B, Braun-Falco O (1987) Schnellhyposensibilisierung mit Hymenopterengiften – Verträglichkeit und Therapieerfolg. Dtsch Med Wochenschr 112:416–424
58. Punnonen J (2000) Molecular breeding of allergy vaccines and antiallergic cytokines. Int Arch Allergy Immunol 121:173–182
59. Rakoski J, Wessner D (2001) A short assessment of sublingual immunotherapy. Int Arch Allergy Immunol 126:185–187
60. Ring J, Bode U, Kadach U, Stix E, Burg G (1983) Gammaglobuline und Allergie. Klinische Ergebnisse einer kontrollierten Studie mit Standard-Immunglobulin G und Plazebo bei Pollinosis. Münch Med Wochenschr 125:289–292
61. Ring J (1987) Spezifische Hyposensibilisierung. Wirkungsmechanismen, Erfolge und Probleme. Allergologie 10:392–403
62. Ring J (1982) Successful hyposensitization treatment in atopic dermatitis: results of a trial in monozygotic twins. Br J Dermatol 107:597–602
63. Ring J (1993) Spezifische Hyposensibilisierung bei atopischem Ekzem. Allergo J 2:1–2
64. Ring J, Przybilla B, Bongardts J (1988) Safety of hyposensitization. In: Proceedings of the annual meeting of the EAACI, Plama de Mallorca, 22–26 April 1987. Abello, Madrid, pp 131–138
65. Schadewaldt H (1979–1982) Geschichte der Allergie, vols 1–4. Dustri, München-Deisenhofen
66. Schramm G, Kahler H, Suck R, et al. (1999) 'Allergen engineering': Variants of the timothy grass pollen allergen Phl p 5b with reduced IgE-binding capacity but conserved T cell reactivity. Immunology 162:2406–2414

67. Sehon AH, Lee WY (1981) Suppression of IgE antibodies with tolerogenic derivates of allergens. In: Ring J, Burg G (eds) New trends in allergy. Springer, Berlin Heidelberg New York, p 294
68. Taylor G, Shivalkar PR (1972) Local nasal desensitization in allergic rhinitis. Clin Allergy 2:125
69. Turkeltaub PC, Marsh DG, Lichtenstein LM, Norman PS (1978) Development of long-lasting immediate hypersensitivity in nonatopic volunteers parenterally immunized with a purified grass pollen extract. J Allergy Clin Immunol 61:171
70. Ulrich JT, Myers KR (1995) Monophosphoryl lipid A as an adjuvant. Past experiences and new directions. In: Powell MF, Newman MJ (eds) Vaccine design: the subunit and adjuvant approach. Plenum Press, New York, pp 495–524
71. Umetsu DT, Hahn JS, Perez-Atayde AR, Geba RS (1985) Serum sickness triggered by anaphylaxis. A complication of immunotherapy. J Allergy Clin Immunol 76:713–718
72. Urbanek R, Karitzky D, Forster J (1978) Die Hyposensibilisierungsbehandlung mit reinem Bienengift. Dtsch Med Wochenschr 103:1656
73. Valenta R, Kraft D (1995) Recombinant allergens for diagnosis and therapy of allergic diseases. Curr Opin Immunol 7:751–756
74. Vervloet D, Khairallah E, Arnaud A, Charpin J (1980) A prospective national study of the safety of immunotherapy. Clin Allergy 10:59–64
75. Wahn U, Rebien W (1979) Ergebnisse der oralen Hyposensibilisierung bei kindlichen Pollenallergikern. Pädiat Prax 21:455
76. Wheeler AW, Woroniecki SR (2001) Immunological adjuvants in allergy vaccines: Past, present and future. Allergology Int 50:295–301
77. Wilson DR, Nouri-Aria KT, Walker SM, Pajno GB, O'Brien F, Jacobson MR, Mackay IS, Durham SR (2001) Grass pollen immunotherapy: Symptomatic improvement correlates with reductions in eosinophils and IL-5 mRNA expression in the nasal mucosa during the pollen season. J Allergy Clin Immunol 107:971–976
78. Wortmann F (1976) Zur oralen Desensibilisierung von Inhalationsallergien bei Kindern. Mschr Kinderheilk 124:218
79. Wüthrich B (1977) Zur spezifischen Hyposensibilisierung der Pollinosis. Schweiz Rundsch Med 66:260
80. Yang WH, Dorval G, Osterland CK, Gilmore NJ (1979) Circulating immune complexes during immunotherapy. J Allergy Clin Immunol 63:305–307
81. Zachariae H, Cramers M, Herlin T, Jensen J, Kragbale K, Ternowitz T, Thestrup-Petersen K (1985) Non-specific immunotherapy and specific hyposensitization in severe atopic dermatitis. Acta Derm Venereol (Stockh) [Suppl] 114:48–54
82. Zimmermann S, Egeter O, Hausmann S, Lipford GB, Röcken M, Wagner H, Heeg K (1998) CpG oligodeoxynucleotides trigger, protective and curative Th1 responses in lethal murine leishmaniasis. J Immunol 160:3627–3630

Positions Papers

83. World Health Organization (WHO) Bousquet J, Lockey RF, Malling HJ, et al. (1998) WHO position paper. Allergen immunotherapy: therapeutic vaccines for allergic diseases. Allergy 53 [Suppl 44]:1–42
84. European Academy of Allergy and Clinical Immunology (EAACI) Bousquet J, Müller UR, Dreborg S, et al. (1987) Immunotherapy with Hymenoptera venoms. Allergy 42:40–413
85. Malling H-J, Abreu-Nogueira J, Alvarez-Cuesta E, et al. (1998) Local immunotherapy. Position paper by the Working Group on Local Immunotherapy of the EAACI Subcommittee and the ESPACI Immunotherapy Subcommittee. Allergy 53:933–944
86. Ärzteverband Deutscher Allergologen (ÄDA) Sennekamp J, Kersten W, Hornung B (1995) Empfehlungen zur Hyposensibilisierung mit Allergenextrakten. Allergo J 4:205–212
87. Deutsche Gesellschaft für Allergologie und klinische Immunologie (DGAI) Kleine-Tebbe J, Fuchs T, Klimek L, et al. (2000) Die spezifische Immuntherapie (Hyposensibilisierung) mit Allergenen. Positionspapier der DGAI, inhaltlich abgestimmt mit dem ÄDA. Allergo J 6 (in press)

6.3.2 Other Immunotherapeutic Procedures

Immunotherapeutic procedures, as well as classic immunosuppression by chemical or biological substances, also include all kinds of active and passive immunizations, and the administration of immunoglobulins (i.m. or i.v.) and immunomodulators [16].

Recently, monoclonal antibodies against certain cell products or surface determinants have opened up a new dimension of immunotherapy with "biologicals." They also comprise gene technologically prepared anti-inflammatory cytokines, soluble receptors, anticytokines, or cytokine antagonists which may be used in allergy [9, 10, 14, 19].

The group of so-called immune response modifiers, which is applied in order to increase the immune response, also belongs to the field of immunotherapy [8]. All these procedures differ markedly from allergen-specific immunotherapy (hyposensitization) by the lack of allergen specificity.

6.3.2.1 Immunosuppressives

Apart from cortisone, the classic immunosuppressives used in severe cases of chronic diseases (asthma or eczema) are methotrexate, cyclophosphamide, azathioprine, and mycophenolate mofetil.

These drugs are commonly used in autoimmune diseases and new developments (from transplantation medicine) with immunophyllin-binding drugs (macrolactams or calcineurin antagonists); the first product was cyclosporin A, later tacrolimus, as well as ascomycin derivatives and rapamycin (Fig. 6.6) [1, 13, 18].

The topically available calcium antagonists tacrolimus and pimecrolimus represent true progress. Tacrolimus seems to be somewhat stronger (approximately comparable to a glucocorticosteroid of class 2). However, with its greasy ointment, it often induces a burning sensation in the first days of treatment. These complaints, however, diminish after continuation.

Pimecrolimus is well accepted by patients with its creamy galenic and can be used in infants and small children especially in the phase where glucocorticosteroids are not wanted.

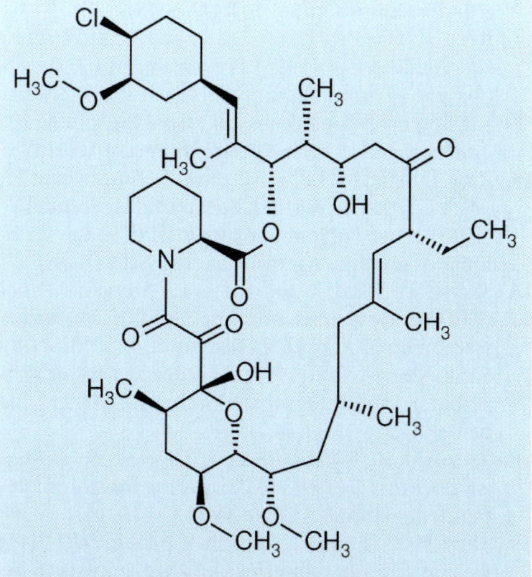

Both substances seem to be well tolerated and do not lead to increased rates of bacterial or viral skin infection as originally suspected. Colonization has even been reduced. There is no atrophy. The future will show how these "corticoids of the year 2000" live up to their hopes.

Special progress in the treatment of atopic eczema has been achieved by the topical application of some of these substances, tacrolimus and pimecrolimus. Little is known about long-term side effects; therefore, careful use is recommended, especially in children (see Sect. 5.5.3 on "Eczema").

6.3.2.2 Monoclonal Antibodies, Cytokines and Cytokine Antagonists

Since the development of hybridoma techniques, monoclonal antibodies have revolutionized medical research and diagnostics. Recently, they have begun to enter the therapeutic regimens for many diseases.

Table 6.15 shows the actual or soon available monoclonal antibodies in antiallergic and antiinflammatory therapy. Of special interest is anti-IgE (monoclonal antibody E25, omalizumab) for bronchial asthma. Anti-IgE has shown efficacy in allergic asthma, especially in reducing corticoids in steroid-dependent asthma [3, 5, 11]. Possibly, it is also effective in hay fever. Studies with anti-IgE and other IgE-mediated diseases are in preparation, maybe also in combination with allergen-specific immunotherapy.

Fig. 6.6. Structural formula of pimecrolimus

Table 6.15. Monoclonal antibodies in the therapy of allergic and inflammatory diseases

Specificity	Example
Cell surface marker	CD4, CD45, LFA-1 (alefacept)
	CD23
Adhesion molecule	ICAM-1
Costimulatory signal	CD40
Transcription factor	GATA-3
Cytokine	IL-5 (mepolizumab)
	TNF-α (infliximab)
Antibody	IgE (omalizumab)

Table 6.16. Cytokines and cytokine antagonists

Receptor antagonists	Mutants of cytokines
IL-4	IL-4
TNFα (etanercept)	
	Antibodies against cytokines
Anti-inflammatory cytokines	IL-5
IL-10	TNF-α
IFN-γ	
IL-18	

A variety of other monoclonal antibodies against cytokines are already available as well as cytokine antagonists (Table 6.16). Antibodies against TNFα (infliximab) as well as a soluble TNFα receptor (etanercept) are new in rheumatoid arthritis and psoriasis. As a side effect of infliximab, activation of tuberculosis has been reported [6].

Other antibodies against surface determinants of cells, especially T cells, represent a modern variant of the old antilymphocyte serum in the beginning of the organ transplantation era [2, 15]. Antibodies against CD4 or against markers of T-memory cells have been successfully used in psoriasis [12].

Antibodies against adhesion or costimulatory molecules also seem promising for allergy therapy. For a long time, various interferons have been used especially in oncology, but also in inflammatory diseases and allergies. The field of chemokines is so complex and its single functions are often redundant, so that very specific antagonists will maybe have only limited effects; the right combination will be the key.

References

1. Abraham RT (1998) Mammalian target of rapamycin: Immunosuppressive drugs uncover a novel pathway of cytokine receptor signaling. Curr Opin Immunol 10:330–336
2. Brendel W, Ring J, Seifert J (1974) Experimental and clinical aspects of ALG. Progr Immunol II 5:245–252
3. Busse W, Corren J, Lanier BQu, McAlary M, Fowler-Taylor A, Della Cioppa G, van As A, Gupta N (2001) Omalizumab, anti-IgE recombinant humanized monoclonal antibody, for the treatment of severe allergic asthma. J Allergy Clin Immunol 108:184–190
4. Hansel TI, Barnes PJ (eds) (2001) New drugs for asthma, allergy and COPD. Karger, Basel
5. Heusser C, Jardieu P (1997) Therapeutic potential of anti-IgE antibodies. Curr Opin Immunol 9:805–814
6. Keane J, Gershon S, Wise RP, Mirabile-Levens E, Kaszica J, Schwieterman WD, Siegel JJN, Braun MM (2001) Tuberculosis associated with infliximab, a tumor necrosis factor α-neutralizing agent. N Engl J Med 345:1098–1104
7. Jardieu PM, Fick RB Jr (1999) IgE inhibitors as a therapy for allergic disease. Int Arch Allergy Immunol 118:112–115
8. Krieg AM (1996) An innate immune defence mechanism based on the recognition of CpG motifs in microbial DANN. J Lab Clin Med 128:128–133
9. Leckie MJ, ten Brinke A, Lordan J, Khan J, Diamant Z, Walls CM, Cowley D, Hansel T, Djukanovic R, Sterk PJ, Holgate S, Barnes PJ (1999) SB 240563, a humanised anti-IL-5 monoclonal antibody: initial single dose safety and activity in patients with asthma. Am J Resp Crit Care Med 159:A624
10. Losman JA, Chen XP, Hilton D, Rothman P (1999) SOCS-1 is a potent inhibitor of IL-4 signal transduction. J Immunol 162:3770–3774
11. Milgrom H, Fick RB, Su JQ, Reimann JD, Bush RK, Watrous ML (1999) Treatment of allergic asthma with monoclonal anti-IgE antibody. N Engl J Med 341:1966–1973
12. Prinz B, Nachbar T, Plewig G (1994) Treatment of severe atopic dermatitis with extracorporal photophoresis. Arch Dermatol Res 287:48–52
13. Reitamo S (2001) Tacrolimus: A new topical immunomodulatory therapy for atopic dermatitis. J Allergy Clin Immunol 107:445–448
14. Renz H, Bradley K, Enssel K, Loader JE, Larsen GL, Gelfand EW (1996) Prevention of the development of immediate hypersensitivity and airway hyperresponsiveness in vivo with soluble IL-4 receptors. Int Arch Allergy Immunol 106:167
15. Ring J, Seifert J, Lob G, Coulin K, Angstwurm H, Frick E, Brass B, Mertin J, Backmund H, Brendel W (1974) Intensive immunosuppression in the treatment of multiple sclerosis. Lancet 2:1093–1095
16. Sacher R, FRCPC, and the IVIG Advisory Panel (2001) Intravenous immunoglobulin consensus statement. J Allergy Clin Immunol 108:S139–146
17. Saint-Remy J-MR (1999) Allergisches Bronchialasthma: Immuntherapie durch Antikörper. Die gelben Hefte 39:59
18. Szczeklik A, Nizankowska E, Dworski R, Domagala B, Pinis G (1991) Cyclosporine for steroid dependent asthma. Allergy 46:312–315
19. Tony H-P, Shen B-J, Reusch P, Sebald W (1994) Design of human interleukin-4 antagonists to inhibiting interleukin-4-dependent and interleukin-13-dependent responses in T cells and B cells with high efficiency. Eur J Biochem 225:659–665

6.4 Unconventional Procedures in Allergy

Like in few other fields of medicine, allergists are confronted with the steadily increasing number of "unconventional, "alternative," or "complementary" methods both in diagnosis and therapy [5, 10, 16, 17, 24]. Especially lay journals and magazines have endless reports about miraculous cures by such methods. Unfortunately, sometimes under economic pressure, some doctors give way to temptation and also practise these methods. The popular argument "who cures is right" ("*wer heilt, hat recht*") is not logical. Clearly thought out, it should mean "who cures does good," but whether he is right is a different question.

Scientific medicine is based on evidence provided by reproducible studies. Scientists are accused of having blinkers on if they argue on the basis of scientific arguments. It is practically impossible to perform reliable and well-controlled studies for all the continuously newly developing and commercialized methods in diagnosis and therapy (Table 6.17). We therefore need to classify according to rather rough criteria of plausibility and arrive at a classification of "complementary" procedures such as:

- Newly developed scientifically sound procedure in clinical trials
- Plausible concept supported by case reports, but exact studies are missing
- Low plausibility, little convincing experience

Table 6.17. Most commonly used unconventional procedures in allergy (according to W. Dorsch)

- Acupuncture
- Autohomologous immunotherapy
- Bach's flower therapy
- Bioresonance
- Diet
- Fasting
- Autologous blood injection
- Electroacupuncture
- Hair mineral analysis
- Homeopathy
- Kinesiology
- Neural therapy
- Fortune-teller's pendulum
- Phytotherapy
- Traditional Chinese medicine

- In spite of scientific studies, no evidence for effect
- The concept is not plausible or dangerous
- Studies are not warranted (e.g., autologous urine injection)

The German Society for Allergology and Clinical Immunology (DGAI) and its subcommittee "Complementary Medicine" (headed by W. Dorsch) is evaluating unconventional procedures from different countries of the world according to scientific criteria [4, 5].

There are a number of so-called complementary methods which may represent a beneficial supplement to classic antiallergic therapy, such as:

- Physical therapy and respiratory training
- Hydrotherapy (according to Kneipp)
- Psychosomatic counseling and relaxation methods (e.g., autogenic training)
- Certain dietetic approaches (see chapter on "Food allergy")
- Climatic therapy
- Certain phytotherapeutic approaches
- (Cum grano salis) acupuncture

On the other hand, there are many "unconventional" methods which cannot be seriously recommended because efficacy is lacking in therapy, or in diagnosis the reliability is worse than throwing dice [9, 10, 12, 18, 21]. Such procedures comprise:

- Autohomologous immunotherapy (reinjection of autologous blood or serum)
- Bach's flower therapy
- Bioresonance
- Injection of autologous blood
- Electroacupuncture
- Kinesiology
- Fortune teller's pendulum
- Hair mineral analysis

Certain procedures are heavily connected with religious-type philosophies (Weltanschauung) and so complex in general methods that the performance of scientific studies is extremely difficult (e.g., anthroposophic medicine, homeopathy). Apart from non-reproducible in vitro studies [2], there have been anecdotal positive reports [22], although in the majority the evaluation has been critical [1, 8, 13]. We have performed a large double-blind controlled study applying all the homeopathy criteria including treatment by an established homeopathist of atopic eczema without any effect [20].

It is important to remember that according to the laws of logic and philosophy, it is difficult or impossible to prove the non-efficacy of a method (Karl Popper)! The proponent of a procedure has to prove that it is efficient. It makes you wonder why some insurance companies pay the costs of these unconventional procedures [13].

Physicians are obliged to advise their patients according to their best knowledge and conscience and be honest; however, we should avoid inducing feelings of guilt in the patient. In such arguments, I usually tell my patient: "Now we are entering the field of religion, and I never discuss religious matters!"

On the other hand, interesting and partly new knowledge for western medicine can be derived from ancient medical experience in foreign countries of the developing world. The history of medicine has plenty of examples that potent drugs have been developed from phytotherapy; this also holds true for allergy [1, 3, 5, 14, 15, 24]; almost all of the current pharmacotherapeutic drugs (see Sect. 6.2) have been derived from plant extracts [5].

From traditional Chinese medicine other than acupuncture, a mixture of Chinese herbs which is applied as tea has shown significant effects in a double-blind study in atopic eczema, but also dangerous side effects [19, 23]. In this area, further research should elucidate the active substance and evaluate the safety.

Who is interested in scientific information about parascientific phenomena can join the "Gesellschaft zur wissenschaftlichen Untersuchung parawissenschaftlicher Phänomene – GWUP (Society for the Scientific Evaluation of Parascientific Phenomena)" and subscribe to the quarterly journal *The Sceptic* (*der Skeptiker*, in German).

References

1. Bock KD (1993) Wissenschaftliche und alternative Medizin. Springer, Berlin Heidelberg New York
2. Davenas E, Beauvais F, Amara J, et al. (1988) Human basophil degranulation triggered by very dilute antiserum against IgE. Nature 333:816–818
3. De Weck AL (2000) From basic science to complementary medicine. ACI Int 13:5–6
4. Dorsch W, Ring J (2002) Komplementärmethoden bzw. sog. "Alternativmethoden" in der Allergologie. Allergo J 11:163–170
5. Dorsch W (1996) Alternative Heilmethoden in der Allergologie? Allergo J 5:388–393
6. Fulder SJ, Munro RE (1985) Complementary medicine in the United Kingdom: Patients, practitioners, and consultations. Lancet II:542–545
7. Fung KP, Chow O, So SY (1986) Attenuation of exercise-induced asthma by acupuncture. Lancet II:1419–1422
8. Köbberling J (1997) Der Wissenschaft verpflichtet. Med Klin 92:171–190
9. Kofler H, Ulmer H, Mechter E, Falk M, Fritsch PO (1996) Bioresonanz bei Pollinose: Eine vergleichende Untersuchung zur diagnostischen und therapeutischen Wertigkeit. Allergologie 19:114–122
10. Kukutsch NA (1997) Darstellung und Diskussion alternativer/komplementärer diagnostischer und/oder therapeutischer Konzepte im Hinblick auf atopische Erkrankungen. Dissertation, Hamburg
11. Lambeck M (2001) Eine Revolution der Physik? Die Unterstützung der Homöopathie und ähnlicher Therapieeinrichtungen durch die Krankenkassen. Skeptiker 14:117–122
12. Lüdtke R, Kunz B, Seeber N, Ring J (2001) Test-retest reliability and validity of the kinesiology muscle test. Complement Ther Med 9:141–145
13. Oepen I, Prokop O (1985) Außenseitermethoden in der Medizin. Wissenschaftl. Buchgesellschaft, Darmstadt
14. Miller MJS, Vergnolle N, McKnight W, et al. (2001) Inhibition of neurogenic inflammation by the Amazonian herbal medicine Sangre del Grado. J Invest Dermatol 117:725–730
15. Ring J, Behrendt H, Vieluf D (eds) (1997) New trends in allergy IV. Springer, Berlin Heidelberg New York
16. Ring J (ed) (1998) Neurodermitis. Expertise zur gesundheitlichen Versorgung und Vorsorge bei Kindern mit atopischem Ekzem. Ecomed, Landsberg
17. Schäfer T, Riehle A, Wichmann HE, Ring J (2002) Alternative medicine in allergies – prevalence, patterns of use, and costs. Allergy 57:684–700
18. Schöni MH, Nikolaizik WH, Schöni-Afolter F (1997) Efficacy trial of bioresonance in children with atopic dermatitis. Int Arch Allergy Immunol 112:238–246

19. Sheehan MP, Atherton DJ (1992) A controlled trial of traditional Chinese medicinal plants in widespread non-exudative atopic eczema. Br J Dermatol 126:179–184
20. Siebenwirth J, Rakoski J (1997) Klassisch-homöopathische Therapie bei Neurodermitis. Hautarzt 48 [Suppl 1]:S22
21. Stiftung Warentest (ed) (1996) Handbuch Die andere Medizin. Nutzen und Risiken sanfter Heilmethoden, 4th edn. Stiftung Warentest, Berlin
22. Wiesenauer M, Gaus W, Häussler S (1990) Behandlung der Pollinosis mit *Galphimia glauca*. Allergologie 13:359–363
23. Wong HCG (2001) Chinese herbal medicine and allergy. ACI Int 13:192–196
24. Wüthrich B (1999) Allergologie: Quo vadis? Schweiz Med Wochenschr 129:905–914

6.5 Allergy Prevention

6.5.1 Definition

Besides activities of "salutogenesis" to improve health ("health promotion"), a variety of procedures are available in order to prevent the occurrence of disease especially in diseases with high prevalence rates such as allergic diseases [2, 42, 43, 49]. One needs to distinguish between primary, secondary, and tertiary prevention [8, 12, 27, 41, 55]:

- *Primary prevention* comprises measures to prevent the occurrence of disease, and eliminate or influence causal factors in disease development or transfer (example: active immunization = vaccination)
- *Secondary prevention* means the earliest recognition of a disease prior to clinical manifestation and prophylaxis of susceptible individuals; this requires screening examinations
- *Tertiary prevention* comprises procedures to prevent sequelae of disease after the manifestation and treatment of an acute disease; this includes rehabilitation and prevention of renewed exacerbations.

6.5.2 Primary Prevention

A rational basis for effective primary prevention requires the definition of risk groups as well as solid knowledge about causal factors of the disease. Unfortunately, in spite of great progress in molecular genetics, there is no reliable "gene test" available to predict safely the allergy risk of an individual. The hopes put into the determination of cord blood IgE or other cellular or humoral parameters (sCD23, T-cell subpopulations, phosphodiesterase concentrations in mononuclear cells, etc.) have not been fulfilled. The only reliable clinical tool is family history (see Sect. 3.1 on "Genetics").

Equally, knowledge about causal factors is limited. Apart from allergens as causal agents, modulating influences of the environment (both natural and anthropogenic) are known (see Sect. 3.3 "Allergy and Environment") including air pollutants in the outdoor and indoor air, nutrition, psychosocial situation, as well as vaccination strategies. It has to be mentioned that concepts and opinions about practical prevention programs differ considerably between experts (refer to the recent discussion about pet-keeping as protection against cat allergy) [38]. In spite of many unsolved problems, some very practical (almost trivial recommendations) can be given on the basis of the current state of knowledge. These recommendations do not harm anybody but may be helpful for children with some likelihood of high risk ("Frankfurt theses" for allergy prevention from 1 December, 1995, updated in 2003) (see Table 6.18) [49]. Common sense should never be forgotten; recommendations should only be changed after convincing and solid new evidence is available. Supplementing the Frankfurt theses, the general recommendation for avoidance of disease-promoting factors (physical, chemical, biological, psychosocial in nature) should be added (see also Sect. 5.1.2 on "Unspecific Irritation Syndrome").

Primary prevention should start in pregnancy; we have developed education programs for women at risk for atopy and pregnant women [14]. During pregnancy smoking should be strictly avoided; the concentration of potent indoor allergens (pets, molds, housedust mites) should be reduced.

Table 6.18. "Frankfurt theses" for primary prevention of allergy in children and adolescents [update by the Aktionsbündnis Allergieprävention (ABAP) (28.06.2002) (Allergo J 2003; 12: 98]

Allergic diseases represent one of the major health problems of our society. The roots for a later development of allergic diseases often occur in infants and small children. Although not all factors responsible for the development of allergic sensitization and disease are known and there is considerable need for research, the actual knowledge allows the following recommendations for prevention:

I. The parents in our country should know that:
1. There is a genetic predisposition for allergic reaction
2. It makes no sense that the mother observes a special diet during pregnancy
3. That strict breastfeeding until the 4th month of life and the late and stepwise addition of solid food in infants can reduce allergic sensitization
4. An environment at home without tobacco smoke can help to reduce the risk of allergy and airway disease
5. An allergen-poor environment can reduce the risk of the development of sensitization and allergy, and strategies to reduce housedust mite growth as well as avoidance of pets makes sense for families with risk of atopy
6. Adequate skin care and avoidance of irritating or frequently sensitizing substances (e.g., nickel containing jewelry or fragrances) may prevent the development of dermatitis
7. Children at risk of allergy and children with allergic diseases can be vaccinated according to general rules in a phase of remission

IIa. Children and adolescents and their parents have a right to:
Get consultation and information regarding risk factors for allergy and possible avoidance strategies

IIb. Children and adolescents suspicious of allergic sensitization have a right to:
1. Individual allergy diagnosis and consultation by a certified specialist
2. A healthy indoor climate at home as well as in kindergartens and schools
3. Qualified allergological consultation for the choice of occupation exceeding the current official laws

III. Children and adolescents and their families affected by allergy with chronic course have a right to:
1. Qualified information and treatment by a certified physician
2. Qualified dietary consultation when there is a risk of food allergy or other adverse food reactions
3. Help with development of own responsibility in coping with the disease by special staff (schooling and education programs) contributing to an improved quality of life and coping with the chronic disease
4. Timely therapy, also regarding secondary and tertiary prevention measures (including pharmacotherapy and immunotherapy)
5. Use of rehabilitation measures as well outpatient and near the living area as well as inpatient in special clinics (including asthma, eczema, swimming and sports groups, rehabilitation in school)
6. Declaration of allergenic substances in foods and in items of daily use

IV. Teachers and education personnel have a right to:
Qualified information in dealing with allergic children

In the prevention and treatment of allergies, lay groups have an important task. Cooperation with experts of different disciplines and lay groups is mandatory
These aims can only be achieved if the qualification of experts and the structural requirements of patient care are improved and allergologic expertise is taken into account by the relevant political committees

Practical recommendations include:

- Nutrition: consistent breast-feeding over 4–6 months, late addition of solid food [44], possibly extensively hydrolyzed hypoallergenic formula [6]. Recent studies show a positive effect regarding the prevalence of atopic eczema in infants by adding probiotics (lactobacillus GG) during pregnancy 2–4 weeks prior to birth [24, 26].
- Reduction of aeroallergen exposure (pets, housedust mites, molds) [1, 3, 25, 26]
- Reduction of exposure to pollutants in indoor air (smoking, chemicals in hobby and occupation) as well as outdoor air (traffic exhaust) [2, 32, 41]
- Avoidance of irritating substances for the airways (e.g., dust) [47] as well as skin (e.g., clothing, skin cleaning and care, jewelry – caveat: ear piercing!)
- Avoidance of disease-promoting factors (physical, chemical, biological, psychosocial in nature) [8, 19]

6.5.3 Secondary Prevention

At this stage, one might discuss immunological or pharmacological approaches; certain studies have been performed in tertiary prevention (early treatment of the atopic child, ETAC) where in many European countries the occurrence of asthma in the following years was significantly reduced by prophylactic administration of an H_1 antagonist cetirizine in infants with atopic eczema and sensitization against grass pollen and/or housedust mites [18]. Similar results have been obtained with the mast cell blocker and H_1 antagonist ketotifen where a reduction of allergic asthma prevalence in patients with allergic rhinoconjunctivitis was observed [33].

Allergen-specific immunotherapy in hay fever also has a preventive effect by reducing the prevalence of asthma in hay fever patients (see Sect. 6.3.1 on "Allergen-Specific Immunotherapy").

6.5.4 Tertiary Prevention

Besides careful causal and symptomatic treatment of allergic diseases, allergen avoidance is at the center of all recommendations for prevention. This is only possible after intensive and competent diagnosis and information of the compliant patient and their surroundings. The patient has to be able to recognize the allergen; this implies the need for better declaration laws (not only for drugs, but also for cosmetics and products in daily use) [2].

Education programs for children and adults can help patients and their families considerably in coping with the allergic disease; they are available for asthma and atopic eczema (Sects. 5.1.3, 5.5.3).

An integral part of tertiary prevention is occupational counseling and information about potential risks through allergens or irritants in certain occupations. Educational programs – which should be monitored for quality ("train the trainer" seminars) – in asthma or eczema "academies" with standard certified protocols [20] should encompass our philosophy that the concept of "patient management" should finally evolve into "self-management" by the patient.

The classic methods of rehabilitation are at the center of tertiary prevention, which can be performed in an outpatient or in severe cases an inpatient setting; sometimes the change of environment not only has allergological but also psychosomatic importance. Specialized hospitals for allergic patients exist in several European countries.

In severe cases, long-lasting rehabilitation can only be achieved under certain climatic conditions including climatherapeutic procedures; North Sea islands as well as climate at high altitude over 1,500 m (e.g., Davos, Switzerland) have been studied in this regard and have shown beneficial effects [7, 14, 54].

Through progress in causal and somatic therapy of allergic diseases and increasing knowledge in prevention, the quality of life of allergic individuals has been improved considerably. Asthma patients can do sports, eczema patients can swim and use the sauna; however, they need to use emollients and follow skin care guidelines before and after sporting activities.

In the many tasks of prevention, lay groups play an important role. By close cooperation between lay groups and experts of different disciplines, the effects can be optimized. Allergologic expertise needs to be heard by political bodies making decisions relevant for allergic individuals [2]. In the following, practical recommendations regarding avoidance of aeroallergens are given.

6.5.5 Strategies for Aeroallergen Avoidance

The biologic basis of aeroallergens has been discussed in Sect. 3.4 on "Allergens."

6.5.5.1 Pollen

The pollen of anemophilous plants is almost ubiquitous during the spring and summer months in central Europe and many countries of the world, except in the desert or at the high altitudes of the alpine regions, where the concentration is lower. Avoidance measures are therefore limited. If the symptomatic period is short, a well-planned vacation in pollen-poor areas can be recommended. At home, allergic

Table 6.19. Reduction of aerogenic pollen exposure in patients with atopic eczema

Recommendations:
- Avoid staying outdoors during peak pollen exposure (see the pollen information service in the media). During cool weather or longer lasting rain, pollen counts are markedly reduced
- Daily peaks (only for rural areas): early morning and evening. During these time periods close the windows. The optimal time for ventilation is between midnight and 4 in the morning
- You can leave the window open if you have fixed a pollen protection foil
- When you have been outdoors, take a shower in the evening (and wash your hair) followed by adequate skin care. Clothes should not be left in the sleeping room since pollen may be transferred there. You should try to keep the bedroom cool and dust poor
- Regular vacuum cleaning (with small particle filter) and moist cleaning of surfaces in the apartment during the pollen season are recommended; however, this should not be done by the affected individual but by other family members
- Use of emollients prior to leaving the apartment on air-exposed skin sites may be recommended
- Do not dry textiles in the outdoor air
- Pets can carry considerable amounts of pollen into the apartment
- Automobile: When your car has been standing some time outdoors, especially under pollinating trees, heavy pollen loads can reach the airways when you turn on the engine and the ventilation. Therefore pollen filters should be used and are available for most cars
- If possible consider your allergy in making your vacation plans by choosing the right time and place of holidays. You might completely avoid allergen exposure

individuals may benefit from certain recommendations for daily life (Table 6.19). Closing the window does not reduce pollen concentration in the indoor air. This only can be achieved by air-conditioning with special filters.

Pollen and mold counts are measured in many countries by different associations or foundations (in Germany "Stiftung Deutscher Polleninformationsdienst" = PID in Bad Lippspringe), which then provide together with meteorologists and phenologists pollen forecasts helpful for allergic individuals in planning their activities and use of prophylactic drugs [3, 32, 42, 48].

6.5.5.2 Mold Spores

Molds grow best in a moist and warm microenvironment. Indoor plants should be reduced, and soil can be covered by aluminum. Moist walls, wallpapers, humid textiles, shower curtains, and humidifiers should be avoided [15, 45].

6.5.5.3 Animal Epithelia

After removal of a pet, the patient has to know that over a longer time (months up to years) small amounts of the respective allergen will still be measurable in indoor air [10, 37, 47, 58].

Washing the cat has reduced cat allergen content in indoor air, but has not been accepted as a practical preventive measure [37]. In occupational animal exposure (farmer, laboratory worker, etc.), wearing a mask or helmet (e.g., airstream) is recommended [3, 47].

6.5.5.4 Housedust Mites

Housedust mites of different species are the most common allergen carrier in the indoor environment [31, 34, 57]. Avoidance measures have to be seen at several levels starting best in the bedroom with the mattress and should be done specifically (it is not necessary to change the apartment into a glass-concrete environment!) [1, 4, 9, 10, 11, 13, 15, 21, 23, 34, 35, 37, 50, 51, 52].

The normal cleaning procedures do not reduce mite allergen content, and normal vacuum cleaners are of little help. During the construction of a house, important measures can be taken (central heating, adequate ventilation, low air humidity, central vacuum cleaner, which is equipped with an adequate filter and blows the air out into the outside environment) [29]

Mites or mite allergen can be detected in environmental samples by a color test which detects the fecal product guanine or by immuno-

Table 6.20. Criteria for quality evaluation of mattress encasings (according to Diepschlag [13])

Criteria	Recommendations
Particle size	0.4–0.6 µm
Water vapor resistance (according to ISO 11092)	$<20 \, m^2 \times Pa/W$
Water vapor permeability (according to DIN 53122/B)	$<6{,}000 \, g/m^2 \times 24 \, h$ (corresponding to ca. $R<74/6 = 12.4$, comfort class "good")
Production	Completely closed around mattress, zip closing
Washing	60 °C and above
Durability	5–10 years
Comfort	Acceptance
Cost	Satisfactory

assays allowing quantification of mite or allergen contents in different areas of the home.

Old mattresses (>5 years) should be replaced and bedding and clothing regularly washed; great progress can be seen in encasings available from different producers with different characteristics which reduce mite allergen exposure in the bed. Quality criteria comprise certain parameters (Table 6.20) [13, 17, 25, 28, 46]. Stuffed animals and small textile items can be put into the deep freeze (once a month over several hours, –20 °C). Washing at 60 °C kills most mites. While there is a consensus that washable floors may be superior to carpeting, new materials and adequate cleaning can save the carpet in the apartment!

Mites may be killed chemically [4, 11, 30] by acaricides such as benzylbenzoate (available as foam, powder, or liquid together with washing powder), tannic acid, highly concentrated saline, as well as liquid nitrogen. Some acarizides do not smell good, but the toxicologic and allergologic risks are low [13]. Sometimes textiles, e.g., in upholstery or old clothing (grandfather's black suit!), can be highly infested with mites. Detailed recommendations for individuals are available in numerous books, brochures, and flyers.

References

1. Arlian LG, Platts-Mills TAE (2001) The biology of dust mites and the remediation of mite allergens in allergic disease. J Allergy Clin Immunol 107:S406–413
2. Behrendt H, et al. (1999) Der Rat von Sachverständigen für Umweltfragen. Umwelt und Gesundheit. Risiken richtig einschätzen. Sondergutachten. Metzler-Poeschel, Stuttgart
3. Bergmann K-Ch (2001) Allergenkarenz bei allergischem Asthma. In: Ring J, Darsow U (eds) Allergie 2000. Dustri, Munich, pp 164–168
4. Bischoff E, Krause-Michel B, Nolte D (1986) Zur Bekämpfung der Hausstaubmilben in Haushalten von Patienten mit Milbenasthma. Allergologie 9:448–457
5. Björkstén B, Sepp E, Julge K, Voor T, Mikelsaar M (2001) Allergy development and the intestinal microflora during the first year of life. J Allergy Clin Immunol 108:516–520
6. Boehm G, Leuschner RM (eds) (1987) Advances in aerobiology. Experientia [Suppl] 51:197–202
7. Borelli S (1997) Deutsche Klinik für Dermatologie und Allergie Davos (Alexanderhausklinik) 1960–1995. Stiftung Derm All Forschung, Davos
8. Bucher H, Gutzwiller F (eds) (1993) Checkliste Gesundheitsberatung und Prävention. Thieme, Stuttgart
9. Cloosterman SGM, Schermer TRJ, Bijl-Hofland ID, et al. (1999) Effects of house dust mite avoidance measures on Der p1 concentrations and clinical condition of mild adult house dust mite-allergic asthmatic patients, using no inhaled steroids. Clin Exp Allergy 29:1336–1346
10. Colloff MJ, Ayres J, Carswell F, Howarth PH, Merret TG, Mitchell EB, Walshaw MJ, Warner JO, Warner JA, Woodcock AA (1992) The control of allergens of dust mite and domestic pets: a position paper. Clin Exp Allergy 22 [Suppl 2]:1–28
11. Colloff MJ, Taylor C, Merrett TG (1995) The use of domestic steam cleaning for the control of house dust mites. Clin Exp Allergy 25:1061–1066
12. DGAI-Stellungnahme: Ring J et al. (1993) Allergie-Prävention. Allego J 2:36–37
13. Diebschlag W, Diebschlag B (2000) Hausstauballergien. Gesundheitliche und hygienische Aspekte, 2nd edn. Herbert Utz Verlag, Munich
14. Disch R, Schöne D (1995) Prävention in der Dermatologie. Präv Rehabil 3:155–160
15. Eggleston PA, Bush RK (2001) Environmental allergen avoidance: An overview. J Allergy Clin Immunol 107:S403–405
16. Ehnert B, Lau-Schadendorf S, Weber A, et al. (1992) Reducing domestic exposure to dust mite

allergen reduces bronchial hyperreactivity in sensitive children with asthma. J Allergy Clin Immunol 90:135–138
17. Ewers U, Kainka E, Umbach KH, Diebschlag W (2000) Methoden zur Überprüfung der Qualitätsanforderungen an milbenallergendichte Matratzen- und Bettbezüge (Encasings). Allergo J 9: 261–269
18. ETAC Study Group (1998) Allergic factors associated with the development of asthma and the influence of cetirizine in a double-blind, randomised placebo-controlled trial: first results of ETAC. Pediatr Allergy Immunol 9:116–124
19. Fröschl M (2000) Gesund sein. Integrative Gesund-Seins-Förderung als Ansatz für Pflege, soziale Arbeit und Medizin. Lucius u. Lucius, Stuttgart
20. Gieler U, Niemeier V, Kupfer J, Brosig B (2001) Psychosomatische Konzepte in der Allergologie. In: Ring J, Darsov U (eds) Allergie 2000. Dustri, Munich, pp 189–192
21. Götzsche PC, Hammarquist C, Burr M (1998) House dust mite control measures in the management of asthma: meta-analysis. BMJ 317:1105–1110
22. Grootendorst DC, Dahlén S-E, van den Bos JW, Duiverman EJ, Veselic-Charvat M, Vrijlandt EJLE, O'Sullivan S, Kumlin M, Sterk PJ, Roldaan AC (2001) Benefits of high altitude allergen avoidance in atopic adolescents with moderate to severe asthma, over and above treatment with high dose inhaled steroids. Clin Exp Allergy 31:400–408
23. Huss K, Squire EN Jr, Carpenter GB, Smith LJ, Huss RJ, Salata K, Salerno M, Agostinelli D, Hershey J (1992) Effective education of adults with asthma who are allergic to dust mites. J Allergy Clin Immunol 89:836–843
24. Isolauri E, Arvola T, Sütas Y, Moilanen E, Salminen S (2000) Probiotics in the management of atopic eczema. Clin Exp Allergy 30:1604–1610
25. Johansson SGO, Haahtela T (eds) (2000) Prevention of allergy and asthma. Interim report. Based on the WHO/IAACI Meeting on the Primary Prevention of Allergy and Asthma. Allergy 55:1069–1088
26. Kalliomäki M, Salminen S, Arvilommi H, Kero P, Koskinen P, Isolauri E (2001) Probiotics in primary prevention of atopic disease: a randomised placebo-controlled trial. Lancet 357:1076–1079
27. Kjellman N-I M, Nilsson L (1999) Is allergy prevention realistic and beneficial? Pediatr Allergy Immunol 10 [Suppl 12]:11–17
28. Kniest FM, Liebenberg B, Ahr A (1992) Mattress-encasings as a barrier for mites and airborne dust. J Aerosol Sci 23 [Suppl I]:S551–554
29. Korsgaard J (1982) Preventive measures in house-dust allergy. Am Rev Respir Dis 125:80–84
30. Kroidl RF (1992) Allergie gegen Hausstaubmilben: Sanierungsmaßnahmen: Konventionell? Mit akariziden Mitteln? Allergologie 15:197–201
31. Lau S, Falkenhorst G, Weber A, Werthman I, Lind P, Buettner-Goetz P, Wahn U (1989) High mite-allergen exposure increases the risk of senzitization in atopic children and young adults. J Allergy Clin Immunol 84:718–725
32. Liccardi G, Custovic A, Cazzola M, Russo M, D'Amato M, D'Amato G (2000) Avoidance of allergens and air pollutants in respiratory allergy. Allergy 56:705–722
33. Medici TC, Radielovic P, Morley J (1989) Ketotifen in the prophylaxis of extrinsic bronchial asthma. A multicenter controlled double-blind study with a modified-release formulation. Chest 96: 1252–1257
34. Müsken H, Wahl R, Franz J-Th, Masuch G, Sauter Ch, Bergmann K-Ch (1996) Häufigkeit von Hausstaubmilben-Sensibilisierung. Allergologie 19: 29–34
35. Nishioka K, Yasueda H, Saito H (1998) Preventive effect of bedding encasement with microfine fibers on mite sensitization. J Allergy Clin Immunol 101:28–32
36. Peat JK, Britton WJ, Salome CM, Woolcock AJ (1987) Bronchial hyperresponsiveness in two populations of Australian school children. III. Effect of exposure to environmental allergens. Clin Allergy 17:291–330
37. Platts-Mills TAE, Rovvey ER, Mitchell EB, Moszoro H, Nock P, Wilkins SR (1982) Reduction of bronchial hyperreactivity during prolonged allergen avoidance. Lancet III:675–678
38. Platts-Mills T, Vaughan J, Squillace S, Woodfolk J, Sporik R (2001) Sensitisation, asthma, and a modified Th2 response in children exposed to cat allergen: a population-based cross-sectional study. Lancet 357:752–756
39. Pürschel W (1973) Dermatologische Klimatherapie an der Nordsee. Dermatologica 146 [Suppl 1]: 1–98
40. Ring J, Abeck D (1996) Vom "Patienten-Management" zum "Selbst-Management": Prävention durch Schulung bei atopischem Ekzem (Neurodermitis). In: Stützner W, Giesler M (eds) Prävention allergischer Erkrankungen im Kindes- und Jugendalter. Kohlhammer, Stuttgart, pp 32–41
41. Ring J, Gfesser M (1997) Atopieprävention. In: Plewig G, Przybilla B (eds) Fortschritte der praktischen Dermatologie und Venerologie, vol 15. Springer, Berlin Heidelberg New York, pp 317–321
42. Ring J, Wenning J (eds) (2000) Weißbuch: Allergie in Deutschland 2000. Urban und Vogel, Munich
43. Ring J, Schäfer T (2001) Vernetzungsansätze in der Allergieforschung. In: Aktionsbündnis Allergieprävention. BMG, Bonn, pp 21–25
44. Saarinen U, Kajosaari M (1995) Breastfeeding as prophylaxis against atopic disease: prospective follow-up study until 17 years old. Lancet 346: 1065–69

45. Schober G (1988) Feuchte und Entwicklung von Wohnungsallergenen. Allergologie 11:229–234
46. Schoenecker I, Grübl A, Bartels P, Ulm K, Bauer CP (2001) Klinische Effekte der Allergenreduktion durch Encasing – eine Metaanalyse. Allergy J 10:95–99
47. Schultze-Werninghaus (1993) Allergenkarenz bei inhalativer Allergie. In: Manuale allergologicum, VII.1, Dustri, Munich, pp 1–9
48. Stiftung Deutscher Polleninformationsdienst (1997) 1. Europäisches Pollenflug-Symposium. Verlag für Medizin und Umwelt, Krefeld
49. Stünzner W, Giesler M (eds) (1996) Prävention allergischer Erkrankungen im Kindes- und Jugendalter. XXIII. Kongreß der Deutschen Zentrale für Volksgesundheitspflege e.V. (DZV). Kohlhammer, Stuttgart
50. Tan BB, Weald D, Strickland I, et al. (1996) Double-blind controlled trial of effect of housedust-mite allergen avoidance on atopic dermatitis. Lancet 347:15–18
51. van Leeuwen S (1926) Allergische Krankheiten. Asthma bronchiale, Heufieber, Urticaria und andere. Dtsch Übers von Verzár F. Springer, Berlin Heidelberg New York
52. Vandenhove T, Soler M, Birnbaum J, Charpin D, Vervloet D (1993) Effect of dry cleaning on mite allergen levels in blankets. Allergy 48:264–266
53. Vervloet D, Penaud A, Razzouk H, Senft M, Arnaud A, Boutin C, Charpin J (1982) Altitude and house dust mites. J Allergy Clin Immunol 69: 290–296
54. Vocks E, Borelli S, Rakoski J (1994) Klimatherapie bei Neurodermitis. Allergologie 17:208–213
55. Wahn U (1987) Möglichkeiten der Allergieprophylaxe bei Säuglingen und Kleinkindern. Allergologie 10:362–364
56. Wahn U, von Mutius E (2001) Childhood risk factors for atopy and the importance of early intervention. J Allergy Clin Immunol 107:567–574
57. Wanner H-U (1994) Biologische Verunreinigungen in der Raumluft. Allergologie 17:526–529
58. Wood RA, Chapman MD, Adkinson NF Jr, Eggleston PA (1989) The effect of cat removal on allergen content household dust samples. J Allergy Clin Immunol 83:730–734
59. Zock JP, Brunekreef B (1995) House dust mite allergen levels in dust from schools with smooth and carpeted classroom floors. Clin Exp Allergy 25:549–553

7 Psyche and Allergy

Psychologic factors influence allergic diseases to considerable extent, this fact being well known to every experienced allergist [8, 19, 26, 32, 48, 62]. However, the nature and importance of this phenomenon are controversial. The term "psychosomatics" itself [2] is interpreted differently: Some regard it only as a general way of looking at the whole sick human being, while others use it more specifically for certain diseases (gastric ulcer, ulcerative colitis, asthma). The term "psychosomatics" in reality is often the source of a new dualism: on the one hand, proponents of the psyche deny the existence of any physicochemical causalities, while on the other hand so-called natural scientific medicine sometimes regards psychosomatic effects only as an unimportant epiphenomenon.

One reason for this situation is that often only the psychologic effects on the induction and maintenance of allergies are considered. It is equally important to study the influence of an existing allergic disease upon the psyche of the patient! This means that we have to study with equal intensity the:
- Somatopsychic influence
- The impairment of quality of life
- Fear of exacerbations

7.1 The Problem of "Allergic Personality Traits"

Since the description of allergic disease, people are tempted to characterize specific personality traits for allergy. Some textbooks describe the "subtle reacting, emotionally easily vulnerable, highly intelligent, but aggressive allergic individual." One sometimes gets the impression that many of these authors have been allergic themselves.

In some studies, characteristic personality profiles have been observed [3, 7, 8, 9, 79]. However, the detailed analysis shows huge discrepancies with characteristic traits such as "longing for contact," "shy," "passive" over "pedantic," "extrovert," "hypercorrect," "hyperactive," "easily contacted" and "impulsive" (cited in [79]).

Psychoanalysis-oriented authors focus on the early infant and sexual conflicts as cause of allergies; they stress the sexual component of itch, the lust sensation in scratching as substitute for orgasm. Swelling of the nasal mucosa in a patient is interpreted as penis envy (the nose as phallic symbol). Occasionally the relation between allergics and compulsive neurotics is mentioned: "Allergens are substitute objects in unconscious libidinous and aggressive phantasies" [40].

The theory of "allergic object relationship" implies that patients become sick when they fear the loss of a strongly emotional object (e.g., mother) or when two objects cannot be reconciled together [40, 49].

Other authors do not agree with the existence of characteristic types of allergic personalities. Rechardt found in a 9 years' longitudinal examination a total normalization of abnormal personality profiles together with improvement of skin symptoms in atopic eczema [55]. In the recent literature, these discrepancies have slowly disappeared. The concepts of acute and chronic stress sequelae are increasingly being recognized [81]. Parent-child interactions seem to be another important field.

7.2 Stress

The term "stress" was put forward 1936 by Hans Selye [69] to mean an "unspecific response of the body to any challenge." Today we know that there is a certain specificity with regard to certain stressors and stress responses. While the phenomenon was regarded as merely biological in the first few decades, recently the psychologic aspects have gained greater and greater recognition. Together with several other authors [69, 76, 78, 80, 81], we want to define stress as:

- *Primary unspecific psychobiological reaction to a challenge of the individual psychochemical or psychic well-being.*

The often used term "stress reaction" is redundant since stress already implies the reaction to the stressor, which can be of variable nature (Table 7.1).

Acute stress is distinguished from chronic stress. Especially chronic stress may give rise to psychopathological sequelae such as anxiousness, instability, loss of activity, reduction of self-confidence, hallucination, hyperventilation, sensory disturbance, or vasovagal reactions [66].

Stress phenomena are complicated by sociocultural influences. Many stressors come from psychosocial exposure. In this context, one could speculate together with Alexander Solzhenitsyn on the adverse effect of a culturally accepted hunt for profit leading to exaggerated competition and finally personal isolation;

Table 7.1. Different types of stressors (examples)

Physical	Trauma
	Pain
	Fatigue
	Exhaustion
	Heat/cold
	Noise
Chemical	Environmental noxious agents (pollutants)
Biological	Nutrition
	Infection
	Allergy
Psychosocial	Life event/sadness
	Anxiety
	Expression
	Emotional arousal

Table 7.2. Methods to quantify stress

Chemical
Measurement of hormones or autacoids (epinephrine, norepinephrine or metabolites, ACTH, CRF, NGF, aldosterone, renin, angiotensin, histamine)

Physiological
Pulse, blood pressure, ECG, muscle tension (EMG), skin temperature, skin blood flow, electric skin resistance, EEG changes

Psychologic
Affect resonance, cognitive activity, various scales, various psychodiagnostic tests (e.g., STAI)

then increased egoistic efforts increase and perpetuate the vicious cycle and lead to stress (cited in [81]).

Stress situations can be recorded and documented by certain psychodiagnostic test procedures such as the "State-Trait-Anxiety Inventory" (STAI) [71] or the "Social Readjustment Rating Scale" [21]. High values in this case often predict future disease. The importance of "life events" for the development of allergic diseases is known. One study found a significant stressful life event in 90% of patients suffering from chronic urticaria prior to the start of the disease [15].

Stress can induce physiologic and pathophysiologic changes via different mechanisms, e.g., via the nervous system (conscious and unconscious), neuroendocrine organs (enterochrome affine cells in the suprarenals and release of adrenaline) as well as endocrinologically via certain hormones (cortisol, aldosterone, hypothalamic CRF, or thyroid hormones). Therefore, stress can be measured by different methods (Table 7.2).

7.3 Influence of Psyche upon Allergy

The well-known psychologic influence upon the allergic reaction can be explained using different concepts. Psychoanalytic models describe situations of conflict by excessive binding to the mother, a disturbed ego feeling in the sense of narcissism. Allergens gain their pathogenic character only through association with certain unpleasant situations; the mediation is unconscious [7, 25].

Table 7.3. Model of conditioned reflexes in allergy

Stimulus	Conditioning	Reaction
Pollen	0	Rhinorrhea
Pollen	Painting of meadow	Rhinorrhea
–	Painting of meadow	Rhinorrhea
Ovalbumin	–	Shock
Ovalbumin	Audiovisual stimulus	Shock
–	Audiovisual stimulus	Shock

On the other hand, behavioristic concepts prefer the model of the conditioned reflex. The somehow conditioned patient no longer needs the allergen for the elicitation of symptoms, but only a certain situation which was previously connected with allergen contact (Table 7.3) [4, 13, 37, 38]. In animal models, elicitation of anaphylaxis through conditioned reflexes has been shown in guinea pigs [47]. In his famous rat experiments, J. Bienenstock used an audiovisual stimulus (flashlight and Rolling Stones music) together with allergen challenge in ovalbumin-sensitized animals; finally rats shocked to the light or musical stimulus alone [13].

Classic psychological elicitors of attacks of allergic diseases (e.g., asthma, itch) include the mention of allergens (often only anecdotal in character!), mentioning the disease (e.g., asthma), the presence of physicians, being at a hospital, anxiety, or a negative experience like personal criticism or lack of acceptance.

Reports describing patients who start sneezing after looking at a painting of a meadow [37] need to be looked at critically. The famous case of a patient of A. Jores who reacted heavily with asthma while standing in front of an oil painting of his mother-in-law, and who on investigation by Karl Hansen was found to have an allergy to the varnish with which the painting had recently been treated, is still open for discussion [29]. In practice, the mechanism of conditioned reflexes may be of importance in the unconscious more than in the conscious field.

Conditioned reflexes may also act in the immune system and have immunosuppressive or immunopotentiating effects [1, 22, 23, 27, 31, 42]. Histamine release can be influenced by conditioning [64].

7.4 Psychoneuroallergology

The recent research area of psychoneuroallergology describes the interactions between psychologic influence and allergic reactions and has developed from work in psychoneuroimmunology [1]. It is surprising how closely the two systems are linked, providing the basis for our interaction with the environment using specific recognition reactions and long-term memory, namely:

- The nervous system (sensory, conscious, fixed tissue structures)
- The immune system (humoral, unconscious)

The important cells of the immune system express receptors for neurotransmitters [1]. Vice versa, cytokines of different immune cells act on nerve cells [1, 22, 37, 53, 56]. A well-known and everyday example is fever after IL-1 and IL-6. Nerve growth factor (NGF) and other neurotrophins act on immune cells and are secreted by immune cells [6, 30, 77]. Substances of the hypothalamic-pituitary axis influence inflammation in the skin [37, 75].

Many reactions of allergic symptoms underlie the control through the autonomic nervous system. Atopics are characterized by an altered reactivity pattern in this system, which can be roughly simplified as increased cholinergic and α-adrenergic together with decreased β-adrenergic sensitivity (β-blockade theory of Szentivanyi) (see Sect. 5.5.3 on "Atopic Eczema").

In cell cultures of nerve cells and intestinal mast cells, it has been shown that synapses are formed between neurites and mast cells, through which mast cells can be activated after electric stimulation [4, 13] (see also Fig. 7.1).

Psychologic factors may influence allergic reactions via stress in different ways and at different levels (Table 7.4).

The influence of stress factors on allergy has to distinguish between the different levels of sensitization and elicitation. In animal experiments, it has been shown that stress induces a transient weakness of the immune system [5, 13, 31, 50, 51, 76, 81]. In a period of disturbed lymphocyte regulation, the switch to TH2 and formation of IgE antibodies might be easier.

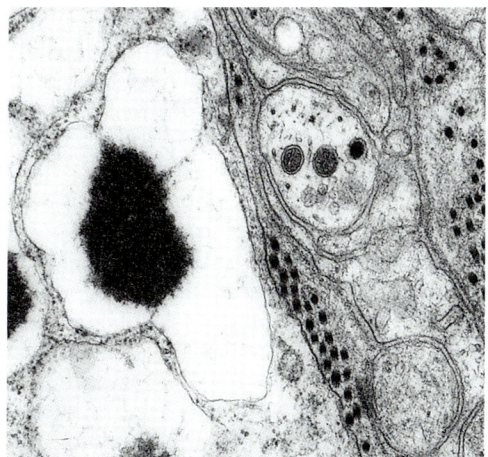

Fig. 7.1. Mast cell and nerve in close proximity in the respiratory mucosa (H. Behrendt)

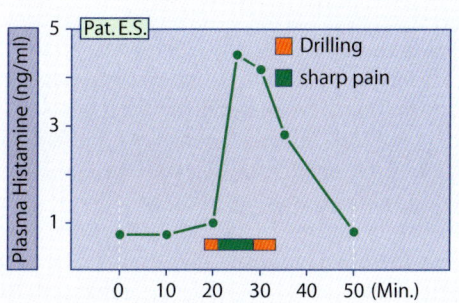

Fig. 7.2. Increase in the histamine concentration in plasma during dental treatment

Besides, stress influences the allergic elicitation reaction via several hormones and autacoids. In animal experiments and humans, increases in plasma histamine have been observed under stress [55, 62] (Fig. 7.2). The hypothalamic pituitary axis also controls vascular changes. It is well known that anxiety can increase vasoconstriction, which can be reversed by hypnosis [3, 14, 82]. Acute anxiety stimulates fibrinolysis, leading to an interaction with the kallikrein-kinin system [1].

The parameter of "stress susceptibility" is crucial and differs from individual to individual. Possibly, this can be explained by the "suggestibility phenomenon" studied in placebo research. Placebo responders are more easily influenced both positively and negatively (improvement or deterioration of an allergic reaction) by suggestion (e.g., allergen provocation) (Bienenstock, pers. comm.).

University students were studied during their final examinations and showed altered cytokine secretion profiles and T-cell subpopulations only in asthmatics; equally, increased IL-5 formation only was observed in asthmatic adolescents during examination [39].

Acute stress does not induce epinephrine release. However, corticotrophin-releasing factor (CRF) is characteristic and can activate mast cells. In experimental stress models (cold, immobilization), gastrointestinal inflammatory reactions are observed [55]. Stress seems to

Table 7.4. Possible concepts for stress influencing allergic reactions

Tissue	Cells/mediators	Clinical consequences
Nervous system	Nociceptors Neurotransmitter Autonomic impulses (weak β-adrenergic, increased cholinergic)	Effect on immune and inflammatory cells as well as manifestation organ
Endocrine system	Hypothalamus (CRF) Suprarenal (catecholamines)	Hormone effects
Immune system	T1 cells NK cells T1/T2 deviation Inflammatory cells (mediator release)	Decreased immunity Tendency to infection IgE formation/atopy
Manifestation organ (airway, skin)	Mucus secretion Bronchoconstriction Vasodilation Itch	Rhinopathy Asthma Urticaria Eczema

lower the threshold for neurotransmitter effects (e.g., tachykinins on the trachea and bronchial muscle).

It has to be admitted that the gap between the exciting new research developments and the practical benefit for today's patients is vague. The sentence of Gronemeyer and Fuchs is still valid: "It is not proven that allergic asthma can be caused by psychic influences; however, there is consensus that exacerbations in asthmatics may be induced, enhanced, or maintained by psychologic influences" [19].

7.5 Clinical Conditions

The practicing allergist often has to deal with psychosomatic problems. There is a wide spectrum of diseases from anaphylactic shock after penicillin (low psychological involvement) to the very much psychologically influenced bronchial asthma and diseases, which are almost merely psychological in nature (Table 7.5).

Besides allergic bronchial asthma (see Sect. 5.1.2), atopic eczema and chronic urticaria are the diseases with the most prominent psychological involvement, sometimes recognizable physiologically (increased sweating after emotional stimulus in lichenified regions, itch during anxiety feelings; cited in [8, 78]).

Sixty to 70% of patients with chronic urticaria suffer from emotional stress, according to many authors, without any specific personality profile or specific stressor. This becomes especially obvious in cholinergic urticaria.

In children with eczema, the parent-child relationship might be a problem area [20]. Psychodiagnostic tests for evaluation of personality profiles have not yielded statistically significant differences between children with eczema and other dermatologically diseased children, neither for neuroticism nor for extraversion. In the Freiburg Personality Inventory (FPI), mothers of children with atopic eczema were more "unspontaneous," "controlled," and less "emotional" than mothers of normal children. Fathers of atopic children did not show significant differences from the controls, but showed a trend to increased "irritability." Compared to the FPI profiles of atopic parents, mothers showed less bodily affect resonance while emotional control was more prominent. In the parental educational style, "rigidity" and "strictness" were more prominent as seen from the view of children with eczema than the criterion "support." There was no difference in the parental educational style of fathers. It was interesting that mothers of eczema children more frequently gratified "adult behavior" of the children while "affective warmth" and "compassion" and "joy" were weaker. In family drawings (family in animals, family in persons), children with atopic eczema did not show a friendly atmosphere. The relationship of mother/father in size was significantly different in that fathers of atopic children were significantly smaller compared to mothers (0.7:1) than in control children (1.1:1) [60, 61] (Fig. 7.3).

In all these considerations, one should never forget that the question regarding cause or sequel of a disease is finally open. Skin diseases are characterized by the fact that disturbances not only lead to impaired function of an organ but always also reflect the psyche of the patient since the skin expresses processes of the soul and has an eminent aesthetic function [8, 9].

We advise parents of children with atopic eczema to know about psychosomatic interactions. Never must these discussions lead to feelings of guilt in the parents! I think that fathers should be integrated more strongly into family affairs and also into the care of the diseased skin of the child, while mothers should be advised to "relax." Skin diseases need patience and can never be managed by force or effort! Compulsory hygienic procedures should be

Table 7.5. Diseases with a strong psychosomatic component in the allergist's office

Often allergic	Often without detectable allergy
Bronchial asthma	Pseudo-allergic drug reactions (e.g., local anesthetics)
Eczema	Dental prosthesis incompatibility
Urticaria	"Eco syndrome" (multiple chemical sensitivity, MCS)

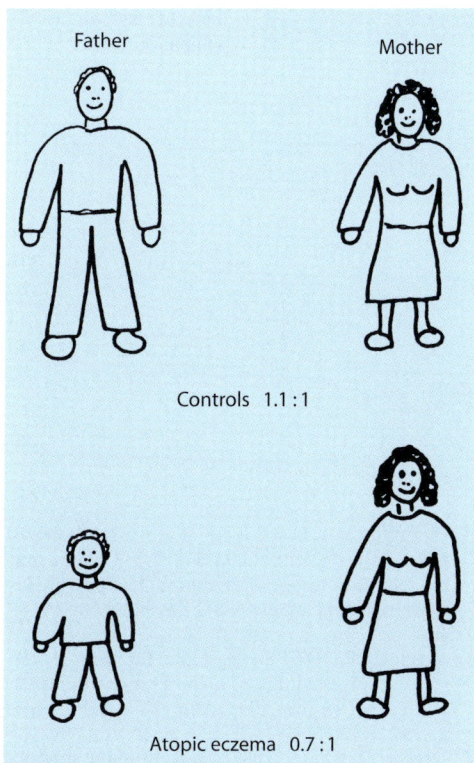

Fig. 7.3. Size ratio of father and mother in drawings made by children with atopic eczema and controls (from [62])

Table 7.6. Abnormal forms of parental affection (often relevant for children with atopic eczema)

Compulsion	No	Care	Yes
Neurotic pressure	No	Consistency	Yes
Dominance	No	Strength	Yes
Exhaustion	No	Stimulation	Yes
Negligence	No	Giving freedom	Yes
Ambition	No	Love	Yes

avoided as well as other abnormal forms of parental affection (Table 7.6).

7.6 Therapy

According to the intensity of psychosomatic interaction, therapeutic procedures should be differentiated and integrated into the somatic medical treatment. Table 7.7 lists several possibilities from placebo treatment to psychoanalysis [8, 14, 17, 24, 26, 44, 48, 49, 54, 59, 63, 72].

Table 7.7. Therapeutic options in psychosomatically influenced allergies (in addition to allergy treatment)

Placebo
Psychopharmacological drugs
(sedatives, sedating antihistamines)
Psychosomatic counseling
Behavioral therapy
Family therapy
Relaxation techniques
Autogenic training
Biofeedback
Hypnosis
Psychotherapy/group therapy
Psychoanalysis

Through the development of new less intense short-term analytic procedures, psychoanalytically oriented psychotherapy may also be helpful [81]. Close cooperation between allergist and psychologist/psychiatrist is an essential prerequisite for success since the exploration of certain emotions may induce severe exacerbation of somatic complaints.

Behavioral therapy comprises:

- Recognition of problem behavior
- Selection of relevant stimuli and consequences
- Intervention
- Evaluation of success [81]

Behavioral therapy in its classic form uses relaxation techniques (e.g., relaxation of large muscles according to Jacobsen [24]) and uses several techniques (Table 7.8) to explain the disease symptoms, the ways to solutions of problems and clinical improvement [20, 81].

Another method of relaxation is biofeedback, which can be performed either indirectly (e.g., electromyogram of frontal muscle) or directly by measuring airway resistance, airway noise (in asthma) or other relevant parameters. However, experience regarding effects in different allergic diseases is limited. It cannot be excluded that some patients suffer exacerbations through use of these techniques.

Similarly limited is our knowledge of hypnosis, which can reduce immediate-type skin reactions in experimental situations as well as clinical exercise-induced asthma [9, 81]. Autogenic training is recommended by many authors as a simple related technique to hypnosis.

Table 7.8. Techniques of behavioral therapy

Conditioning	Examples
Classic	• Desensitization" (e.g., "reciprocal inhibition" with relaxation techniques after priorization of stimuli in a hierarchy) • Flooding (exposure to an excessive dose of stimulus) • Training of self-defense (training of the capacity to express own desires and feelings without hurting others) • Communication therapy (pairs)
Operative	• *Positive reinforcement* • Negative reinforcement • Punishing • Ignorance (e.g., "time out") • Overdosing ("satiation")
Observational Cognitive	• Model learning (exemplary situations) • Development of a new view of interactions • Bibliotherapy • Paradoxical communication

In modern educational programs (for asthma or atopic eczema), psychosomatic concepts are integrated (see Sect. 6.5 on "Prevention"). Above all is the classical *"primum nil nocere,"* which also holds true for psychosomatic exploration and therapy. It is so much easier to recognize emotional difficulties and conflicts than to solve them.

References

1. Ader R, Felton DL, Cohen N (eds) (2001) Psychoneuroimmunology, 3rd edn. Academic Press, London
2. Alexander F (1950) Psychosomatic medicine. Norton, New York
3. Bell IR, Jasnoski ML, Kagan J, King DS (1991) Depression and allergies: survey of a nonclinical population. Psychother Psychosom 55:24–31
4. Bienenstock J, Perdue Blennerhassett M, et al. (1987) Inflammatory cells and epithelium: mast cell/nerve interactions in lung in vitro and in vivo. Am Rev Respir Dis 138:S31–S34
5. Black S (1969) Mind and body. Kimber, London
6. Bonini S, Lambiase A, Bonini S, et al. (1996) Circulation nerve growth factor levels are increased in humans with allergic diseases and asthma. Proc Natl Acad Sci U S A 93:10955–10960
7. Boor C de (1965) Über psychosomatische Aspekte der Allergie. Psyche (Stuttgart) 19:365
8. Borelli S (1967) Psyche und Haut. In: Gottron HA (ed) Handbuch der Haut- und Geschlechtskrankheiten, vol 8. Springer, Berlin Heidelberg New York, 264–568
9. Bosse KA, Gieler U (eds) (1987) Seelische Faktoren bei Hautkrankheiten. Huber, Bern
10. Castagliuolo I, Wershil BK, Karalis K, Pasha A, Nikulasson ST, Pathoulakis C (1998) Colonic mucin release in response to immobilization stress is mast cell dependent. Am J Physiol 274:G1094–1100
11. Csermely P (1997) Stress of life: From molecules to man. Proceedings of a conference. Budapest, Hungary, 1–5 July, 1997. Ann N Y Acad Sci 851:1–547
12. Darsow U, Ring J (2001) Neuroimmune interactions in the skin. Curr Opin Allergy Clin Immunol 1:435–439
13. Djurie VJ, Bienenstock J (1993) Learned sensitivity. Ann Allergy 71:5–14
14. Ewer TC, Stewart DE (1986) Improvement in bronchial hyperresponsiveness in patients with moderate asthma after treatment with a hypnotic technique: A randomised controlled trial. Br Med J 293:1129–1132
15. Fava GA, Perini GI, Santonastaso PI, Veller FC (1980) Life events and psychological distress in dermatologic disorders: Psoriasis, chronic urticaria and fungal infections. Br J Med Psychol 53:277–282
16. Fischer A, McGregor GP, Saria A, Philippin B, Kummer W (1996) Induction of tachykinin gene and peptide expression in guinea pig nodose primary afferent neurons by allergic airway inflammation. J Clin Invest 98:2284–2291
17. Gieler U, Stangier U, Ernst R (1988) Psychosomatische Behandlungskonzepte im Rahmen der klinischen Therapie von Hautkrankheiten. Praxis Klin Verhaltensmed Rehabil 1:50–54
18. Grant EN, Wagner R, Weiss KB (1999) Observation on emerging patterns of asthma in our society. J Allergy Clin Immunol 104 [Suppl 2]:S1–9
19. Gronemeyer W, Fuchs E (1967) Krankheiten durch inhalative Allergeninvasion. In: Hansen K, Werner M (eds) Lehrbuch der klinischen Allergie. Thieme, Stuttgart, p 122

20. Hölscher K (1998) Psychosomatische Aspekte. In: Ring J (ed) Neurodermitis. Ecomed, Landsberg, pp 29–44
21. Holmes TH, Rahe RH (1967) The social readjustment rating scale. J Psychosom Res 11:213–218
22. Iamandescu IB (1998) Psychoneuroallergology. Romcartexim, Bucharest
23. Jabaaij L, Grosheide PM, Heijtink RA, Duivenvoorden HJ, Baillieux RE, Vingerhoets AJ (1993) Influence of perceived psychological stress and distress on antibody response to low dose rDNA hepatitis B vaccine. J Psychosom Res 37:361–369
24. Jacobsen E (1938) Progressive relaxation. University of Chicago Press, Chicago
25. Jores A, v Kerekjarto M (1967) Der Asthmatiker. Huber, Bern
26. Kämmerer W (1987) Die psychosomatische Ergänzungstherapie der Neurodermitis atopiea – Autogenes Training und weitere Maßnahmen. Allergologie 10:536–541
27. Kang DH, Coe CL, McCarthy DO (1996) Academic examinations significantly impact immune responses, but not lung function, in healthy and well-managed asthmatic adolescents. Brain Behav Immun 10:164–181
28. Kaptchuk TJ (1998) Powerful placebo: the dark side of the randomised controlled trial. Lancet 351:1722–1725
29. Katsch G (1955) Psychologische und chemische Allergie beim Asthma. Dtsch Med Wochenschr 80:1125
30. Kerschensteiner M, Gallmeier E, Behrens L, et al. (1999) Activated human T cells, B cells, and monocytes produce brain-derived neurotropic factor in vitro and in inflammatory brain lesions: a neuroprotective role of inflammation? J Exp Med 189:865–870
31. Kiecolt-Glaser JK, Garner W, Speicher C, Penn GM, Holliday J, Glaser R (1984) Psychosocial modifiers of immunocompetence in medical students. Psychosom Med 46:7–14
32. Kleinsorge H (1964) Allergie, eine psychosomatische Erkrankung? Med Klin 59:1193
33. Kunkel G (2001) Neurogene Aspekte der allergischen Entzündungsreaktion. In: Ring J, Darsow U (eds) Allergie 2000. Dustri, Munich, pp 179–181
34. Kupfer, J, Gieler U, Braun A, et al. (2001) Stress and atopic eczema. Int Arch Allergy Immunol 124:353–355
35. Laube BL, Curbow BA, Fitzgerald ST, Spratt K (2003) Early pulmonary response to allergen is attenuated during acute emotional stress in females with asthma. Eur Respir J 22:613–618
36. Luger TA, Kalden D, Scholzen TE, Brzoska T (1999) Alpha-melanocyte-stimulating hormone as a mediator of tolerance induction. Pathobiology 67:318–321
37. MacKenzie JN (1886) The production of the so-called "rose cold" by means of an artificial rose. Am J Med Sci 91:44–57
38. MacQueen G, Marshall J, Perdue M, Siegel S, Bienenstock J (1989) Pavlovian conditioning of rat mucosal mast cells to secrete rat mast cell protease II. Science 243:83–85
39. Marshall GD, Agarwal SK, Lloyd C, Cohen L, Henninger EM, Morris GJ (1998) Cytokine dysregulation in healthy medical students associated with exam stress. Brain Behav Immunol 12:297–307
40. Marty P (1974) Die allergische Objektbezeichnung. In: Brede K (ed) Einführung in die psychosomatische Medizin. Athenäum-Fischer, Frankfurt
41. McAlexander MA, Undem BJ (1997) Enhancement of tachykinin-induced contractions of guinea pig isolated bronchus by corticotropin-releasing factor. Neuropeptides 31:293–299
42. McEwen BS, Stellar E (1993) Stress and the individual. Mechanisms leading to disease. Arch Intern Med 153:2093–2101
43. McEwen BS (1998) Protective and damaging effects of stress mediators. N Engl J Med 338:171–179
44. Michel FB (1994) Psychology of the allergic patient. Allergy 49:28–30
45. Miller BD (1987) Depression and asthma: a potentially lethal mixture. J Allergy Clin Immunol 80:481–486
46. Niebel G (1995) Verhaltensmedizin der chronischen Hautkrankheit. Interdisziplinäre Perspektiven der atopischen Dermatitis und ihre Behandlung. Huber, Bern
47. Noelpp-Eschenhagen I, Noelpp B (1954) New contributions to experimental asthma. Progr Allergy 4:361
48. Nolte D (1985) Asthma – Atemnot – Atemfunktion. Gedon & Reuss, Munich
49. Overbeck G (1987) Psychosomatische Aspekte bei Asthma bronchiale. Zur Frage der allergischen Objektbeziehung. Allergologie 10:498–502
50. Panconesi E (1984) Stress and skin diseases: psychosomatic dermatology. In: Parish LC (ed) Clinics in dermatology. Philadelphia, Lippincott
51. Parker CW (1991) Environmental stress and immunity: possible implications for IgE-mediated allergy. Perspect Biol Med 34:197–212
52. Petermann F (ed) (1995) Verhaltensmedizin in der Rehabilitation. Ansätze in der medizinischen Rehabilitation. Hogrefe, Göttingen
53. Pothoulakis C, Castagliuolo I, Leeman SE (1998) Neuroimmune mechanisms of intestinal responses to stress. Role of corticotropin-releasing factor and neurotensin. Ann N Y Acad Sci 840:635–648
54. Prochazka P (1994) Sensibilität und Abgrenzung bei Neurodermitkern. Porch, Wiesen (CH)
55. Rechardt E (1970) An investigation in the psychosomatic aspects of prurigo Besnier. Psych Klinik d Univ, Helsinki
56. Reimann H-J (1981) Stress and histamine. In: Ring J, Burg G (eds) New trends in Allergy. Springer, Berlin Heidelberg New York, p 50

57. Braun A, Lommatzsch M, Lewin GR, Virchow JC (1999) Neurotrophins: A link between airway inflammation and airway smooth muscle contractility in asthma. Int Arch Allergy Immunol 118: 163–165
58. Richter R, Dahme B (1987) Psychosomatische Aspekte des Asthma bronchiale. Prax Klein Pneumol 41:656–660
59. Richter R, Ahrens S (1990) Psychosomatische Aspekte der Allergie. In: Fuchs E, Schulz KH (eds) Manuale allergologicum, VIII. Dustri, Munich, pp 1–16
60. Ring J, Palos E, Zimmermann F (1986) Psychosomatische Aspekte der Eltern-Kind-Beziehung bei atopischem Ekzem im Kindesalter. I. Psychodiagnostische Testverfahren bei Eltern und Kindern und Vergleich mit somatischen Befunden. Hautarzt 37:560–567
61. Ring J, Palos E (1986) Psychosomatische Aspekte der Eltern-Kind-Beziehung bei atopischem Ekzem im Kindesalter. II. Erziehungsstil, Familiensituation im Zeichentest und strukturierte Interviews. Hautarzt 37:609–617
62. Ring J (1993) Allergieforschung: Die Kluft zwischen Grundlagenforschung und klinischer Realität. Allergo J 2 [Suppl 1]:S5–S11
63. Ring J (ed) (1998) Neurodermitis. Ecomed, Landsberg
64. Russell M, Dark KA, Cummins RW, Ellmann G, Callaway E, Peeke HVS (1984) Learned histamine release. Science 225:733–734
65. Santos J, Saunders PR, Hanssen NP, Yang PC, Yates D, Groot JA, Perdue MH (1999) Corticotropin-releasing hormone mimics stress-induced colonic epithelial pathophysiology in the rat. Am J Physiol 277:G391–399
66. Sapolsky R (1992) Stress, the aging brain, and the mechanisms of neuron death. MIT Press, Cambridge, MA, pp 1–429
67. Saunders PR, Kosecka U, McKay DM, Perdue MH (1994) Acute stressors stimulate ion secretion and increase epithelial permeability in rat intestine. Am J Physiol 267:G794–799
68. Schäfer T, Staudt A, Ring J (2001) Entwicklung des Deutschen Instruments zur Erfassung der Lebensqualität bei Hauterkrankungen (DIELH). Hautarzt 52:492–498
69. Selye H (1936) A syndrome produced by diverse nocuous agents. Nature 113:32
70. Smyth JM, Stone AA, Hurewitz A, Kaell A (1999) Effects of writing about stressful experiences on symptom reduction in patients with asthma or rheumatoid arthritis: a randomized trial. JAMA 281:1304–1309
71. Spielberger C, Gorsuch R, Lushene R (1970) The STAI manual. Consulting Psychologists Press, Palo Alto, CA
72. Stangier U (1987) Verhaltenstherapie bei dermatologischen Erkrankungen. Dt Derm 35:206–227
73. Szentivanyi A (1968) The beta adrenergic theory of the atopic abnormality in asthma. J Allergy 42:203
74. Szczepanski R, Gebert N, Hümmelink R, Könning J, Schmidt S, Ründe B, Wahn U (1996) Ergebnis einer strukturierten Asthmaschulung im Kindes- und Jugendalter. Pneumologie 50:544–548
75. Teofoli P, Frezzolini A, Puddu P, et al. (1999) The role of proopiocortin-derived peptides in skin fibroblast and mast cell function. Ann N Y Acad Sci 885:268–276
76. Udelman DL (1982) Stress and immunity. Psychother Psychosom 37:176–184
77. Undem BJ, Kajekar R, Hunter DD, Myers AC (2000) Neural integration and allergic disease. J Allergy Clin Immunol 106:S213–220
78. Von Eiff A (1984) Zur Psychology und Klinik des Stress. Therapiewoche 34:7192–7196
79. Whitlock A (1976) Psychophysiologic aspects of skin disease. Saunders, Toronto
80. Wright RJ, Rodriguez M, Cohen S (1998) Review of psychosocial stress and asthma: an integrated biopsychosocial approach. Thorax 53:1066–1074
81. Young StH, Rubin JM, Daman HR (eds) (1986) Psychobiological aspects of allergic disorders. Praeger, New York
82. Zachariae R, Jorgensen MM, Egekvist H, Bjerring P (2001) Skin reactions to histamine of healthy subjects after hypnotically induced emotions of sadness, anger, and happiness. Allergy 56:734–740

Chapter 8

Outlook

At the end of this book dedicated to allergy in practice, one may be allowed a look into the future:
- What themes will be of interest for allergists in the coming years?
- What new knowledge can we expect?
- Which controversies will we struggle with?
- What can our patients hope for?

8.1 Pathophysiology

The great problems of immunological research in the past 30 years have been practically solved: the basis of antibody diversity by the gene rearrangement, the characterization of the T-cell receptor in its analogy to the antibody molecule, the mechanisms of isotype switching in the production of different antibody classes (from IgG to IgE) as well as the importance of innate immunity in the often common end phase with the sequelae of specific adaptic immune responses.

The IgE-mediated immediate-type reaction with its bridging of receptor-bound molecules on the surface of mast cells, basophils and other cells with consecutive liberation of proinflammatory mediators and cytokines is quite well understood. Nevertheless, many questions remain open, e.g., the interaction of various mediators in physiologic and pathophysiologic homeostasis over and above allergic reactions (what role do mast cells play in antigen presentation or eosinophils in cardiac disease?).

The genetic basis of the altered immune response has been discovered within a short space of time. Many of the associated gene loci do not have a known function. After the identification of the human genome and the era of "proteomics," we can expect a renaissance of exact clinical description ("phenomics").

Mechanisms of signal transduction after allergen contact with surface receptors are being characterized and will offer new therapeutic options. An era of receptor research might open many options through new methods such as immunochemical detection methods or the recombinant production of defined molecules.

When the second edition of this book (in German) appeared, the histamine H3 receptor was brand new; today, we are excited about the H4 receptor. Histamine and histamine antagonists remain actual and important for allergists as well as the many other mediators and their potential antagonists and inhibitors.

Toll-like receptors – first described in *Drosophila* as mediators of many effects of the innate immune system after contact with endotoxin or bacterial nucleotides – will also be recognized as important structures in the human and give rise to new therapeutic considerations.

"Suppressor cells," which were once so famous and then were completely forgotten in the 1980s (there was a poem: "If killer, helper or suppressor, for each one there is a professor"!), have reappeared under a new name, T3 cells or regulatory T cells. They are characterized by secretion of interleukin-10 and might help to explain the natural disappearance and decrease of allergic reactions over the lifetime.

Psychoneuroallergology, for a long time filled with excitement for researchers, has not yet really yielded any relevant advances for practical life. This might be achieved by better clinical studies maybe by using modern techniques like positron emission tomography (PET) or evoked potentials together with psychodiagnostic tests performed under allergic provocation conditions.

Experimental allergology should not only look inside the organism but should also consider the environment, from whence the only causal factors of allergy come, namely the allergens. Without allergens there is no allergy! Here the progress has been immense; data banks contain all known structures and conformational epitopes of the most important allergens. Many are available in recombinant form and may soon be used in clinical routine. However, the question regarding the nature of "allergenic potency" remains unanswered. What makes an allergen an allergen? So far there is no chemical correlate, neither the amino acid sequence nor a tertiary or quarternary structure, nor functional properties such as enzyme character – which could explain the allergenic potency of a certain protein. It may be possible that completely other factors perhaps coming from the microenvironment of the allergen, play a role in the early phase of allergen liberation. The exciting new findings describing the liberation of not only allergens but also highly active proinflammatory substances with eicosanoid-like effect (pollen-associated lipid mediators, PALMS, or pollotrienes) (H. Behrendt) are only a beginning and open a new dimension of understanding for the interaction between environment and the genetically shaped individuum.

8.2 Clinical Studies

Only a few allergic diseases have been investigated with exact epidemiologic trials for estimating prevalence and incidence in the general population as atopic diseases and this also only in childhood. We do not have enough data for all the other allergic diseases or for other age groups.

Each epidemiological trial, even when equipped with the most modern molecular genetic techniques, is only as good as the clinician making the diagnosis of the phenotype. There will be a renaissance of clinical research.

It will need to better define subpopulations of disease entities (e.g., in eczema IgE-associated and "intrinsic" (non-atopic) variants, different morphologies, different clinical courses, different age groups for onset of disease). New allergic disease entities may evolve; naturally, they will be met with much criticism. While the etiology of drug reaction is fairly clear, this seems to be very difficult in the much less well defined conditions with hypersensitivity reactions against environmental influences. The disease of "eco-syndrome" or "multiple chemical sensitivity" MCS or "idiopathic environmental intolerance" (IEI) remains an enigma for scientists and its existence is questioned by many people; however, many patients in modern societies suffer tremendously from this condition. We may hope that by unprejudiced and in its best sense psychosomatic research, it may be possible to find objective parameters for this syndrome, thus helping to establish a rational diagnosis.

Of course new allergens will be described, not only of anthropogenic but also of natural origin: just think of the epidemic of natural rubber latex allergy at the end of the 1980s! Allergists need to approach each single patient without ideology; we have to believe the patient, even if his or her story might sound absurd; otherwise, we would never detect anything new!

The interplay between different external and internal factors in the development of a clinical symptom has for many years obscured the understanding and diagnosis of anaphylactic and other allergic reactions. The fact that certain stimuli have to act together and at the same time, which we have called "summation anaphylaxis," is not an exception but may be the rule (e.g., infection plus exercise or stress plus allergen or allergen plus allergen or allergen plus allergy-promoting drug). All these phenomena are much more common than we previously thought and they are difficult to diagnose. We have to admit that there are false-negative provocation tests in allergy diagnosis!

HIV infection has, similarly to syphilis 500 years ago, led to a multitude of very impressive and partly new dermatologic entities; similarly, the colorful spectrum of drug reactions with exanthematous eruption, immunologically and non-immunologically mediated hypersensitivity reactions (formerly called "pseudo-allergic") is only beginning to be understood. Only better knowledge about the pathophysiological mechanism will allow new methods of therapy and prevention.

Granulomatous inflammation has only recently been discovered as a potential allergic disease. The increasing interest in natural killer cells with T-cell properties (NKT cell) might help to understand many so far unknown granulomatous inflammatory reactions in their pathophysiology.

The role of allergy in bronchial asthma has been known for a long time. However, pneumologists seem to forget this in the adult age or underestimate it. This also holds true for atopic eczema, where many dermatologists still believe it to be only a disease of dry skin and psychosomatic interaction. However, many patients know that contact with aeroallergens or certain foods is able to trigger heavy eczema flares, which we can now prove and measure in the atopy patch test.

The classic paradigm of TH1 and TH2 in a kind of ying-yang theory like "good" and "evil" may be soon outdated. TH2 is perhaps only the characteristic of acute phase while in chronic inflammation TH1 reactions and maybe later autoimmune phenomena play a role. TH2 and IgE should also be regarded as neutrally as parameter like blood pressure, which is not good or bad but may lead to disease when it is too high or too low.

8.3 Diagnosis

The taking of the history will remain the domain of the experienced allergist. In skin test procedures, standardization of test solutions will be improved; but we have to fear that the selection of allergens will be reduced dramatically by the increased demands of allergists for better purification and standardization (for economic reasons). So maybe in 10 years we will be back again to the days of Cooke and Coca, making our own extracts for skin tests. In the field of in vitro allergy diagnosis, specificity and sensitivity of IgE detection will be further improved. The relevance of specific antibodies of other classes like IgG4 or IgA2 (for instance in mucosal secretions) is still unclear; some of them might be helpful for prognostic evaluation or for therapy control in routine diagnosis. It might be that the relation of IgG4/IgE is the crucial parameter when we believe that the mass effect law also holds true for allergic reactions (Kurt Blaser).

The atopy patch test should leave the phase of research tool and become a routine diagnostic procedure; only the high costs of production of allergen preparations argue against. Also food allergens will be used in the atopy patch test and may save provocation tests.

It should be the aim of modern allergology to improve considerably the armamentarium of provocation testing and maybe achieve the diagnosis without it. Every provocation implies exposure of a sensitized organism with the specific pathogen, namely the allergen. Still, I think in the coming years professionally monitored provocation tests will be necessary in allergen diagnosis, at least in order to allow a comparison of new diagnostic techniques. Otolaryngologists and dermatologists should help – like pneumologists a long time ago – to develop a reproducible test for measuring hyperreactivity of the nasal mucosa or of the skin for clinical routine.

Apart from the detection of specific antibodies or cells or cellular mediators, the detection of inflammatory mediators will be more important. Cellular tests will be increasingly used in allergy diagnosis, especially basophil degranulation and activation markers.

In immunoblot techniques, allergen-specific sensitization against single proteins in allergen mixtures can be detected, which will help to evaluate the relevance of certain allergens and allow individual "pattern diagnosis."

The diagnosis of drug allergy should be improved considerably. Unfortunately, the only reliable skin test modality, namely the penicillin polylysine (PPL) conjugate (Alain de Weck), might be lost for economic reasons.

The quantitative detection of specific allergen in the environment of the patient is a new dimension for allergy diagnosis, which seems to be limited to housedust mites and some indoor allergens. There will be considerable progress made on outdoor air by measuring pollen allergens instead of pollen grains and correlating them to dose response exposure and clinical symptoms. Contact allergens and food allergens will also be detected with simple methods maybe to be performed by the patient with simple dipstick tests.

Microchip techniques (arrays) may detect activated gene expression profiles but also secretion products of cells in high quantity and with minute amounts of material.

Using modern functional genomic studies, it may be possible to diagnose certain allergy or atopy risk parameters in early life or in the collected blood.

8.4 Therapy

Apart from allergen avoidance, causal therapy in allergy means the induction of specific tolerance. This may be achieved by classic allergen-specific immunotherapy (hyposensitization), but only for some allergens and some IgE-mediated allergic diseases. Most of the allergic diseases at this time cannot be treated causally. A lot of work will have to be done and hopes are pinned on the induction of tolerance through regulatory T cells, through interference with the second signal in the T/B interaction (blockade of costimulatory molecules) as well as for new specific antagonists and inhibitors of mediators and cytokines.

So-called "biologicals" are of great scientific interest and are already undergoing the first clinical trials so that they may soon be used routinely (like anti-IgE, anticytokines, inhibiting cytokines, isoforms of cytokines, soluble cytokine receptors, etc.). However, the true place of these new substances in the allergy management of the future cannot be evaluated today. It will depend upon the ratio of effect and safety, but also on economic questions. Thus we might find ourselves with a real "cost explosion."

In the field of chemical pharmacology, further improvements with regard to more specific or complementary effects and the reduction of side effects can be expected such as new antihistamines, new glucocorticosteroids or new immunosuppressives. Allergists know – contrary to pharmacology textbooks – that patient individuality is tremendous with regard to the effects and side effects of drugs. In certain individual patients, only certain substances of a certain class are effective. The same holds true for side effects. Therefore, the supreme law in allergy therapy is individuality in pharmacotherapeutic management. There may be patients where the uncritical use of generics is not good or even dangerous.

New anti-inflammatory drugs with fewer side effects and new immunosuppressive or immunomodulatory substances will enrich the therapeutic armamentarium.

Allergen-specific immunotherapy will be improved by new adjuvants. Apart from phospholipids, also bacterial oligonucleotides (e.g., CpG motifs) or mykobacterial or other microbial lipoproteins may be used.

Also the route of administration seems to be critical. Apart from classic subcutaneous administration of allergen extracts, sublingual/oral allergen-specific immunotherapy is on the march, although the mechanism of this type of immunotherapy is not yet clear. By using recombinant allergens in diagnosis and therapy, new methods of individually tailored allergy treatment may be possible (B. Valenta).

8.5 Prevention

For decades the only recommendations for primary prevention of allergy were rather boring or "negative" (avoidance, avoidance, avoidance). It is time to think of active prevention strategies! A first step seems to be the use of probiotics (lactobacillus G), which needs to be validated in future studies and different modalities. Active prevention also means true vaccination of infants with common (mixed recombinant) allergen epitopes. From mouse and dog experiments we know that there is a "window of opportunity" when tolerance may be induced. Such studies, however, require careful planning, a multicentric modality and very careful ethical considerations. I believe that the time has come for such studies. They should be performed under the umbrella of international organizations such as academies of allergy or the World Allergy Organization.

In the environment, primary prevention not only includes agricultural and city planning under allergy considerations (why do we have to plant birch trees in the schoolyard?). Also new gene-technology procedures may help to develop hypoallergenic foods, plants or animals (let us clone a hypoallergenic cat!).

By better integration of allergologic expertise into the political decision-making process (not only in declarations and regulations), we might help in primary allergen prevention by changing the construction of houses, apartments and cars.

New products for effective skin and mucosal protection could be developed in which the precise effects of barrier disruption in the epithelium are elucidated.

8.6 Controversies

Progress in the above-mentioned fields might help the most important current controversies, which are:

- Buy a cat or kill the cat?
- Consequences of the hygiene hypothesis: should we vaccinate or let children experience the infectious disease? Which diseases? Should allergic parents send their children into farm and stable?
- Immunotherapy in asthma and atopic eczema?
- Sublingual/oral versus subcutaneous immunotherapy?
- Epinephrine when and how in the treatment and prevention of anaphylaxis?
- Breast-feeding or hypoallergenic formula for infants?
- And many more

8.7 Role of Allergology

Regarding professional politics, allergology as the science of allergic diseases is the science of understanding and treating allergic diseases – since its origin in the early 20th century it has had to fight its corner between practical general medicine and the powerful established medical specialties such as pneumology/internal medicine, dermatology, pediatrics, and otolaryngology. The training for an allergy specialist differs widely in different countries of the world. In some countries, allergy training is based on internal medicine or pediatrics (United States), whereas other countries train their allergists in clinical immunology laboratories and only later in different clinical disciplines (e.g., southern Europe). In central Europe (e.g., Germany), a 2-year additional training period in an allergy department follows the complete training in an allergy-relevant specialty like pneumology, dermatology, pediatrics or otolaryngology. In some countries, there are no allergy specialists at all.

Regarding the high prevalence of allergic diseases, we have to admit that the often heard postulate "every allergic patient has to be seen by an allergist" will simply not be possible. We therefore need to include the general practitioner in the primary prevention and diagnosis of allergy. At the next step, different organ-related specialists can deal with routine allergic disorders. The complex conditions, specific

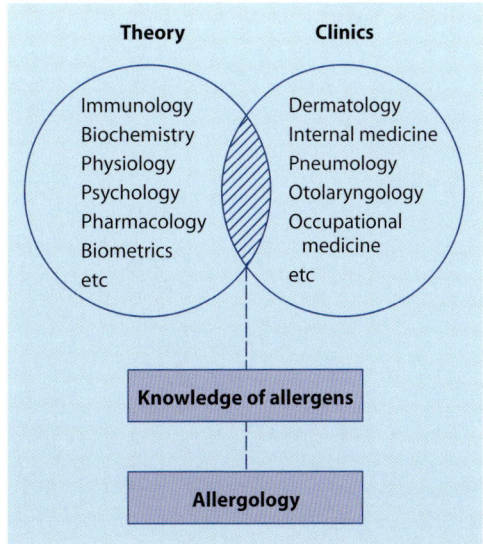

Fig. 8.1. Interdisciplinary relationships in the field of allergology

provocation tests, drug allergies, food allergies, anaphylaxis, the indication and formulation of allergen-specific immunotherapy as well as the first injections up to the maintenance dose are the true domain of allergists.

However, well-trained allergists need interdisciplinary training and cooperation between different specialties. We need improvement of medical education at university, improvement of residency and training, and improvement of training facilities by clear-cut criteria and certification.

Allergology – by definition – is interdisciplinary in character (Fig. 8.1). It is a clinical discipline gaining knowledge from several theoretical specialties, which then is used in different clinical fields. The common strand keeping allergy specialists together and defining them is the profound knowledge of the more and more numerous and difficult to know causal (allergens) and modulating factors (adjuvants) in the environment.

Appendix

9.1 Societies

WAO/IAACI (World Allergy Organization/International Association of Allergology and Clinical Immunology), WAO Secretariat, 611 East Wells Street, Milwaukee, WI 53202, USA; Tel.: +1-414-2761791, Fax +1-414-2763349, www.worldallergy.org; current president: Carlos Baino-Cagnani, Cordoba, Argentina

Collegium Internationale Allergologicum (CIA), 611 East Wells Street, Milwaukee, WI 53202, USA; current president: Johannes Ring, Munich, Germany

American Academy of Allergy, Asthma and Immunology (AAAAI), 611 East Wells Street, Milwaukee, WI 53202, USA

American College of Allergists (ACA)

EAACI (European Academy of Allergology and Clinical Immunology), PO Box 24140, 10451 Stockholm, Sweden; www.eaaci.org; current president: Ulrich Wahn, Berlin, Germany

Asian Pacific Society for Allergy and Clinical Immunology (APACI)

Japanese Society for Allergology; current president: Hisao Tomioka

Interasthma Community of Independent States; current president: Revaz Sepiashvili

DGAI (German Society for Allergology and Clinical Immunology), DGAI-Geschäftsstelle, Postfach 70 04 64, 81304 Munich, Germany; Tel.: +49-89-54662968, Fax: +1-89-583824; www.dgai.de; current president: Gerhard Schulze-Werninghaus, Bochum, Germany

Brazilian Society for Allergy and Clinical Immunology

Other national allergy societies (see website of the WAO)

9.2 Allergy Journals

Allergo Journal

Allergologie

Allergology International

Allergy

Allergy Clinical Immunology International/ The Journal of the World Allergy Organization

Annales d'Allergologie

Annals of Allergy, Asthma and Immunology

Clinical and Experimental Allergy

Contact Dermatitis

Current Allergy Reports

Current Opinions in Allergy and Clinical Immunology

Dermatosen in Beruf und Umwelt

International Archives of Allergy and Immunology

Journal of Allergy and Clinical Immunology

Journal of Investigational Allergology

Pediatric Allergy and Immunology

9.3 Position Papers of the European Academy of Allergology and Clinical Immunology (EAACI)

Authors	Title	Source
Malling HJ (1988)	EAACI Position Paper: Immunotherapy	Allergy 43 [Suppl 6]:25–35
Dreborg S, Backman A, Basomba A, Bousquet J, Dieges P, Malling HJ (1989)	Skin tests used in type I allergy testing	Allergy 44 [Suppl 10]:1–59
Müller U, Mosbech H, Blauw P, Dreborg S, Malling HJ, Przybilla B, Urbanek R, Pastorello EA, Blanca M, Bousquet J, Jarisch R (1991)	Emergency treatment of allergic reactions to Hymenoptera stings	Allergy 21:281–288
Frolund L, Bonini S, Cocco G, Davies RJ, de Monchy JG, Melillo G, Pauwels R (1993)	Allergen extracts. Standardization of preparations for bronchial provocation tests. A Position Paper of the EAACI Subcommittee on Bronchial Provocation Tests	Clin Exp Allergy 23:702–708
Malling HJ, Weeke B (1993)	EAACI Position Paper: Immunotherapy	Allergy 48 [Suppl 14]:7–35
Müller U, Mosbech H (1993)	EAACI Position Paper: Immunotherapy with Hymenoptera venoms	Allergy 48 [Suppl 14]:36–46
Dreborg S, Frew AJ (1993)	EAACI Position Paper: Allergen standardization and skin tests	Allergy 48 [Suppl 14]:48–82
Terho E, Frew AJ (1995)	Type III allergy skin testing. Position Statement of the EAACI Subcommittee on Skin Tests and Allergen Standardization	Allergy 50:390–394
Bruijnzeel-Koomen C, Ortolani C, Aas K, Bindslev-Jensen C, Björkstén B, Moneret-Vautrin D, Wüthrich B (1995)	Adverse reactions to food	Allergy 50:623–635
Moscato G, Godnic-Cvar J, Maestrelli P, Malo JL, Burge Sherwood P, Coifman R (1995)	Statement on self-monitoring of peak expiratory flow in the investigation of occupational asthma	Allergy 50:711–717
Müller U, Mosbech H, Aberer W, Dreborg S, Ewan P, Kunkel G, Malling HJ, Przybilla B, Vervloet D (1995)	Adrenaline for emergency kits. EAACI Subcommittee on Insect Venom Allergy	Allergy 50:783–787
D'Amato G, Spieksma FT (1995)	Aerobiologic and clinical aspects of mold allergy in Europe	Allergy 50:870–877
Rueff F, Przybilla B, Müller U, Mosbech H (1996)	The sting challenge test in Hymenoptera venom allergy. Position Paper of the EAACI Subcommittee on Insect Venom Allergy	Allergy 51:216–225
Charpin D, Sibbald B, Weeke E, Wüthrich B (1996)	Epidemiologic identification of allergic rhinitis	Allergy 51:293–298
Molina CI (on behalf of the EAACI Computing Group of the Audiovisual Subcommittee) (1996)	Information technology and media in allergy	Allergy 51:603–607
Passalacqua G, Bousquet J, Bachert C, Church MK, Bindslev-Jensen C, Nagy L, Szemere P, Davies RJ, Durham SR, Horak F, Kontou-Fili L, Malling HJ, van Cauwenberge P, Canonica GW (1996)	EAACI Position Paper: The clinical safety of H1-receptor antagonists	Allergy 51:666–675

Authors	Title	Source
Buscaglia S, Palma-Carlos AG, Canonica GW (1997)	EAACI guidelines for continuing medical education. Essentials for accreditation, standards for commercial support and system of credits	Allergy 52:490–503
Melillo G, Bonini S, Cocco G, Davies RJ, de Monchy JG, Frolund L, Pelikan Z (1997)	EAACI provocation tests with allergens. EAACI Subcommittee on Provocation Test with Allergens	Allergy 52:1–35
Kontou-Fili K, Borici-Mazi R, Kapp A, Matjevic LJ, Mitchel FB (1997)	EAACI Position Paper: Physical urticaria: classification and diagnostic guidelines	Allergy 52:504–513
D'Amato G, Chatzigeorgiou G, Corsico R, Giolekas D, Jäger S, Kontou-Fili K, Kouridakis S, Liccardi G, Mariggi A, Palma-Carlos AG, Palma-Carlos ML, Pagan Aleman A, Parmiani S, Puccinelli P, Russo M, Spieksma FT, Torricelli R, Wüthrich B (1997)	Evaluation of the prevalence of skin prick test positivity to *Alternaria* and *Cladosporium* in patients with suspected respiratory allergy	Allergy 52:711–716
Müller UR; Bonifazi F, Przybilla B, Youlten L, Mosbech H, Fernandez Sanchez J, Vervloet D (1998)	Withdrawal of the Medihaler-epi/adrenaline Medihaler: Comments of the EAACI Subcommittee on Insect Venom Allergy	Allergy 53:619–620
D'Amato G, Spieksma FT, Liccardi G, Jäger S, Russo M, Kontou-Fili K, Nikkels H, Wüthrich B, Bonini S (1998) Pollen-related allergy in Europe	Pollen-related allergy in Europe	Allergy 53:567–578
Malling HJ, Abreu-Nogueira J, Alvarez-Cuesta E, Björkstén B, Bousquet J, Caillot D, Canonica GW, Passalacqua G, Saxonis-Papageorgiou P, Valovirta E (1998)	Local immunotherapy	Allergy 53:933–944
Bousquet J, Lockey R, Malling HJ (1998)	WHO Position Paper on allergy immunotherapy: therapeutic vaccines for allergic diseases	J Allergy Clin Immunol 102:558–562 Allergy 53:44–48
Demoly P, Kropf R, Bircher A, Pichler WJ (1999)	Drug hypersensitivity; Questionnaire. EAACI Interest Group on drug hypersensitivity	Allergy 54:999–1003
Ortolani C, Bruijnzeel-Koomen C, Bengtsson U, Bindslev-Jensen C, Björkstén B, Host A, Ispano M, Jarisch R, Madsen C, Nekam K, Paganelli R, Poulsen LK, Wüthrich B (1999)	EAACI Position Paper: Controversial aspects of adverse reactions to food	Allergy 54:27–45
Passalacqua G, Albano M, Bachert C, Davies RJ, Durham SR, Kontou-Fili K, Horak F, Malling HJ, van Cauwenberge P, Canonica GW (2000)	Inhaled and nasal corticosteroids: safety aspects	Allergy 55:16–33
van Cauwenberge P, Bachert C, Passalacqua G, Bousquet J, Canonica GW, Durham SR, Fokkens WJ, Howarth PH, Lund V, Malling HJ, Mygind N, Passali D, Scadding GK, Wang DY (2000)	Consensus statement on the treatment of allergic rhinitis	Allergy 55:116–134
Dubois AE, Palma Carlos AG, Ewan PW, de Monchy JG (2000)	European specialist care in allergology and clinical immunology in the new millennium	Allergy 55:338–339

Authors	Title	Source
Johansson SG, Hourihane JO, Bousquet J, Bruijnzeel-Koomen C, Dreborg S, Haahtela T, Kowalski ML, Mygind N, Ring J, van Cauwenberge P, van Hage-Hamsten M, Wüthrich B (2001)	A revised nomenclature for allergy: An EAACI position statement from the EAACI nomenclature task force	Allergy 56:813–824
Matricardi PM, Bjorksten B, Bonini S, Bousquet J, Djukanovic R, Dreborg S, Gereda J, Malling HJ, Popov T, Raz E, Renz H, Wold E, for the EAACI (2003) Task Force 7	Microbial products in allergy prevention and therapy	Allergy 58:461–471

9.4 Allergy Textbooks

Ader J, Felten DL, Cohen N (eds) (2001) Psychoneuroimmunology, 3rd edn, vols 1, 2. Academic Press, San Diego

Bergmann KC/Stiftung Deutscher Polleninformationsdienst (2001) (ed) Pollenbestimmungsbuch der Stiftung Deutscher Polleninformationsdienst. Takt, Paderborn

Borelli S, Düngemann H (eds) (1981) Fortschritte der Allergologie und Dermatologie. IMP-Verlag, Basel

Branen AL, Davidson PM, Salminen S, Thorngate JH (eds) (2002) Food additives, 2nd edn. Marcel Dekker, New York

Brent L (1997) A history of transplantation immunology. Academic Press, San Diego

Cantani A (2000) Allergologia e Immunologia Pediatrica dall' Infanzia e Aduleszenza. Verduci Editore, Rome

Cooke RA (1947) Allergy in theory and practice. Saunders, Philadelphia

Cox CS, Wathes CM (1995) Bioaerosols handbook. CRC Press, Boca Raton

Denburg JA (ed) (1998) Allergy and allergic diseases, the mechanisms and therapeutics. Humana Press, Totowa, NJ

Der Rat von Sachverständigen für Umweltfragen, Behrend H, Ewers HJ, Hüttl RF, Jänicke M, Plaßmann E, Rehbinder E, Sukopp H (1999) Umwelt und Gesundheit: Risiken richtig einschätzen. Sondergutachten. Metzler-Poeschel, Stuttgart

Deutsche Forschungsgemeinschaft, Eisenbrand G et al. (eds) (1996) Food allergies and intolerances. Verlag Chemie, Weinheim

Diebschlag W, Diebschlag B (2000) Hausstauballergien. Gesundheitliche und hygienische Aspekte, 2nd edn. Herbert Utz, Munich

Ferencik M, Rovensky J, Matha V, Jensen-Jarolim E (2005) Wörterbuch Allergologie und Immunologie. Springer, Berlin New York

Fröschl M (2000) Gesundsein. Integrative Gesund-Seins-Förderung als Ansatz für Pflege, soziale Arbeit und Medizin. Lucius, Stuttgart

Fuchs E, Schulz KH (eds) (1988ff) Manuale Allergologicum. Dustri, München-Deisenhofen

Fuchs E (1992) Allergie. Was tun? Piper, Munich

Fuchs T, Aberer W (eds) (2002ff) Kontaktekzem. Dustri, München-Deisenhofen

Grevers G, Röcken M (eds) (2001) Taschenatlas der Allergologie. Thieme, Stuttgart

Hansel TT, Barnes PJ (eds) (2001) New drugs for asthma, allergy and COPD. Karger, Basel

Hansen K (ed) (1957) Allergie, 3rd edn. Thieme, Stuttgart

Hausen B, Vieluf IK (1997) Allergiepflanzen, Pflanzenallergene. Handbuch und Atlas der allergieinduzierenden Wild- und Kulturpflanzen, 2nd edn. Ecomed, Landsberg

Heppt TW, Bachert FC (1998) Praktische Allergologie: Schwerpunkt HNO-Heilkunde. Thieme, Stuttgart

Heppt TW, Renz H, Röcken M (eds) (1998) Allergologie. Springer, Berlin Heidelberg New York

Holgate ST, Church MK, Lichtenstein LM (2001) Allergy, 2nd edn. Mosby, London

Iamandescu IB (1998) Psychoneuroallergology. Romcartexim, Bucharest

Jäger L, Merk HF (1996) Arzneimittelallergie. Gustav Fischer, Jena

Jorde W (ed) (2000) Schimmelpilzallergie. Dustri, München-Deisenhofen

Kämmerer H, Michel H (1956) Allergische Diathese und allergische Erkrankungen, 3rd edn. Bergmann, Munich

Kay AB (ed) (1997) Allergy and allergic diseases, vols I, II. Blackwell, Oxford

Kemp SS, Lockey RF (eds) (2000) Diagnostic testing of allergic disease. Marcel Dekker, New York

Konietzko J (2001) Arbeitsbedingte Erkrankungen. Ecomed, Landsberg

Koppelman G (2001) Genetics of asthma and atopy. Proefschrift, Groningen

Korenblat PE, Wedner HJ (eds) (1992) Allergy: Theory and practice, 2nd edn. Saunders, Philadelphia

Leung DM, Greaves MW (eds) (2000) Allergic skin disease. Marcel Dekker, New York

Lieberman PL, Blaiss MS (eds) (2001) Atlas of allergic diseases. Current Medicine, Philadelphia

Lockey RF, Bukantz SC (eds) (1999) Allergens and allergen immunotherapy, 2nd edn. Marcel Dekker, New York

Marone G, Lichtenstein L, Galli SJ (eds) (2000) Mast cells and basophils. Academic Press, San Diego

Marquardt H, Schäfer SG (eds) (1994) Lehrbuch der Toxikologie. Wissenschaftliche Verlags-Gesellschaft, Mannheim

Middleton E, Reed CE, Ellis IS, et al. (eds) (1993) Allergy: Principles and practice, 4th edn. Mosby, St. Louis

Mygind N (1986) Essential allergy. Blackwell, Oxford

Peter H, Pichler W (eds) (1996) Klinische Immunologie, 2nd edn. Urban & Schwarzenberg, Munich

Przybilla B, Bergmann KC, Ring J (eds) (2000) Praktische allergologische Diagnostik. Steinkopff, Darmstadt

Rietschel RL, Fowler JF (2001) Fisher's contact dermatitis, 5th edn. Lippincott Williams & Wilkins, Philadelphia

Ring J, Burg G (eds) (1981) New trends in allergy. Springer, Berlin Heidelberg New York

Ring J, Burg G (eds) (1986) New trends in allergy, II. Springer, Berlin Heidelberg New York

Ring J, Przybilla B (eds) (1991) New trends in allergy, III. Springer, Berlin Heidelberg New York

Ring J, Behrendt H, Vieluf D (eds) (1997) New trends in allergy, IV. Springer, Berlin Heidelberg New York

Ring J, Behrendt H (eds) (2002) New trends in allergy, V. Springer, Berlin Heidelberg New York

Ring J, Fuchs Th, Schultze-Werninghaus G (eds) (2000) Weißbuch Allergie in Deutschland, 2nd ed. Urban & Vogel, Munich

Ring J (1998) Neurodermitis. Expertise zur gesundheitlichen Versorgung und Vorsorge bei Kindern mit atopischem Ekzem. Ecomed, Landsberg

Ring J, Ruzicka Th, Przybilla B (eds) (2005) Handbook of atopic eczema. 2nd ed. Springer, Berlin Heidelberg, New York

Roitt IM (1998) Essential immunology, 9th edn. Blackwell, Oxford

Ruzicka T, Ring J, Przybilla B (eds) (1991) Handbook of atopic eczema. Springer, Berlin Heidelberg New York

Rycroft R, Menné T, Frosch PJ, Lepoittevin JP (eds) (2001) Textbook of contact dermatitis, 3rd edn. Springer, Berlin Heidelberg New York

Schadewaldt H (1980ff) Geschichte der Allergie, vols I–IV. Dustri, München-Deisenhofen

Schopf R (ed) (1997) Allergologie systematisch. Uni-Med, Bremen

Schultze-Werninghaus G, Bachert C, Kapp A, Wahn U (eds) Manuale allergologicum. 2nd. ed. Dustri, Munich

Schwanitz HJ, Szliska C (2001ff) Berufsdermatosen. Dustri, München-Deisenhofen

Sennekamp HJ (1998) Exogen allergische Alveolitis, 2nd edn. Dustri, München-Deisenhofen

Simon HU (ed) (2000) CRC desk reference for allergy and asthma. CRC Press, Boca Raton

Simon E (ed) (2002) Histamine and H1-antihistamines in allergic disease. Marcel Dekker, New York

Stanley RG, Linse HF (1974) Pollen: Biology, biochemistry, management. Springer, Berlin Heidelberg New York

Stüntzner W, Giesler M (eds) (1996) Prävention allergischer Erkrankungen im Kindes- und Jugendalter. Kohlhammer, Stuttgart

Thomson AW (ed) (1998) The cytokine handbook, 3rd edn. Academic Press, San Diego

Turner MW, Natvig JB (ed) (1999) Immunology nomenclature. Hogrefe-Huber, Seattle

UCB Institute of Allergy (ed) (1997) European Allergy White Paper. UCB Institute of Allergy, Braine-l'Alleud

Urbach C (1935) Klinik und Therapie der allergischen Krankheiten. Wilhelm Maudrich, Vienna

Vaughan WT, Black JH (1948) Practice of allergy. Mosby, St. Louis

Wahn U, Wichmann HF (eds) (2000) Spezialbericht Allergien. Statistisches Bundesamt. Metzler-Poeschel, Stuttgart

WHO (1999) Environmental Health Criteria 212: Principles and Methods for Assessing Allergic Hypersensitization Associated with Exposure to Chemicals. WHO, Geneva

Wichmann HE, Schlipköter HW, Füllgraff G (eds) (1992ff) Handbuch der Umweltmedizin. Ecomed, Landsberg

Williams HC (ed) (2000) Atopic dermatitis: The epidemiology, causes and prevention of atopic eczema. Cambridge University Press, Cambridge

Wüthrich B (ed) (1999) The atopy syndrome in the third millennium. Karger, Basel

Zürcher K, Krebs A (1992) Cutaneous drug reactions. An integral synopsis of today's systemic drugs, 2nd edn. Karger, Banel

Illustration Credits

(if not already credited)

Archiv der Klinik und Poliklinik für Dermatologie und Allergologie am Biederstein, Technische Universität Munich: Figs. 4.1, 5.19, 5.24, 5.27, 5.28, 5.36, 5.67, 5.68, 5.71, 5.73, 5.81

Archiv der Dermatologischen Klinik und Poliklinik der Ludwig-Maximilians-Universität Munich:
Figs. 4.1d, 5.31–34, 5.39a, 5.47, 5.50, 5.51, 5.53, 5.58, 5.65, 5.69, 5.72, 5.74–80, 5.83

Archiv der Hautklinik, Universitätskrankenhaus Eppendorf, Hamburg: Figs. 5.6–11, 5.14–18, 5.22, 5.35, 5.37, 5.38, 5.43–46, 5.49, 5.54, 5.57, 5.63, 5.64, 5.66, 5.82a

Subject Index

AAC rule 102
Acaricides 55
acetylcysteine 223
acetylsalicylic acid (ASA) 182, 185
- idiosyncrasy 186, 190
actinic reticuloid 171
actinomycete 53
active immunization 227
acute
- severe asthma 81
- urticaria 90
adhesion molecule 14
adrenergics
- a-adrenergics 222
- b adrenergics 222
adverse drug reaction 175
- additives 191
- provocation test 179
adverse food reaction 104
aeroallergen 44, 82, 98
- avoidance 243
- occupational 57
AIDS 61, 194
air pollutant 37
- gaseous 37
- indoor 40
- particulate 37
airborne contact dermatitis 147
airway resistance 70
allergen 42
- airborne 47
- avoidance 43, 60
- carriers 42
- detection 44
- exposure 32, 36
- extract 44, 230
- - toxicity 233
- natural allergen 45
- origins 42
- terminology 44
allergenic potency 43
allergen-specific immunotherapy 116, 117, 227, 260
- pregnancy 231
- side effects 233
allergic
- agranulocytosis 18, 128

- bronchial asthma 137
- bronchopulmonary mycosis 141
- conjunctivitis 122
- contact dermatitis 6, 19, 145
- cytotoxic organopathies 130
- cytotoxicity 126
- eye disease 122
- hemolytic anemia 128
- personality traits 248
- rhinitis 76, 78
- - pharmacotherapy 79
- - prevalence 34
- thrombocytopenia 129
- thrombocytopenic purpura 127
- vasculitis 133, 134
- - hemorrhagic type 134
- - necrotic type 135
- - papulonecrotic type 134
- - therapy 135
allergology 261
- definition 261
- role 261
allergotoxicology 36
allergy
- classical genetics 30
- classification 5
- clinical manifestation 2
- conditioned reflexes 250
- definition 2, 4
- diagnosis 259
- environmental factors 34
- history 60, 61
- immediate type 76
- passport 179
- prevalence 35
- prevention 218, 241, 260
- psyche 248
- tests 61, 62
- - complications 62
- therapy 260
- to coins 146
- treatment 218
- unconventional procedures 239
Ambrosia artemisiifolia 51
amphotericin B 95
ampicillin exanthema 195

analgesics 181
anaphylactic shock 101, 252
anaphylatoxin 25
anaphylaxis 57, 76, 97
- augmentation anaphylaxis 99, 100
- classic anaphylaxis 16
- elicitors 99
- factitia 100
- idiopathic 98
- summation anaphylaxis 100
Anderson sampler 48
animal epithelia 54, 244
antiallergic
- drug 219, 225
- - pregnancy 225
- pharmacotherapy 220
antibiotics 87
antibody-mediated cytotoxicity 125
anticholinergics 87
antigen interaction 8
antihistamine 78, 79, 86, 95, 220, 224
anti-idiotypic antibody 229
aquagenic urticaria 92
aqueous rhinorrhea 77
arachidonic acid 20
Artemisia vulgaris 49
Arthus reaction 63, 183
ascomycin derivative 237
aspergillosis 141
Aspergillus fumigatus 53
asthma 79, 185
- acute severe asthma 81
- attack 81
- bronchial asthma 80
- IgE-mediated 82
- infect-allergic asthma 83
- intrinsic asthma 81, 82
- irritative toxic asthma 82
- psychogenic asthma 83
- schools 87
- symptoms 81
asthmatic inflammation 84
atopic
- cataract 122
- conjunctivitis 122
- diathesis 65
- disease
- eczema 5, 20, 33, 151, 252
- - diagnosis 154
- - genetics 157
- - prurigo 154
- - *Staphylococcus aureus* 158
- - stigmata 152
- - therapy 159
atopy
- candidate genes 31, 32
- definition 18
- history 1
- IgE 17
- latent atopy 18

- patch test (APT) 61, 157, 158
- risk factors 30
augmentation anaphylaxis 99, 100
autacoid 251
autogenic training 253
autoimmune
- disease 210
- thyreoiditis 210
autonomic nervous system dysregulation 158

B cell 8
- maturation 14
B memory cells 10
bacterial toxin 104
basidiospores 53
basophil
- degranulation test 67
- leukocyte activation test 68
bee venom 119
behavioral therapy 253, 254
beta$_2$ adrenergics 86, 95
beta-lactam antibiotics 181
beta-lactoglobulin 106
Betula verrucosa 44
biofeedback 253
biological activity unit (BAU) 44
biological unit (BU) 44
biotinylation 67
birch pollen grain 43
bird allergen 55
blepharitis 123
blood eosinophilia 130
body plethysmography 70
bovine collagen hypersensitivity 108
brain-derived nerotrophic factor (BDNF) 83
bronchial
- asthma 80
- - avoidance measures 85
- - classification 81
- hyperreactivity 83
- provocation test 69
bullous drug eruption 20, 196, 204
Burkard trap 48
butylhydroxyanisol (BHA) 149
bypass activation 25

cadmium 39
cAMP 17
Candida 55
carboxypeptidase B 25
CAST-ELISA 178
cat allergen 54
celery 106
celery-mugwort-spice syndrome 44
cellular
- allergen stimulation test (CAST) 68, 190
- hypersensitivity 19
- test 259
cephalosporin 181
cereal allergy 106

cGMP   17
Charcot-Leyden's crystals   83
chemical pharmacology   260
chemokine   13
cholinergic
– hyperreactivitiy   85, 223
– urticaria   91
chronic
– obstructive bronchitis   85
– obstructive pulmonary disease (COPD)   85
– urticaria   91
cicatricial pemphigoid   123
classic anaphylaxis   16
climate therapy   86
clonal anergy   12
cluster of differentiation (CD)   11
cold urticaria   91
colonic allergen provocation (COLAP)   72, 109
comedo formation   167
complement system   24
conjunctival provocation test   68
conjunctivitis
– cicatricial   123
– giant papillary   123
– microbial-allergic   123
contact
– allergy   169
– – epidemiology   35
– – time (CAT)   147
– anaphylaxis   92
– dermatitis   143, 144
– – airborne   51
– lenses   123
– stomatitis   146
– urticaria   92
contact-allergic conjunctivitis   123
Coomb's test   128
corticosteroid   78
corticotrophin-releasing factor (CRF)   251
coupling allergy   145
cow's milk allergy   106, 110
cradle cap   152
crossed radioimmunoelectrophoresis (CRIE)   230
cross-sensitization   44
crusta lactea   151
cumulative toxic hand eczema   146
Curschmann's spirales   83
cutaneous
– atrophy   169
– drug eruption   202
– lymphocyte antigen   145
– lymphoma   171
cyclooxygenase (COX)   23, 191
cyclophosphamide   135
cyclosporin   95, 237
cytokine   9
– antagonist   238
– secretion   12
cytoplasm   49
cytotoxic

– antibody   125
– reaction
– – autoimmune type   127
– – hapten type   127
– – immune complex   127
cytotoxicity
– allergic cytotoxicity   126
– antibody-mediated   125

danazol   95
Darier's sign   92
demographic urticaria   91
dendritic cell (DC)   9
depot penicillin   191
dermatitis   143
– contact dermatitis   143, 144
– diaper dermatitis   144
– irritant contact dermatitis   144
– perioral rosacea-like dermatitis   168
– seborrheic dermatitis   144
– therapy   149
dermatopathology   200
Dermatophagoides
– *farinae*   55
– *pteronyssinus*   55
dextran anaphylaxis   6, 19
diaminoxidase (DAO)   26
diaper dermatitis   144
dinitrochlorbenzene   61
disodium cromoglycate (DSCG)   220
double-blind placebo-controlled food challenge (DBPCFC)   71
doxepin   95, 224
drug
– allergy   176, 259
– – HIV infection   183
– – hyposensitization   180
– – risk factors   177
– – skin test   178
– eruption
– – bullous drug eruption   20, 196, 204
– – cutaneous drug eruption   202
– – erythematovesicular drug eruption   194
– – hemorrhagic drug eruption   194
– – macular drug eruption   195
– – maculopapular drug eruption   195
– – psoriariform drug eruption   204
– – urticarial drug eruption   194
– exanthema   196
drug-induced
– erythema nodosum   196
– hepatitis   130
– nephropathy   130
dry skin   159
dual reaction   63
dyshidrotic hand eczema   145
dyspnea   80, 81, 101

early treatment of the atopic child (ETAC)   243
eco-syndrome   212, 213

- pathophysiology 214
eczema 143
- itch 224
eicosanoid 20
elbow eczema 153
endogenous
- autoimmune uveitis 124
- psychoses 214
endotoxin 211
environmental
- noxious agent 214
- pollution 36
environmentophobia 37
enzyme deficiency 104, 187
eosinophil
- cationic protein (ECP) 25, 66
- protein X (EPX) 67
eosinophilia myalgia syndrome (EMS) 130
epidermolyis 202
epinephrine 101, 222
erythema
- exsudativum multiforme 123
- multiforme 197
erythematovesicular drug eruption 194
etanercept 238
ethylnitrosourea (ENU) mutagenesis project 32
exanthematous drug eruption 193
exercise-induced urticaria 91
exfoliative dermatitis 195, 196
exogenous allergic alveolitis 136, 139
experimental allergology 258
extrinsic allergic alveolitis 209

Fab fragment 15
farmer's lung 136, 139
Fc fragment 15
Fcg receptor 131
feather allergy 55
fingertip eczema 145
Finn chambers 147
fish allergy 107
food allergy 105
- allergens 105
- beta-lactoglobulin 106
- celery 106
- cereal 106
- cow's milk 106
- cross-reactions 105
- diet 109
- fish 107
- gastrointestinal tract 107
- gene technology 105
- hen's eggs 106
- hidden allergen 107
- seafood 107
- therapy 110
- vegetable/fruit 106
foot eczema 146
force exspiratory volume (FEV) 70
Frankfurt theses 241, 242

Freiburg Personality Inventory (FPI) 252
friction test 61
fungal allergic rhinitis 79
fungi taxonomy 53

gametophyte 49
gammaglobulin 188, 229, 233
gastrin 107
gelatine volume substitute 188
gene technology 105
giant papillary conjunctivitis 123
glucocorticoid 101
- application 166
glucocorticosteroid 79, 87, 164, 221
- side effects 167
glycoprotein 43
graft versus host reaction 124
granuloma 233
- anulare 209
granulomatous
- hypersensitivity 20
- inflammation 259
- reaction 6, 207
- - therapy 209
grass pollen 52
gravimetric collection 48
Greaves test 94
group allergy 145
guanine 68

hay fever 33, 77
health promotion 241
Helicobacter pylori 94
helminths 57
hematologic disease 5
hemorrhagic drug eruption 194
hen's eggs allergy 106
heparin 183
heparin-induced thrombocytopenia (HIT) 129, 183
hepatitis, drug-induced 130
hereditary angioneurotic edema (HANE) 93
Herxheimer's trias 83
Hevea brasiliensis 57
hidden allergen 107
histamine 20, 21, 66, 77, 89, 257
- equivalent potency (HEP) 44
- release reaction 16
- structural formula 22
- synthesis 220
HIV infection 61, 120, 183, 194, 258
Hoigné syndrome 191
hormone 251
horse epithelia 54
housedust mite 55, 244
- allergy 78
human
- eosinophilic leukocyte 22
- immune system 8
- leukocyte antigen (HLA) 31

- mast cell   22
- serum albumin   97
hydroa vacciniformia   172
hydrocortisone   166
hydroxyethyl starch (HES)   185
hygiene hypothesis   35
Hymenoptera   114
hyperacute rejection   125
hyper-IgE syndrome   12, 158
hyperimmunoglobulin   119, 233
hypersensitivity   18
- cellular   19
- granulomatous   20
- pneumonitis (HP)   43, 53, 136–138, 209
- - allergens   140
- - diagnosis   138
- - therapy   141
- reaction   76
- stimulating/neutralizing   6, 20
- syndrome   175, 183
hypnosis   253
hypocapnia   83
hyposensitization   86, 117, 180, 218
- methods   232
hypotension   102
hypothalamic pituitary axis   251

ichthyosis hands   155
idiopathic
- anaphylaxis   98
- environmental intolerance (IEI)   213
- thrombocytopenic purpura (ITP)   129
- urticaria   93
IgE   211
- antibodies   99, 228
- autoantibodies   211
- increased production 157
IgE-mediated
- asthma   82
- immediate-type reaction   257
- reaction   16
IgG-blocking antibody   228
immune
- complex anaphylaxis   6, 131
- response
- - modifier   236
- - primary   9
- - secondary   9
- system   250
immunity
- acquired   8
- innate   8
immunodeficiency   61
immunoglobulin   15
- E   2
- Fab fragment   15
- Fc fragment   15
immunosuppressives   237
immunotherapy   236
- allergen-specific   86, 116, 117, 227, 260

- - pregnancy   231
- - side effects   233
- oral/sublingual   233
in vitro
- allergy test   64
- histamine release test   67
infect allergy   12, 124
- asthma   83
infectious rhinitis   78
infliximab   238
inhalation allergen   82, 122
insect venom allergy   56, 67, 114
- diagnosis   115
- risk factors   116
- sting provocation   116
insulin allergy 182
interface dermatitis   202
interleukin (IL)   10
intolerance syndrome   190
intradermal test   61, 62
intragastral provocation under endoscopic control (IPEC)   109
intravenous anesthetics   188
intrinsic asthma   81, 82
iodine allergy   188
ipratropium bromide   79
irritant contact dermatitis   144
irritative contact eczema   146
isotype switch   18
itch   159
- eczema   224
- prurigo   224
- wheal   224

Jarisch-Herxheimer reaction   191

kallikrein-kinin system   25
Kveim test   62

late cutaneous reaction   63
latent atopy   18
latex milk   57
lepromin   207
leukocytoclastic vasculitis   133, 139, 183
leukotrienes   23, 221
- antagonists   86, 95
Lewis' triad   89
lichen planus   204
lid eczema   123
light urticaria   92
lipatrophy   182
lipocortin   164
lipopolysaccharide S (LPS)   211
lipoxygenase   23
- inhibitor   221
local anesthetics   189, 190
localized heat urticaria   91
long-acting thyroid-stimulating factor (LATS)   210
lupus erythematosus   204
Lyell's syndrome   124, 198

- diagnosis 201
- drug-induced 198–200
lymphocyte transformation test (LTT) 68, 178
lymphohistiocytic reaction 196

macular drug eruption 195
maculopapular drug eruption 195
major
- basic protein (MBP) 25
- histocompatibility complex (MHC) 8
malignant hyperthermia 189
mast cell 17
- activation 16
- blockers 86
- stabilizers 218, 220
- tryptase 66
mastocytosis 92
- aggressive type 92
meadow grass dermatitis 173
mediator substance 21
melittin 115
methylhistamine 67
microbial-allergic conjunctivitis 123
microchip techniques 260
Micropolyspora faeni 139
minimal erythema dose (MED) 172
Mitsuda test 62
mold spores 44, 52, 244
- asexual 52
- sexual 52
molecular genetics
- association studies 31
- candidate gene analysis 31
- coupling analysis 31
- single nucleotide polymorphism (SNP) 31
monoaminooxidase (MAO) inhibitor 220
monoclonal antibody 236, 237
monophosphoryl lipid (MPL) 230
Montelukast 95
mucous membrane pemphigoid 124
multiple chemical sensitivity (MCS) 212, 213
multi-subunit immune recognition receptor (MIRR) 12
Münchhausen's syndrome 100
muscle relaxant 189
myasthenia gravis 210

N-acetyl-aspartyl-glutamic acid 223
N-acetyltransferase (NAT) 176
nasal
- hyperreactivity 77
- provocation test 69
natural rubber latex allergy 57
nematode larvae 57
nephropathy, drug-induced 130
nerve growth factor (NGF) 83, 250
nervous system 250
neurasthenia 215
neuropeptide 26
neutrophil granulocyte 25

nickel allergy 146, 147
NK cells 208
non-allergic vasomotor rhinitis 79
non-infectious vaginitis 55
non-ionizing electro-magnetic radiation 170
non-steroidal anti-inflammatory drug (NSAID) 190
nystatin 95

olfactory sensitivity 214
omalizumab 237
opipramol 95
oral
- cromoglycate 111
- provocation test (OPT) 71, 179, 182
- - for idiosyncrasy (OPTI) 94, 109
organic dust toxic syndrome (ODTS) 138
otitis media 79
ozone 38

paper-radioimmunosorbent test (PRIST) 65
papillary hyperplasia 122
paraneoplastic retinopathy 124
parasitosis 57
parenteral provocation 72
passive cutaneous anaphylaxis (PCA) 72, 211
patch test 147, 178
peak exspiratory flow (PEF) 70
penicillin 97
- allergy 180, 181
penicilloyl polylysine (PPL) 178
peptidase 26
peptide 10
perioral rosacea-like dermatitis 168
persistent light reaction 172
phenology 47
Phleum pratense 49
phosphodiesterase inhibitor 223
phospholipase 16, 26, 164
- A2 115
photoallergic contact dermatitis 171
photoallergy 51, 170, 171
- diagnosis 173
photohypersensitivity 171
photo-patch test 173
photo-prick test 173
photosensitization 170, 172
physical
- provocation test 94
- test 63
- urticaria 91
phytotherapeutics 223
pimecrolimus 160, 237
Plantago lanceolata 49
plasma protein solution 132, 188
platelet drop 23
platelet-activating factor (PAF) 23
pneumonia 199
pollen 44, 243
- agglomerations 39

- calendar   47
- counts   48, 49
- differentiation   51
- forms   51
- grains   39
pollen-associated lipid mediator (PALM)   40
pollinosis   49, 60, 77
pollotrienes   40
polymorphic light eruption photoprovocation   172
porphyria   171
Prausnitz-Küstner test   72
pregnancy   241
pressure urticaria   92
prick test   61, 62, 181
procaine polyvinylpyrrolidone (PVP)   207
properdin   25
prostaglandin   22, 23
provocation test   68, 259
prurigo itch   224
pruritis   159
pseudo-allergic
- drug reaction   185
- mechanisms   4
- reaction (PAR)   20, 76, 191
psoriariform drug eruption   204
psychodiagnostic test   252
psychogenic asthma   83
psychoneuroallergology   250, 257
psychosomatics   248
purpura   134
- chronica progressiva   195
- pigmentosa progressiva   6
pyrazolone   182

Quincke's edema   89, 90
quinine   129

radioallergosorbent test (RAST)   64, 67, 230
- inhibition   230
radiographic contrast media   188
ragweed   51
rapamycin   237
rebound phenomenon   166
recombinant hirudin   183
red midge larvae   56
rehabilitation   243
relaxation techniques   253
releasability   99
repeated open application test (ROAT)   148
reverse
- anaphylaxis   6, 211
- placebo provocation   190
rhinitis
- allergic rhinitis   76, 78
- - pharmacotherapy 79
- classification   78
- infectious rhinitis   78
rhinomanometry   69
rush hyposensitization   182

salina   63
saliva   54
Samter's triad   83, 186
sarcoidosis   208
scabies mite   56
Schamberg's disease   195
sclerosiphony   137
scoring system atopic dermatitis (SCORAD)   155, 156
scratch test   61
seafood allergy   107
seasonal allergy   232
seborrheic dermatitis   144
sebostasis   159
secretolysis   87, 223
serine esterase   16
serotonin   24
serum
- nephritis   130
- sickness   19, 131, 132
shock fragment   76
signal transduction   257
silent lung   81
silkworm   57
single nucleotide polymorphism (SNP)   31
sinusitis   79
skin test   61, 178
slow-reacting substance of anaphylaxis (SRS-A)   23
smoking   40
Social Readjustment Rating Scale (SRRS)   249
solar urticaria   172
soluble bovine collagen   208
somatization disturbance   215
specific IgE antibodies   64
sperm allergy   55
spongiosis   158
stanazolol   95
staphylococcal scalded skin syndrome (SSSS)   198, 200
Staphylococcus aureus   158
State-Trait-Anxiety Inventory (STAI)   249
status asthmaticus   81, 87
steroid acne   167
Stevens-Johnson syndrome   123, 197, 198
stimulating/neutralizing hypersensitivity   6, 20
sting provocation   116, 118
stomatitis medicamentosa   204
storage mites   55
stress   249
- protein   43
- susceptibility   251
striae distensae   168
sulfidoleukotriene antagonist   221
sulfido-leukotrienes   68
sulfite   39
sulfur dioxide   39
summation anaphylaxis   100, 258
sun allergy   171
superoxid dismutase (SOD)   25
suppressor

– cells   257
– T cells   229
sympathetic ophthalmia   124
sympathicomimetics   222
syndroma muco-cutaneo-oculare Fuchs   123
syndrome of burnt skin   198
systemic photo-provocation test   173

T cell   8
T regulator cells   10
tachykinin   26
tachyphylaxis   166, 229
tacrolimus   160, 237
teleangiectasia eruptiva macularis perstans   92
terbutaline   95
tetracyclin   95
TH1/TH2
– balance   229
– reaction   14
theophylline   101, 223
thrombocytopenia   18, 126
thyreoiditis   6
tobacco smoke   40
toll-like receptor   257
toluidine-blue staining   67
toxic
– agent   36
– antibody   131
– epidermal necrolysis (TEN)   124, 198, 200
– – pathophysiology   203
– – therapy   201
– granulocytopenia   128
– shock syndrome (TSS)   203
tricyclic antidepressant   95
5-OH-tryptamine, see serotonin
tuberculin reaction   207

unguentum emulsificans aquosum   160
unspecific irritation syndrome   86
urtica dioica   92
urticaria   57, 89, 185

– acute type   90
– aquagenic   92
– cholinergic   91
– chronic type   91
– cold   91
– contact   92
– dermographic   91
– diagnosis   93
– exercise-induced   91
– factitia   91
– idiopathic   93
– light   92
– localized heat   91
– physical   91
– pigmentosa   92
– pressure   92
– solar   172
– therapy   95
– vasculitis   93, 134
urticarial drug eruption   194
urticariogen   98
UV therapy   96, 160

vaccination   227
vegetable/fruit allergy   106
Venn diagram   30
vernal keratoconjunctivitis   122

wasp venom   119
Western blotting   67
wheal itch   224

xanthine derivative   86, 223
xenogeneic
– protein   132
– serum therapy   6

yin yang theory   14

zirconium granuloma   207

RC
584
.R56
2005

SOUTH UNIVERSITY
709 MALL BLVD.
SAVANNAH, GA 31406